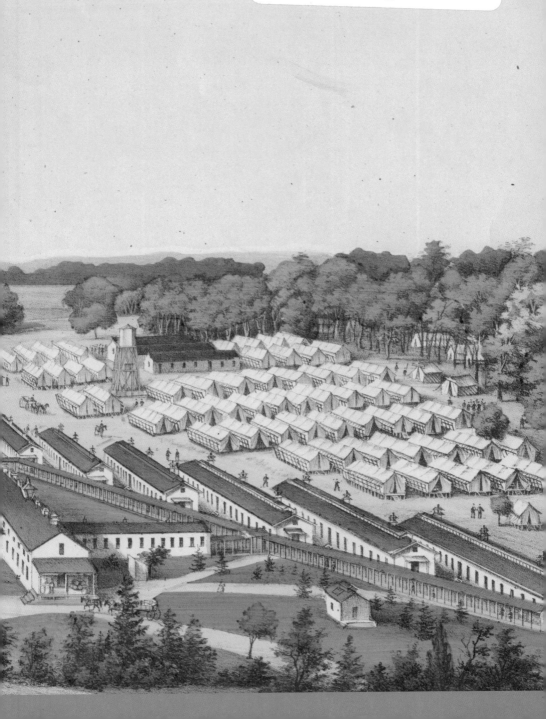

HEALING A DIVIDED NATION

HEALING A DIVIDED NATION

HOW THE AMERICAN CIVIL WAR
REVOLUTIONIZED WESTERN MEDICINE

CAROLE ADRIENNE

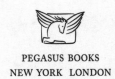

PEGASUS BOOKS
NEW YORK LONDON

HEALING A DIVIDED NATION

Pegasus Books, Ltd.
148 West 37th Street, 13th Floor
New York, NY 10018

Copyright © 2022 by Carole Adrienne

First Pegasus Books cloth edition August 2022

Interior design by Maria Fernandez

Front endpapers: Harewood Hospital, Washington, D.C.
Back endpapers: Soldiers Rest, Alexandria, Va.
Both images courtesy of The Library Company of Philadelphia.

Library of Congress Cataloging-in-Publication Data is available.

ISBN: 978-1-63936-185-4

10 9 8 7 6 5 4 3 2 1

Printed in the United States of America
Distributed by Simon & Schuster
www.pegasusbooks.com

This work is dedicated to

Rose DeWolf

Gretchen Worden

Alfred Jay Bollet

CONTENTS

INTRODUCTION

The term "Civil War medicine" familiarly conjures images of ragtag hospital tents, open-air amputations, and frantic, crude, assembly-line surgeries. It evokes the stoic faces of long-dead soldiers staring somberly from small velvet-and-gold-framed mementos and of heart-wrenching photographs of amputees and prison camp starvation victims.

In actuality, the footprint of Civil War medicine stretched from Solferino, Italy, to towns and cities across America. It spanned the miles to Geneva, Switzerland, and throughout Europe. This war was a pivotal event of not only the greatest carnage on American soil, but also of the upending of long-held social and scientific norms. It was the crucible of modern medicine and revolutionary societal change, and it laid the foundation for the future of Western health care and medical education.

Upon embarking on this research, the outer rings of the story revealed an incredible width and breadth to the effects of Civil War medicine. The story was about elevating medicine to a science and promoting women to be powerful participants in business, management, and the medical field. Female physicians and the first degreed African American doctors made their professional public debuts in the U.S. It was the beginning of a humanitarian movement that encompassed the compassionate, devoted efforts of untold tens of thousands of volunteers. Civil War medicine contributed to the creation of the original Geneva Convention of 1864, highlighting the need for protocols to protect wartime wounded and their caretakers. It is inherent in the founding of the International and American Red Cross and encompassed the publication of the six-volume compendium *The Medical and Surgical History of the War of the Rebellion*, considered by Europeans of the time to be America's greatest contribution to medical science. This text highlighted the exhausted, blood-soaked efforts of medical personnel over four painful years. It was about a huge field of heroes beyond the battlefields and it was a story about hope, endurance, and tenacity.

In 1861, America's population was 29 million. Twenty million resided in the Northern states that would become known as the "Union." Transportation was provided by horses, trains, and steamer ships, and the Republican Abraham Lincoln had been inaugurated as the sixteenth president of the United States. This innovative leader with a history of personal tragedies and physical ailments would help to change the culture of health care in the West. American medicine of 1860 was almost identical to the medicine of 1760—a time before X-rays and antibiotics, before diagnostic techniques of any sophistication. It was a time before knowledge and acceptance of the germ theory of disease or any effective treatments for infection.

While the field of medicine had long remained static, the mid–19th century technology of armaments was advancing rapidly. A new and highly effective generation of weapons and ammunition appeared on America's battlefields. Rifled gun barrels, huge elliptical bullets, cannon shot, and the first repeating guns all caused horrific types of never-before-seen wounds. The new weapons ran directly up against old medicine. At the Battle of Antietam, in Maryland, in 1862, there were 23,000 casualties in only ten hours. The 1863 Battle of Gettysburg, Pennsylvania, resulted in 53,000 casualties in three days of fighting. American medicine, just beginning to transcend a scientific darkness, was faced with hundreds of thousands of grievously wounded men and only primitive medical understanding, tools, and techniques.

The violence claimed lives at a fantastic rate of speed. Tens of thousands would lose limbs and virtually all surgeries were followed by dangerous infections. The wounds were devastating, although more men actually died of disease and sepsis. As the Civil War raged in America, Dr. Louis Pasteur, the chemist and microbiologist in France, was working on his germ theory of disease, an idea familiar to many of his European colleagues. By the end of the war, Pasteur would prove that disease is caused by microorganisms, and that the organisms do not arise by spontaneous generation. Pasteur's discoveries would lead to methods for preventing mass contagion, but that knowledge was not disseminated through the American medical community in time to save the hundreds of thousands of Union and Confederate soldiers who died of diseases ranging from malaria to measles.

The American Civil War marks the pivotal moment in time when medicine emerged from the "medical Middle Ages," a time when the medicine of 1860 was regarded as an "art," not a "science." This was America in the shocking grip of a four-year epidemic of disease and violence. It was the young men of the country dying by the thousands not only of gunshot wounds and infections, but of diarrhea, malnutrition, and chicken pox. It was a time in this country before the acceptance of the English Dr. Joseph Lister's discoveries in combating infection. Sterilization was unheard of, and ambulance service and skilled nursing care did not exist.

The Civil War casts a huge shadow on the history of the United States, shocking a government that was unprepared for a massive and lengthy conflict and a military that was not organized to manage casualties on a gigantic scale.

The Library of the College of Physicians of Philadelphia boasts among its holdings the notes, letters, and publications of Dr. William Williams Keen. His writings shine with a brilliant intellect and a clever, dark sense of gallows humor. Keen would enter army service in the Civil War at age twenty-three with less than two years of medical training, and serve again in uniform at age eighty in World War I. The writings of Dr. Keen and his 19th-century colleagues create a stunning picture of deficiencies in the areas of medical knowledge and equipment. They also bring to life many very young men with extremely limited experience, tools, and training, who were suddenly thrust into a hideous swirling eddy of smoke, screams, blood, and gunfire from which they were expected to save the lives of other young men. Keen looked back on his wartime service:

> We surgeons in 1861–65, utterly unaware of bacteria and their dangers, committed grievous mistakes which nearly always imperiled life and often actually caused death. May Le Bon Dieu forgive us our sins of ignorance. We operated in old blood and pus-stained coats, the veterans of a hundred fights. We operated with undisinfected hands.

A newly lethal age of warfare was heralded by the American Civil War, although, tragically, advances in medicine lagged far behind. The new arms were highly efficient and caused extensive damage. The combination of new weaponry and old medicine resulted in 1.2 million casualties and at least 620,000 deaths, more than the total number of American deaths in World Wars I and II and Vietnam combined. The familiar swords, sabers, and bayonets were still carried into battle, but bladed weapons inflicted few Civil War wounds: only 2 percent of the casualties were attributed to these instruments. The massive carnage of this conflict was caused by far more powerful arms.

The smoothbore musket was replaced by superior guns with rifled barrels that could project spinning ammunition with much greater range, accuracy, and penetration, allowing troops to kill at distances of 500 yards. European armies had introduced the Minié ball (named for its inventor, French army officer Claude-Étienne Minié), a large ellipsoid with a hollow base. The Minié ball tore an enormous wound on impact. The ball was so heavy that a head or abdominal wound was almost always fatal; wounds to the extremities shattered the bones.

Another 19th-century invention, the percussion cap, was extremely important to the efficiency of guns, providing more reliable ignition and simplified loading. The percussion cap made possible the development of the self-contained "fixed" brass cartridge, which led to the repeating magazine. American inventor Richard Gatling patented his rapid-fire gun in 1862. It was the source from which modern semiautomatic and automatic weapons descended. Some repeating magazine rifles were used in the Civil War, as were the new manually operated machine guns. Battle had become far more sophisticated and deadly.

A Manual of Military Surgery was written in 1861 by the esteemed physician, surgeon, and teacher Dr. Samuel D. Gross, conceived as "a kind of pocket companion for the young surgeons who were flocking into the army." Dr. Gross described common wounds received in battle:

> The most formidable wounds of the kind are made by the conical rifle and musket balls and by cannon balls, the latter often carrying away the greater portion of a limb, or mashing and pulpifying the muscles and viscera in the most frightful and destructive manner; while the former commit terrible ravages among the bones, breaking them into numerous fragments.

Union statistics showed that 71 percent of all gunshot wounds were to the extremities and that amputation was the fastest and most common lifesaving treatment. Those wounded in the head, neck, chest, and abdomen were the least likely to live and frequently no treatment was administered; those with abdominal wounds usually died of peritonitis if they did not bleed to death first. It is to the credit of the surgeons and nurses that an estimated 75 percent of the amputees survived the crude surgical and convalescent procedures.

The Civil War casualties are the symbols of lives devastated, bodies and families torn apart, and of unimaginable suffering. They are the human reminders of prison camps like Andersonville in Georgia and Camp Douglas in Chicago, Illinois, the survivors of limb loss, of disease, of the wide range of warfare's vicious assaults. They are a manifestation of the bloody birth of modern medicine and, from an additional perspective, they are the tangible record of a sweeping revolution of health care and social evolution that would extend across the Western world.

Every large-scale conflict following the American Civil War has been fought with the advantage of understanding Pasteur's germ theory of disease and Lister's work on sepsis. When violence first erupted in 1861, the Union Army had fewer than ninety doctors. By 1865 their numbers had swollen to 12,000 in the Union and more than 3,000 in the Confederate Army. In a terrible irony, although Lister and Pasteur were conducting their work during this time, the Civil War doctors were not able to benefit from the important discoveries of the Europeans until quite some time after the end of the war.

The Northern and Southern doctors of 1861–1865 came from a kaleidoscopic array of backgrounds. Many had been educated in the two-year American medical schools; some from affluent families had attended four-year institutions in Europe. U.S. medical education was woefully behind that of its Continental colleagues—many states still prohibited human anatomical dissection in their medical schools. A large number of the doctors who served had learned their skills from apprenticeships to older physicians, or from family members who worked as doctors, and some of those who served as wartime surgeons had originally trained as dentists.

The first degreed African American doctors in the country made their initial public engagements in the Civil War. Thirteen of these physicians served, most having acquired their educations in Canada as American medical schools, with the exception of a very few institutions including Oberlin College in Ohio, would not allow them to attend.

Born to free people of color in Virginia and refused admission to the University of Pennsylvania, Dr. Alexander Thomas Augusta received his medical training at Trinity Medical College in Toronto. After the start of the Civil War, Dr. Augusta wrote to Union president Abraham Lincoln and offered his services to the U.S. Army as a doctor to work with the "colored regiments" that were being created during the Civil War. He was given a presidential commission in 1862, receiving a major's commission as surgeon for African American troops. The Contraband Hospital in Washington, D.C., was designated for the care of free blacks and former slaves, and Dr. Augusta became the surgeon-in-charge at the hospital, and later the regimental surgeon for the Seventh Infantry of the United States Colored Troops in Maryland. When he joined his new regiment, objections to his appointment were raised by several white surgeons refusing to accept a superior officer who was black. Their actions led to his reassignment to a recruiting station for black troops.

Dr. Augusta's proud wearing of the Union Army uniform provoked a heated reaction from both whites and blacks. He was attacked on a train in Baltimore and forced off a streetcar in Washington, D.C. The violent discrimination of the latter incident led to an outraged response by Republican senator Charles Sumner of Massachusetts, who requested that the United States Congress extend to black passengers the same rail privileges granted to whites. Within a year, seats on streetcars in the Capitol were opened to both blacks and whites. When Dr. Augusta left the service, he held the rank of brevet lieutenant colonel, and subsequently became the first black hospital administrator and the first black professor of medicine in the United States.

In a field that had traditionally been male, women began to appear as nurses and unofficial medics in the hospitals and on the battlefields. Barred entrance to most medical schools, an estimated 200–300 American women may have possessed medical diplomas at the onset of the Civil War. Across the country, numbers of women had studied and worked with their physician husbands or fathers, and many served in the war as medical volunteers. Untold thousands more women surged into the fray, volunteering as nurses—another area that had always been exclusively male.

The Confederacy's Dr. Orianna Moon Andrews, from a wealthy family in Virginia, was only the third woman from the Southern states to attend the Female Medical College of Pennsylvania, having studied the prerequisite science and mathematics. She graduated in 1856, and, moving outside the comfort zone of most mid-19th-century women, spent the next two years in Europe and the Middle East. At the start of the American hostilities she offered her medical services to the Confederate Army and vowed "to follow the army and seek the wounded on the field of battle," stating that she had "the will and the nerve to witness and relieve the suffering" of the soldiers. She met Dr. John Andrews at the bedside of his wounded brother at Charlottesville General Hospital after the Battle of Bull Run in 1861. Dr. Andrews was both shocked and enchanted with the confident and competent female physician and they were soon married and worked together throughout much of the war.

President Abraham Lincoln of the Union, fascinated by advancements in science and technology, permitted and encouraged some revolutionary actions during the Civil War, including allowing Dr. Jonathan Letterman, medical director of the Army of the Potomac, the leeway to create an ambulance corps, and, breaking long-held racial barriers, commissioning the African American Dr. Alexander Thomas Augusta as a surgeon and major in the Union Army.

Personally, Lincoln had a checkered medical history, his earliest known emergency having occurred at age nine when he was kicked in the head by a horse. Unconscious for hours, the young boy recovered from the accident, but was dealt a huge emotional blow that same year when his mother and a close aunt and uncle died.

The Lincoln family was known for its many sufferers of mental illness, and Abraham Lincoln himself fought a lifelong battle with depression that may have been genetic, but was surely compounded by multiple tragic losses in his life, including two of his sons, Eddie and Willie, who died as children. It's possible that the president may have suffered from mercury poisoning due to the "blue pills" he took to combat syphilis and constipation, and some speculate that he may also have had a rare genetic disease, either Marfan syndrome or multiple endocrine neoplasia type 2B. His medical history includes at least two bouts with malaria and a case of smallpox contracted in 1863.

Estimates are that at least 225,000 Union troops perished from disease. The American medical community of the early 1860s was not aware of the causes or cures for the contagious spread of most diseases. One huge culprit was the filth of the Army camps, where bacteria and viruses proliferated through the foul and contaminated water, poor diet, exposure to the elements, and terrible sanitary conditions. The number of those who may have died from their wartime ailments following the cessation of the hostilities is unknown.

About one half of Civil War deaths are attributed to intestinal disorders including typhoid fever, diarrhea, and dysentery. Thousands died from pneumonia and tuberculosis and one million cases of malaria were reported by the Union Army during the war. Young soldiers from rural areas were particularly susceptible to the common contagious "childhood" diseases and many died from measles, chicken pox, mumps, and whooping cough. Data suggests that one third of all men who died in Union and Confederate veterans' homes succumbed to late stages of venereal disease. Prostitutes and camp followers contributed to the loss of thousands of lives during and after the war by sexually transmitted diseases including gonorrhea and syphilis.

Americans had a long familiarity with disease epidemics, including yellow fever. One of the most dreaded was the highly contagious and frequently fatal smallpox, which, ironically, was the only disease for which inoculation was available. One strange episode from among the thousands of pages of memoirs, letters, and notes from the Civil War physicians in 1863 was haunting and unforgettable.

The first known mass inoculation of the Civil War era occurred in New Bern, North Carolina, in a Union Army encampment. The origins of the vaccine stretched back many centuries and arrived in America with a man stolen from Africa.

The practice of "variolation" or "inoculation" may have developed in 8th-century India or 10th-century China, and apparently existed in parts of Africa at least by the 17th century. The technique involved making a cut in the skin and rubbing it with pus or scab material from a victim of the disease. Those who underwent the process were then free from the danger of smallpox contagion.

Variolation first appears in America in the early 18th century. Cotton Mather, a New England Puritan minister, is known primarily as a powerful figure in the Salem Witch trials. In 1706, his congregation purchased for him an enslaved West African man whom he renamed Onesimus. Mather had a strong scientific curiosity, and in conversations with Onesimus learned that the man had been inoculated against smallpox by the variolation process as a child in Africa. Onesimus's shared information would later save countless American lives.

In 1721 a smallpox epidemic swept Boston, infecting about half of its residents and killing more than 14 percent of them. Cotton Mather and Boston physician Zabdiel Boylston, who also supported the variolation theory, sprang into action. Boylston inoculated 242 people. Of those he treated, only one in forty died, as opposed to one in seven in the uninoculated population. By 1796, an effective vaccine had been developed by English physician Edward Jenner. Civil War doctors had access to a long-proven prophylactic procedure for smallpox.

The wartime mass inoculation in North Carolina was a shocking collision of degradation and salvation. Union doctor Daniel Hand was in charge of the Army medical department in North Carolina in 1863. A community of several thousand free blacks and some white refugees had congregated there for protection, and the Army provided quarters and rations for them, including medical care.

Smallpox broke out in the impoverished community, with 200 people suddenly in need of physicians' attention. It was apparent that a massive epidemic was imminent. Young Northern doctors volunteered their service to New Bern, and Dr. Hand requested a large quantity of vaccine virus from Washington. After some difficulty, the virus arrived from the surgeon general and Hand ordered it ground up and mixed with glycerin. Surgeon Daniel Hand never forgot that day.

> Collecting all the medical officers who could be spared,—some twenty or more,—we had the provost guard one Sunday morning drive all the negroes in town out on a long bridge over the Trent River. The doctors then vaccinated each one as he or she was let off. Many of them kicked and screamed, and the whole garrison turned out to see the performance. Altogether we vaccinated six thousand that day, and following this up we very soon checked the spread of smallpox.

Before the Civil War, Americans convalesced at home. There were few hospitals in the country, many of which were small eight- or ten-bed infirmaries, frequently attached to almshouses. There were a handful of military hospitals in the U.S. and U.S. territories; Fort Leavenworth in Kansas was considered a large facility, having forty beds.

By 1864 there would be about 400 hospitals in the United States, comprising approximately 400,000 beds. Huge, newly designed "pavilion hospitals" had begun to appear, structured like spokes on a wheel, and supplies and services moved more smoothly through them. Philadelphia hosted the two largest military hospitals in the North: Satterlee with 3,519 beds;

Mower Hospital with 3,100. The Confederacy boasted a number of new or expanded facilities including Chimborazo Hospital in Virginia, which had 8,000 beds and a reputation for a low death rate. Specialty hospitals were designated: orthopedic, contagious disease, amputee, eye, and ear.

Owing to the huge number of casualties, the hospitals also served as research laboratories, allowing for the observation of symptoms and similarities that were documented and preserved for the future of medical education and practice. The vast number of gunshot wounds and amputations began to show patterns in recovery, and the phenomenon of "phantom limb" was noted and studied by Dr. Silas Weir Mitchell and his colleagues at Turner's Lane Hospital in Philadelphia. This hospital for "nervous injuries" provided rich resources for the foundation of neurology as traumatic nerve injury became regarded as a specific area of medicine for the first time.

Although the Civil War hospitals predated the concept of sterilization, they were clean, ventilated, and contagion-contained. They were actually close to modern hospitals, a great similarity being hospital hierarchies. As institutions, they were basically military wards and strictly regimented. Today's hospitals still operate on that model of military power structure: follow the doctors' orders.

The Civil War signaled a huge shifting of the tectonic plates of caste, ending slavery in America and forever changing the societal position of women. In the stinking vat of violence and disease that was the war in America, another movement was stirring. The suffering mass of humanity that constituted the armies began to arouse the citizens' nonpartisan concern, inspiring the creation of solutions and salves. Women, shaking off their mantles of second-class citizenship, led the way, presenting a strong new image of female ability and worth. Women streamed onto the battlefields and into the hospitals, took over running businesses, and organized training for skilled nurses. A culture that had not previously welcomed them suddenly found their support to be invaluable. Women, in their wartime work, challenged the sentimental domestic image of weak and frail beings, and continued to do so after the war.

In a society that did not invite women to the frontlines of business or management, charity work was a socially sanctioned activity. There was a long religious tradition of women engaging in philanthropy as volunteers. On April 29, 1861, about two weeks after the start of the Civil War, Dr. Elizabeth Blackwell, one of the country's first degreed female physicians, and Louisa Lee Schuyler, a leader in charitable work, organized a meeting of women in New York City at The Cooper Union for the Advancement of Science and Art. They were there to create an organization called "Women's Central Association of Relief for the Sick and Wounded of the Army" with goals of making clothing, bandages, and food, and furnishing nurses (who had always previously been male) for the soldiers of the Union Army.

In a world without telephones, email, or texts, word spread among the women of New York and between three thousand and four thousand women showed up in a watershed moment of coordination and humanitarian aid. The effort would eventually evolve to the United States Sanitary Commission, the huge national organization that would provide the services and support that the government could not.

The United States Sanitary Commission was a massive and highly effective volunteer organization that grew from the small groups of women who originally met in parlors to roll bandages, sew clothing, and prepare food for the soldiers. In a country plagued with one million casualties from disease and violence, the Commission provided medical supplies, food, camp inspection, and other services including a huge fundraising campaign. Many women's aid societies in the South provided valuable relief, but the Confederacy had nothing that could equal the North's huge U.S. Sanitary Commission, created to augment the government's effort. The Commission's main focus was the sanitary and hygienic condition of the troops, and it sought to bring supplemental relief in a variety of ways.

Patterned on the British Sanitary Commission, which had been formed in the 1850s to clean up the horrible refuse of the Crimean War, the U.S.S.C. organized volunteer branches in many cities, arranged for examinations of troops, camp, and medical facilities, and found unsanitary conditions and poor diet everywhere. They began a traveling outpost with the Army of the Potomac to speed the delivery of sanitary supplies to its field hospitals. The Commission provided the majority of medical supplies to the battlefields of Antietam, Fredericksburg, Chancellorsville, and the Second Battle of Bull Run. It sent hospital ships to transport the sick and wounded, and responded to thousands of civilian letters inquiring about dead, hospitalized, and missing soldiers. Members collected food, clothing, bedding, and financial contributions, and commissioned and distributed pamphlets on sanitation and hygiene. During its existence, the United States Sanitary Commission raised cash estimated at more than $15 million (equal to more than $400 million in today's dollars) and untold amounts in valuable supplies.

The outpouring of compassion gave rise to vast relief efforts including "Sanitary Fairs" such as the ones held in Philadelphia, New York, Chicago, Cincinnati, and other cities. The expo-like multi-week fairs raised millions of dollars to improve the hygienic habits of the troops and the deplorable condition of the camps. The volunteer Western Sanitary Commission in St. Louis established and equipped hospitals. The Northwestern branch rushed carloads of fresh vegetables to prevent scurvy among the soldiers.

In 1862 and 1864, the Commission provided and staffed hospital ships to evacuate the sick and wounded of the Army of the Potomac, breaking naval tradition by allowing the assistance of two nuns from the Holy Cross order, Sister Adela and Sister Veronica, aboard one ship as the first women nurses on those vessels. In response to thousands of civilian letters inquiring about dead, wounded, and missing soldiers, members of the Commission began a hospital directory that included the names of the patients in every general hospital. Paired with the humanitarian effort sparked by Swiss businessman Henri Dunant's traumatic experience of witnessing the 1859

Battle of Solferino, Italy, and its day of 40,000 casualties, the relief movement became international. By the end of the Civil War, the effort would contribute to the institution of the Geneva Convention, which sought to protect the rights of the wounded and their caretakers in times of war. The American Civil War would provide a great deal of the impetus, inspiration, and participation for the Geneva Convention, and extend to the direction of the International Committee of the Red Cross and the American Red Cross.

This war touched American emotions in a way no other conflict has. It pitted American against American, it ended the practice of slavery in this country, and it established the United States as one nation, indivisible. It also created one million casualties.

The weight of the deadly effects of the war was borne by a powerful network of heroes, many of them surprising or unlikely. This is the story of their tenacity, vision, courage, and skill. The marathon lifesaving race featured a diverse group of dedicated participants: professional physicians, medical students, and neophyte volunteers. The movement was supported by empathetic leaders who championed some innovative solutions and a fiercely devoted citizenry that threw itself passionately into support for the sick and wounded. Compassion and care were wielded in a frequently bipartisan manner as the cast included men and women, black and white, Northern and Southern, all in shockingly new and demanding roles.

The Civil War marks an epic turning point in the history of medicine, when scientific understanding evolved dramatically. When the war ended, medicine was transformed by the birth of neurology as well as advances in surgical technique, anesthesiology, medical record-keeping, prosthetic design, plastic surgery, and the evacuation of wounded. Women and African Americans became an integral part of medicine and responsible management, and both the military and the public became aware of the importance of sanitation and hygiene. A huge international volunteer humanitarian movement arose and would revolutionize the protection of wartime wounded and medics.

In 1860 in the United States, ambulance service and skilled, trained nursing care did not exist. It is estimated that prior to the war, approximately three hundred doctors in the entire country had ever witnessed surgical operations or seen gunshot wounds. There was no understanding that invisible organisms could transmit disease, or that infection could be fought with alcohol or vinegar. Anesthesia was a daring new field in dentistry, not surgery. The period is a touchstone in time for Americans and an important model of courage and caring.

This story is an incredible example of Americans at their best. It is a story about human triumph over the devastation of war. Our country is presently in the process of reexamining our global reflection, and America needs a reminder of our magnificent strengths and the inclusive kindness of our hearts right now. *Healing a Divided Nation: How the American Civil War Revolutionized Western Medicine* illustrates the stamina and diversity of Americans and the power of compassionate dedication. It demonstrates selfless contributions and noble behavior from a population working through a fog of grief. It is about heroism in the face of seemingly unending horror.

This book holds the hope that in experiencing this part of our history, Americans will regain a sense of pride in our abilities and potential; that we will see the possibility of ourselves unified in a country dedicated to fairness and equality, to diversity; an inclusive place of wonderful, endless opportunity to those who seek it; that Americans will embrace the beauty of our national character in its myriad shapes and colors.

CHAPTER ONE

THE STATE OF AMERICAN MEDICINE IN 1861

T he genesis of modern Western health care can be traced to the Civil War period, the war that is widely considered to mark the moment in time when medicine emerged from the "Medical Middle Ages." Medicine had remained much the same for the previous 100 years and was considered to be an "art" rather than a "science" in the year 1860, an era before the common use of anesthesia, the understanding of sepsis, or awareness of the germ theory of disease. At the beginning of the Civil War, possibly as few as three hundred doctors in America had ever witnessed surgery or seen a gunshot wound and then, in a shockingly sudden nightmare, a million devastating casualties occurred.

"In 1861, neither North nor South was medically prepared for the vast casualties the war would produce. Sick or injured people were treated at home. Medicine was practiced with virtually no governmental regulation. No ambulances took people to hospitals, and hospitals were for poor people who were about to die": observed Robert D. Hicks, PhD, senior consulting scholar, William Maul Measey Chair for the History of Medicine, and director emeritus of the Mütter Museum of the College of Physicians of Philadelphia.

The technology of Western medicine of the period is exemplified by a telling suggestion from the esteemed British physician and author Sir Thomas Longmore, who advised:

> Of all instruments for conducting an examination of a gunshot wound, the finger of the surgeon is the most appropriate.

Fortunately for the Civil War doctors, although the field of medicine remained tied to primitive techniques, pathology had advanced during the previous two centuries. The increasing practice of the dissection of cadavers in the Western world had opened new windows to understanding disease and abnormalities, although the medical schools were popularly regarded with some measure of suspicion and disdain. Owing to the shortage of readily available bodies for autopsy examinations, American medical students had acquired a reputation akin to that of marauding ghouls for "body snatching" from fresh graves. In 1861, several states still prohibited dissection by medical students. No rules or laws had been established for the donation of a body "to science," and it would be many years before organizations like the American Medical Education and Research Association (AMERA) would provide standards and accreditation for non-transplant organizations dealing with whole-body donation, university anatomical programs, and the use of human tissue.

American physicians of the mid–19th century frequently trained through an apprenticeship with an older doctor, who passed along his own fund of knowledge, both good and bad, and sometimes the mentor or "preceptor" sponsored the student's admission to a formal medical college. The average medical student in the United States trained for two years rather than the European requisite of four, and received little clinical and laboratory experience. Doctors of the Civil War, with minimal relevant training and equipment, faced an onslaught of grievously wounded and sick men.

Clinical medicine was only a part of the story, as record-keeping and data analysis were not, by any means, standard practices at the time.

The thirteen original American colonies relied on a single educational institution for instruction in the medical arts—the University of Pennsylvania, founded in 1740—that opened the doors of its School of Medicine in Philadelphia in 1765, offering students lectures on anatomy and "the theory and practice of physic." Led by John Morgan, a young physician from the city, the trustees organized a medical faculty that was structured separately from the existing collegiate faculty. Dr. Morgan and most of the professors had received their medical educations at the University of Edinburgh and many had also attended advanced studies in London, where a more hands-on approach to the learning process was applied.

Prospective students at Penn's new School of Medicine faced no prerequisite classes or preparation for their admission. They were not required to take a qualifying exam. In exchange for a large entrance fee, classes or lectures were given for a two-year course of study, with the second year a repetition of the first. A faculty panel decided on the conferring of degrees upon graduating students, and few professional standards were in place. Upon going into practice, most doctors prescribed and compounded their own pharmaceutical preparations and medications.

The more intensive European educations of Penn's medical professors contributed two novel concepts to the training of American physicians: the new medical school was established within an existing institution of higher learning, and the school emphasized the importance of clinical practice and bedside teaching in addition to lectures. Penn prevailed as the leader in medical education in America for decades, and the requirements and standards originally set by the School of Medicine remained mostly intact for the next one hundred years.

Women were not permitted to enroll in the University of Pennsylvania's School of Medicine or in most American medical schools for many decades, until the Female Medical College of Pennsylvania was granted a charter in

1850 that allowed the school to grant degrees to women. The New England Female Medical College was given the authority to confer medical degrees in 1856. It was an outgrowth of the Female Education Society, which had been founded in 1848 to provide women's medical training, although the Society did not have the ability to award medical degrees. By the start of the Civil War, at least three medical schools for women existed and some other institutions had become coeducational. Most American medical schools continued to bar women, some maintaining the gender discrimination for decades. In 1945, eighty-eight women were finally admitted to Harvard Medical School, the first coeducational class in its history.

Mid–19th century African Americans faced seriously difficult roads to gain medical educations, even more so for people from Southern states with laws that made it illegal for enslaved or free people of color to learn to read. In some startling instances, a few daring and dedicated souls managed to run a gauntlet of obstacles and attain brilliant goals. The first African American to receive an M.D. degree from an American medical school was David Jones Peck of Carlisle, Pennsylvania, the son of prominent minister and abolitionist John Peck, a free man of color. Young David Peck interned for two years with a white anti-slavery physician and was accepted to Rush Medical College in Chicago, Illinois, graduating in 1847. His achievements were held up by activist abolitionists to promote the concept of full citizenship for blacks. Most of the thirteen African American doctors who served in the Civil War had graduated from medical schools in Canada, where a more liberal and inclusive attitude existed.

By the onset of the Civil War in 1861, the School of Medicine of the University of Pennsylvania was typical of other medical teaching facilities: there were no laboratories in which to conduct tests or prepare medications. The School had no hospital of its own, but it did conduct a dissecting room and gave clinical instruction in a neighboring hospital. The country then had more than eighty medical schools, many of which operated independently of large universities, and very little surgery was performed. Most schools were merely faculties of professors who delivered lectures for which they sold tickets usually ranging from $10 to $25 (roughly $330–$825 today) per course. Most medical schools conducted lectures for only four to five months of the year and second-semester lectures were a repeat of the first. Courses in anatomy, surgery, midwifery, and other subjects were available, but optional. A panel of professors usually determined whether a given student was entitled to a degree after two years of study—no national examining boards or requirements existed. Many independent medical schools had sprung up in the United States, and the mere possession of a diploma granted the right to practice. Reform of the licensing system did not occur until many years after the war.

America's first medical school sent more surgeons to both the Union and Confederate armies than any other collegiate institution in the country, but Penn and the other schools, unaware of the gigantic, chaotic conflict ahead, weren't prepared to take an organized part in the war effort—a war that would be far larger and last much longer than anyone had anticipated.

The famed American surgeon, educator, and author Dr. William Williams Keen developed an unusual perspective throughout his ninety-five years. Keen's writings and letters sparkle with astute observations, dark humor, and witty commentary. He began his military medical career in the Civil War as a twenty-three-year-old surgeon with less than two years of training, and followed his service with a long and brilliant career in medicine. Dr. Keen served his country again in uniform at age eighty in World War I. In his later years he marveled at the primitive state of medicine during his earliest experiences as a doctor:

> There were practically no clinical thermometers in our armies in 1861–1865. Imagine the plight of a surgeon, physician, obstetrician, or even of the mother of a family today without a clinical thermometer. Hemostatic forceps, retractors and dilators, now in

constant use, were utterly unknown. Instruments for examining all the accessible hollow organs, the ear, the nose, the bronchial tubes in the interior of the lung, the stomach, bladder, ureter and kidney, were not so much as dreamed of. The chemistry and physics of the blood and the various devices to study the blood pressure was unknown.

Some of the most difficult surgical challenges faced by Civil War surgeons were locating and tying bleeding blood vessels. One of the only tools available for seizing and holding arteries was a sharp, slender hook attached to a handle and called a "tenaculum."

Frequently the surgeons were forced to utilize household utensils, odd pieces of wood or metal, and other unlikely items as makeshift surgical instruments. Confederate surgeon Dr. Hunter Holmes McGuire was General Stonewall Jackson's medical director and personal physician. A brilliant student whose education had begun in Philadelphia prior to the war, McGuire was noted as sometimes attempting neurosurgery in the field. A colleague once observed him breaking off one prong of a table fork, bending the point of the other prong, and using it to elevate the bone in a depressed fracture of the skull. The patient was reported to have survived.

In mid-19th-century wartime America, surgeons did not have regular access to some of the most important diagnostic tools to have been developed. Since ancient times, man has sought to see a magnified version of those things too tiny for the human eye to distinguish. Some knowledge dates back two thousand years, when it became known that glass bends light. Spectacle makers were producing lenses by the end of the 13th century, and the close of the 16th century brought the revelation that combining lenses could create far more advanced optical instruments.

During the Civil War, most of the microscopes used in Union military hospitals were provided by Joseph Zentmayer, a German optical worker who had immigrated to America in his early twenties. In 1858 he opened a shop in Philadelphia at Eighth and Chestnut Streets and continued to improve upon the design and workmanship of the microscope, being awarded in 1875, among other accolades, the Elliott Cresson Medal of the Franklin Institute "for some discovery in the Arts and Sciences, or for the invention or improvement of some useful machine, or for some new process or combination of materials in manufactures, or for ingenuity, skill, or perfection in workmanship."

Virtually all of the microscopes in use at the beginning of the Civil War were privately owned; the United States Army Medical Department did not stock them until 1863.

Civil War Lieutenant Colonel Joseph Janvier Woodward, who served as an Army assistant surgeon, experimented with photographing objects as seen under a microscope while using direct sun as the light source. Woodward became a pioneer in photomicroscopy and was known worldwide for helping to prepare the foundation for modern surgical pathology. He performed the autopsies on President Abraham Lincoln and on Lincoln's assassin, John Wilkes Booth, and wrote the reports on both. After the war, Woodward was a coauthor of the six-volume *Medical and Surgical History of the War of the Rebellion* and a curator of sections of the Army Medical Museum. He is regarded as the first scientist to initiate photomicrography as an invaluable tool for medical and scientific applications.

In the six information-packed volumes of *The Medical and Surgical History of the War of the Rebellion*, it is clear that Civil War surgeons were familiar with using stethoscopes to assist in diagnoses. By the early 1800s, it had become apparent to physicians that auscultation—listening to the sounds of the heart and lungs—bore much valuable information about the health of a person. Before they had access to instruments designed for listening, it was common for doctors to put an ear to the chest of a patient. In an 1816 effort to avoid impropriety with a female patient, French physician Dr. René Theophile Hyacinthe Laënnec rolled sheets of paper into a tube and used it instead of his ear to listen to the woman's chest. His observations led to a remarkable discovery:

I recalled a well-known acoustic phenomenon: if you place your ear against one end of a wood beam the scratch of a pin at the other end is distinctly audible. It occurred to me that this physical property might serve a useful purpose in the case I was dealing with. I then tightly rolled a sheet of paper, one end of which I placed over the precordium [chest] and my ear to the other. I was surprised and elated to be able to hear the beating of her heart with far greater clearness than I ever had with direct application of my ear. I immediately saw that this might become an indispensable method for studying, not only the beating of the heart, but all movements able of producing sound in the chest cavity.

Impressed with the quality of the application, Dr. Laënnec later created a wooden tubular device, which he called a stethoscope—from the Greek "stethos" for chest and "skopein" for view or observe—to explore the concept further. The early instruments were monaural, meant for one ear, and in common use by the doctors of the Civil War. The state of American medical training was revealed as still far behind that of European institutions: despite the long existence of two important tools, the stethoscope and the microscope, even Harvard Medical School did not possess these devices until after the Civil War.

The hypodermic syringe, designed to deliver medication beneath the skin, may have its origins in ancient weapons like poison darts and blowpipes that were designed to introduce toxic substances into the body of an enemy. The device is basically a simple pump, and early medical versions of the instrument were called "clysters" and used for giving enemas. The tool was also useful for wound irrigation and douches. The 1850s appear to have introduced hypodermic syringes made of various materials including metal, glass, and wood.

The Civil War version of the instrument lacked a sharp needle, but was still used to deliver medications under the skin. A doctor would make a small incision in the skin and insert the point of the syringe to administer medicine. The syringes were frequently cumbersome to use, and if they weren't easily available in the field, an incision was made and a medic used his finger to dust morphine powder into the wound or push it into the open cut, using his saliva to make the powder stick.

Considering all of the bullet wounds occurring on the battlefields of America, a particular French invention of 1862 was a dangerous but very useful tool for the Civil War surgeons. Dr. Auguste Nélaton of Paris, also credited with the invention of the rubber catheter, created his famous probe for locating and identifying bullets within the human body. The probe was a long, slender, sturdy but flexible wire tipped with unglazed porcelain in the form of a bulb. The probe could be inserted into a wound until it hit something solid. If the instrument had located a bullet, the lead of the projectile would leave a mark on the porcelain tip of the probe. If no mark appeared, it was likely to have touched bone. Despite the unknown but almost certain danger of carrying dirt and germs farther into the wound, the tool was a welcome addition to Civil War diagnostic techniques.

The Nélaton probe made an appearance at one of the most famous bullet wounds in American history, which occurred with the assassination of President Abraham Lincoln. After the doctors spent some hours of probing Lincoln's wound with a finger and keeping it free of clots to allow it to discharge freely, Army Surgeon General Joseph K. Barnes conducted an examination using a Nélaton probe. He was assisted by the first physician to reach the president in his theater box after the shooting, twenty-three-year-old Charles Leale, M.D., of New York City.

> An examination was made by the Surgeon General and myself who introduced the probe to a distance of about two and a half inches, where it came in contact with a foreign substance . . . at first supposed to be the ball, but as the white porcelain bulb of the probe did not indicate the mark of lead, it was generally thought

to be another piece of loose bone. The probe was introduced the second time and the ball was supposed to be distinctly felt.

Rows of archived surgical kits from the Civil War are featured in the holdings of two outstanding American collections, the Mütter Museum of the College of Physicians of Philadelphia and the Thomas Jefferson University Center City Archives and Special Collections. Many of the boxes that hold the instruments are handsomely constructed and frequently embellished with engraved metal plates or carved designs and are sometimes personalized with the owner's initials or monogram. Inside the surgeons' kits are compartments commonly lined with velvet and featuring an array of instruments used for amputations involving arms or legs. Many of the tools have handles made of ivory, wood, or metal, and it is clear that sterilization of them would not have been possible.

Amputation was the most common surgery performed during the Civil War, estimated at three quarters of all operations, and it saved many thousands of lives. Amputating a badly damaged limb changed the situation from a very complex operation to a far simpler procedure. Wounds that involved a joint or bone or were complicated by a large amount of tissue damage were usually candidates for amputation. The battlefields were a fertile classroom and laboratory for the procedure—with practice, an amputation could be completed by an experienced surgeon in about six minutes. The doctors learned to cut as far from the heart as possible and never to slice through joints.

A scalpel was used to slit the skin, and a Caitlin or Catlin knife—a long, double-bladed knife used in amputations since the 17th century—was used to cut through the muscle and separate tissue from the bone. A variety of saws was available to cut through the bone; one of the most common was a flexible chainsaw with detachable handles. The surgeon positioned the saw, then pulled the handles back and forth until the bone was severed. Another common variation of the amputation saws were the single-bladed backsaw type of tool with a pistol grip handle. Civil War surgeons utilized a multitude of knives, lancets, tweezers, and suturing needles, none of which were sterilized or even thoroughly cleaned between patients during an onslaught of wounded.

Patients receiving surgery, known as a "primary amputation," within 48 hours after being wounded had the best chance of survival. After an amputation, patients were usually transferred to a general hospital, where the procedure might be revised or re-amputated if infection had occurred in the bone or tissue.

If a soldier survived his wound and subsequent surgery, he wasn't necessarily healed, as he still faced the looming specter of infection. Almost every soldier who received surgical treatment in the war suffered postoperative infections. American surgeons unknowingly passed dirt and bacteria from one patient to the next, operating with reused instruments and bandaging wounds with septic dressings. Although surgeons were aware of a correlation between cleanliness and a low infection rate, most battlefield conditions didn't permit even a cursory attempt at cleanliness. Doctors unwittingly contaminated injuries from one patient to another as they reused bloodied instruments without even washing their hands. Bullets were also responsible for carrying dirt and bacteria directly into wounds.

After probing a laceration with unsterilized tools or fingers to remove pieces of bullet, shell, or bone, doctors sprinkled morphine powder into the wound, packed it with moist lint or unsterilized cotton, and bandaged it with wet, unsterile bandages. Inflammation and quantities of pus were expected as part of the "healing" process.

A former medical student, Dr. William Williams Keen, remembered witnessing surgical demonstrations during his training at the Jefferson Medical College in Philadelphia. He attended classes with the revered surgeon, teacher, and author Dr. Samuel D. Gross, who incorporated practices that were then perfectly acceptable and are now known to invite and encourage infection:

Before an operation nothing was rendered sterile by antiseptics, or by heat. I have seen more than once, my old teacher, Professor S.D. Gross, give a last fine touch to his knife on his boot—even on the sole—and then at once use it from the first cut to the last. When threading a needle, all of us pointed our silk by wetting it with germ laden saliva and rolling it between germ laden fingers . . . naturally every wound suppurated so that in the little hospital of only eight or ten beds then attached to the Jefferson Medical College, pus was always on tap. "Tomorrow, Hugh," I have often heard Professor Gross say to the orderly, "I shall lecture on suppuration. Get me half a tumbler of pus from the hospital!" And Hugh was always successful!

The postoperative infections were one of the most serious problems in the pre-antibiotic era of the mid–19th century. "Laudable pus" was the thick, creamy excretion that was associated with a more positive healing outcome than "malignant pus," a thin, bloody liquid that oozed from wounds and frequently heralded a terminal condition. The exact organisms that caused the Civil War infections remain unknown, but speculation includes the possible presence of *Streptococcus* bacteria and the nefarious *Clostridia*, which can cause a variety of conditions from tetanus to botulism.

America's war illuminated some terrible ironies: At the time, surgeon Dr. Joseph Lister of the University of Glasgow was experimenting with the theory that contamination by invisible organisms caused the infection of surgical wounds. In 1865, Dr. Lister successfully used carbolic acid to prevent wound infection. He would become known as the "father of antiseptic surgery," but not in time to help the Civil War victims. If the Americans had been aware of the European's work, the use of even simple vinegar as an antiseptic would have dramatically reduced the infections and the suffering.

Erysipelas and hospital gangrene were two of the most feared infections, usually preceding death. Hospital gangrene, seen mostly in wounds and amputation stumps, caused tissue to die and blacken. It spread quickly, sometimes a half-inch per hour, and was jarringly evident to patients and doctors. Forty-five percent of patients with this form of gangrene died, usually in the larger, more crowded hospitals. Dr. Keen remembered:

> Hospital gangrene—a disease now banished I hope, forever—whose very name is a bit of sarcasm, was very common. Often did I see a simple gunshot wound, scarcely larger than the bullet which made it, become larger and larger until a hand would scarcely cover it, and extend from the skin downward into the tissues until one could put half his fist into the sloughing wound.

Erysipelas was a common disease during the Civil War; its symptoms included fever and intense local inflammation of the skin. The infection could spread below the skin and pass into the bloodstream, causing what was known as "pyemia" or "blood poisoning." Physicians who owned microscopes were able to observe these tissue changes, but the instruments were rarely available, as the Army Medical Department didn't stock them until 1863.

William Williams Keen, M.D., who became an illustrious surgeon, professor, and author, reflected on the standard practices of the time:

> We used undisinfected instruments from undisinfected plush-lined cases, and still worse, used sponges which had been used in prior pus cases and had been only washed in tap water. If a sponge or an instrument fell on the floor it was washed and squeezed in a basin of tap water and used as if it were clean.
>
> Our silk to tie blood vessels was undisinfected. We dressed the wounds with clean but undisinfected sheets, shirts, tablecloths, or other old soft linen rescued from the family ragbag. We had no sterilized gauze dressings.

Our dressings consisted of simple ointments, often only cold unboiled water. Little did we dream that our patients recovered in spite of our encouragement of infection. The healing power of good old Mother Nature is often almost past belief.

Army physicians treated their patients with the most advanced care available, but those treatments were frequently ineffective and sometimes harmful. They applied preparations like croton oil, which burned the skin, in the belief that a "counter irritant" would increase blood flow. It didn't work. Soldiers weak from diarrhea were dosed with emetics to induce vomiting in the belief that "cleaning out one's insides" was beneficial—a treatment that probably only worsened the existing condition.

Castor oil was used as a laxative during the Civil War. It is a vegetable oil made by pressing castor beans; a pale yellow liquid with a very distinct taste and odor. Considered to be safe in small doses, larger amounts or dosages given to patients with weakened systems can cause nausea, abdominal cramping, vomiting, and diarrhea. The Union Army purchased 220,000 quarts of castor oil during the war.

Quite a few Civil War treatments had a folkloric history, including some for the care of burns, which have been and remain a common and complicating factor in the realm of combat injuries. War burns have been described throughout more than five thousand years of military history, one of the savage types of results stemming from the invention of gunpowder and sophisticated explosives. Dr. Samuel D. Gross observed:

Among the accidents of war are burns; produced by ordinary fire or by the explosion of gunpowder.

Various remedies have been proposed for these injuries. I have myself always found white-lead paint, such as that employed in the arts, mixed with linseed oil the consistency of very thick cream, and applied so as to form a complete coating, the most soothing and efficient means.

The application of white-lead paint to burns was actually a precursor to some modern treatments. Many burn patients were successfully treated with paint during the Civil War—the paint was soothing, and it diminished fluid loss from burn surfaces. There was a danger of lead toxicity when the burned surface was very large, and a susceptibility to infection, as none of the ointments were sterile.

Few effective medications existed at the time but many available and widely advertised treatments were dangerous and actually contained lethal ingredients like arsenic and mercurous chloride. One of the only pharmaceuticals that was widely embraced for the successful treatment of malaria and some other ailments was quinine.

Quinine, one of the most effective medicines available for treating the challenging disease of malaria, was known in Europe at least since the 17th century and had likely been used in South America for far longer. It was used to address fevers of all kinds but was especially helpful in treating the chills and fever of the dreaded malaria.

Extracts from the bark of the Peruvian cinchona tree were brought to Spain by returning Jesuit missionaries and appeared almost miraculous in malaria treatment. Quinine, considered one of the most important medical discoveries of the period, is a component of the bark, which was also referred to as "sacred bark," "cardinal's bark," or "Jesuits' bark."

Prior to the 19th century, the bark of the tree was administered by being dried, ground to a powder, mixed with wine or another liquid, and drunk. In 1820, French chemists Joseph Caventou and Pierre-Joseph Pelletier, the codiscoverers of caffeine and strychnine, were able to extract and isolate quinine from the bark. The standard treatment for malaria then evolved to replacing the raw bark with the purified quinine.

The private civilian wartime organization, the United States Sanitary Commission, authorized a report on "Quinine as a Prophylactic Against

Malarial Diseases" in 1861, recommending regular preventive doses for troops, and thousands of soldiers lined up for whiskey-laced measures of the drug. The Union Army purchased more than nineteen tons of quinine and nine tons of cinchona fluid extract during the Civil War; Powers and Weightman, a Philadelphia-based firm, was the nation's largest supplier of quinine.

Northern soldiers in Confederate territory were faced with the onslaught of the South's tropical diseases for which the drug was the optimal treatment. The Union's need for increasing quantities of quinine drove the industrial manufacture of its production, with a new attention to testing and quality control. The amplified need for the drug inspired the creation of laboratories and large-scale manufacturing for the first time in the country.

Unfortunately for the quinine needs of the Medical Corps of the Confederacy, the U.S. naval blockade was extremely effective. Blockade running was the best hope for procuring some of their desperately needed medications, and U.S. inspectors found the precious quinine secreted in numerous innocuous-appearing products including dolls and slaughtered animals. Quinine could be sold on the black market in the South for $400–$600 per ounce (approximately $13,000–$19,000 in 2021 U.S. dollars).

Although quinine could have serious adverse effects including cardiovascular reactions, kidney failure, anaphylactic shock, vomiting, diarrhea, and abdominal pain, it was the primary treatment for malaria during the Civil War, staying in popular use until synthetics became available in the 1920s. It endured as a go-to treatment for malaria in many parts of the world, remaining on the World Health Organization's List of Essential Medicines into the 21st century, although it was removed from the list in 2006 and replaced by other drugs with fewer side effects but comparable success.

When quinine wasn't available to them during the Civil War, Confederate surgeons frequently substituted turpentine, treating the soldiers with "friction of turpentine to the spine and twenty drop doses internally."

Turpentine was routinely prescribed for oral and topical use in America and Europe. It was applied to wounds to discourage maggots and mixed with castor oil to treat diarrhea. Made from distilled pine resin, the flammable turpentine, usually associated with solvents, paint thinner, lamp oil, and preserving the wood of ships, has a long and storied history of its use as medicine. Turpentine was used internally as a treatment for depression by the Romans, and as a cure for intestinal parasites like tapeworms. It was mixed with animal fat and applied topically for chest ailments, and inhaled to address nasal and throat problems. Unfortunately, the ingestion of turpentine can be extremely toxic, causing bleeding in the lungs, kidney damage, and numerous other dangerous side effects.

When the Confederate Army's access to adequate supplies of quinine was severely curtailed, turpentine was still readily available as it was one of the South's largest exports after cotton and rice. Its production had begun in the Colonial era in the pine forests of the Carolinas and moved farther and farther south, propelled by the availability of slave labor for the grueling process of collecting the sap. Turpentine camps stretched from North Carolina to Florida and many remained in production into the 20th century. It was clear to the medical staff that turpentine was not as effective as quinine, but it was considered the best of the substitute pharmaceuticals and was certainly accessible to the Confederate Army.

There was some supposition at the time of the war that certain substances might actually be able to fight infection. Iodine, discovered in 1811, was sometimes used as an antiseptic to treat infection during the Civil War. The substance occurs naturally in the form of iodide ions in fish, oysters, certain seaweeds, seawater, dairy products, and some vegetables grown in iodine-rich soil. It was in common use during the Civil War in the form of Lugol's Solution, a combination of elemental iodine and potassium iodide together with distilled water, developed in 1829 by a French physician as a cure for tuberculosis. Although Civil War doctors did not know the science behind the antimicrobial properties and effectiveness of the preparation, they did acknowledge that it was sometimes very helpful in treating wounds and it remained a fairly standard medication for surgical site infections.

Many thousands of Civil War soldiers suffered severe gastric and intestinal disorders, largely owing to their frequent lack of solid nutrition and clean drinking water. Diarrhea was extremely common among the troops, and calomel, or mercurous chloride, was the usual prescription. When it occurs, mercury toxicity presents in a high concentration of mercury in saliva, which can lead to a loss of teeth and gangrene of the mouth and cheeks in some patients. There are many recorded cases of toxic reactions to the drug during the wartime period, including that of Louisa May Alcott, the famous author of many popular books and novels including *Little Women*, who volunteered to serve as a nurse during the Civil War, but contracted typhoid pneumonia six weeks into her first assignment. Alcott came close to death and was returned to her home and treated with calomel. The medication left her with permanent pain for the rest of her life and she wrote, "I was never ill before this time and never well afterward."

"Blue mass" and "blue pills" both contained the toxin mercurous chloride. They were used to treat many ailments, sometimes causing severe reactions. Union President Abraham Lincoln used "blue pills" reportedly to combat depression, chronic constipation, and/or syphilis. The mercury-based medication was in common usage from the 17th century and well into the 19th for treating venereal disease, tuberculosis, toothaches, intestinal parasites, and the pain of childbirth.

Blue mass medications were very varied in strength and purity as they were "magistral preparations"—mixed independently and individually by the pharmacists who dispensed them, a widespread practice in the mid-1800s. The main ingredient was mercury, in its elemental or compound form (such as mercury chloride, also called calomel), but the compounds could also contain glycerol, rose honey, licorice, or hollyhock. Sold in the various form of pills, a claylike substance, or sometimes a syrup, each blue pill usually contained about one grain (64.8 milligrams) of mercury; the color being provided by blue dye or blue chalk.

Abraham Lincoln was known to have suffered deeply from chronic "melancholia" and lengthy depressions. For several years prior to his election as president, Lincoln used blue mass pills to relieve his gloom, as they were commonly prescribed at the time. There is serious speculation that he may have suffered from mercury poisoning, as the dosage he ingested would have been almost nine thousand times the current safety standard issued by the Environmental Protection Agency.

Lincoln was known earlier as a friendly, compassionate, and fairly even-tempered person, despite the tragic and devastating losses he suffered throughout his life, but his personality appears to have changed after he began using the blue pills. He was said to sometimes fly into rages with occasional physical ramifications—once grabbing and shaking another politician until a third person broke his grip on the man. He is also reported to have experienced symptoms including tremor attacks, insomnia, forget-fulness, and outbursts of angry and bizarre behavior, all of which may have been caused by the neurological effects of mercury poisoning and certainly attributable to the massive doses he was consuming.

It's possible that Lincoln may have suspected a correlation between his medications and his new behavioral aberrations—at the onset of the Civil War he apparently stopped taking the pills, stating that they made him "cross." Mercury poisoning can be reversible, and he seems to have then reverted to his more dignified, calm, and composed demeanor, commanding respect for his wartime leadership and the ability to function well under pressure.

The narcotics opium and morphine were used to treat pain and diarrhea. The liberal use of these drugs was criticized after the war for the proliferation of addiction, often called "Old Soldier's Disease." The rising consump-tion of opium in the United States peaked in the 1880s, with commercial opium preparations that were available without a prescription.

Opium was used to treat diarrhea, the most common disease affecting the Civil War soldiers. The drug was widely available in patent medicines, including the popular "laudanum," usually as a tincture of 10 percent opium in alcohol. Effective methods of pill manufacturing had been known for decades, and opium in pill form was a convenient way to store, transport, and administer the drug.

Morphine, an opium alkaloid, was available in pill or powder form and could also be dissolved in liquid for injections. Dr. Henry S. Hewitt, medical director of the Army of the Ohio, issued a standing order for its use during the Atlanta campaign in the summer of 1864:

> The insertion of morphine into wounds of the chest, attended by pain and dyspnea, has been of the utmost advantage. I made the insertion of morphine into all painful wounds a standing order of the medical department, and it has acted so admirably as to enlist every surgeon in favor of the practice. Its good effects are especially remarkable in painful wounds of the joints, abdomen, and chest.

Opiates were extremely popular as treatments and were used liberally as their effects were rapid and visibly evident. It is estimated that the Union army used approximately ten million opium pills, almost three million ounces of opium in powder and tincture form and almost thirty thousand ounces of morphine during the war. Opiates were prescribed for a huge range of ailments including dysentery, typhoid fever, headaches, syphilis, and hemorrhoids, in addition to their application for postoperative pain or for cough suppression in pneumonia patients. There was some resistance to the overuse of narcotics, but as expressed by Union Captain Oliver Wendell Holmes Jr., an honored place among medicaments remained for opium,

> which the Creator himself seems to prescribe, for we often see the scarlet poppy growing in cornfields, as if it were foreseen

that where there is hunger to be fed there must also be pain to
be soothed.

By the end of the war and for many years afterward, an epidemic
of addiction was made apparent from the rising opium consumption
in the United States. The condition called "Old Soldier's Disease" was
common in veterans' homes and in the public. A huge number of women
were addicted to opiates, possibly more women than men, especially in
the postwar period. Narcotics and cocaine were openly sold over the
counter and recommended for a wide range of ailments and "female
complaints." The widespread availability of the drugs continued until
1906, with the passing of the Pure Food and Drug Act in the United
States. An investigation into the drugs revealed that opium, morphine,
and heroin were to be found in a huge variety of commercial pain
relievers, pneumonia cures, teething treatments, and cough syrups. It
has been argued that the Civil War gave the first evidence of rampant
drug addiction in America.

Civil War doctors usually included among their medicaments a drug
called belladonna, made from an extremely toxic plant of the nightshade
family. Belladonna was a common medication used during the Civil War;
its name, "beautiful woman" in Italian, came from a time when women used
it in eye drops to dilate their pupils, believing it to make their appearance
more seductive. Liquid extract of belladonna was included in the United
States Army Standard Supply Table, carried in the doctors' medical kits,
and utilized in hospitals and in the field. The drug was used to treat a wide
variety of ailments, from intestinal cramps or diarrhea to whooping cough,
asthma, sciatica, and scarlet fever. It was also compounded as a topical
ointment by mixing it with lard and applying it to an afflicted area two or
three times a day.

This powerful drug was described in the 1858 publication of the *United
States Dispensatory* as a potent narcotic and anodyne.

Among its first obvious effects, when taken in the usual dose, and continued for some time, are dryness and stricture of the faeces and neighboring parts, with slight uneasiness or giddiness of the head, and dimness of vision. In medicinal doses, it may also occasion dilatation of the pupil, decided frontal headache, slight delirium, colicky pains and purging, and a scarlet efflorescence of the skin; but this last effect is rare. In large quantities, belladonna produces the most deleterious effects. It is in fact a powerful poison, and many instances are recorded in which it has been taken with fatal consequences.

Belladonna is still used in medicine, particularly its derivatives atropine and scopolamine, which have useful properties. Atropine continues to be used in eye drops and also as an antidote for some insecticides and chemical warfare agents.

A few blessedly effective drugs for pain relief were available to Civil War physicians—the anesthetics ether and chloroform were routinely administered. The war prompted wider use of these agents, which had actually been available in America for more than a decade. The uses of ether as an anesthetic had been lauded in a report on surgery to the College of Physicians of Philadelphia fifteen years before the start of the war. Although myths abound of Civil War surgeries performed while patients were fully conscious, of soldiers biting on bullets to bear the pain, of men rendered unconscious with large doses of alcohol, in actuality, both Northern and Southern armies had access to anesthetics throughout the war and they were used in virtually all surgeries that were carried out.

Anesthesia was given to keep a patient unconscious during his surgery. At the time, a standard dose of anesthesia gave surgeons an estimated window of nine minutes to work, but with imprecise quality, methods, or amounts administered, soldiers sometimes woke up at the end of the operation while still on the operating table, surrounded by the gore of previous operations and the sound of other surgeries.

Although anesthesia was almost always used during surgical procedures, a good number of reports from witnesses who saw soldiers thrashing
in apparent pain on operating tables have been circulated. A phenomenon
now known as "second-stage anesthesia" was noted by many wartime
surgeons: in this interim stage of consciousness, the patient is physically
restless and active before the body reaches complete unconsciousness.
Surgery was often performed outdoors, where passing soldiers may have
witnessed the writhing and moaning of the patient and assumed that no
anesthesia was being used.

Ether was indispensable as an anesthetic, but, due to its highly flammable nature, it could also be extremely dangerous to use, especially indoors.
Dr. Keen recounted a terrifying incident in surgery:

> I particularly remember a gunshot wound just above the inner
> end of the right clavicle. The hemorrhage was profuse.
>
> I etherized the man and proceeded to search for the wounded
> vessel. My only light was a square block of wood with five auger
> holes, in each one of which was placed a candle. It was before
> even the days of petroleum, which had then just been discovered
> in Pennsylvania. As the wound was so near the mouth, of course
> the light had to be near the ether cone. I have often wondered
> why I did not have the sense to use chloroform. Suddenly the
> ether took fire and the etherizer flung away both cone and bottle.
> Luckily the bottle did not break or we might have had an ugly
> fire in a hospital constructed wholly of wood. I was fortunate
> enough finally to secure the vessel after much searching and a
> large loss of blood. The patient recovered.

On the battlefield, chloroform was preferred over ether because it had
less bulk, more rapid induction, and was nonflammable. For reasons then
unknown, it occasionally performed unpredictably in certain patients, and

could cause sudden death. If a patient breathed too deeply he might inhale an overdose of chloroform, which could stop the heart.

The Confederacy was concerned with having low reserves of chloroform, but an invention by Dr. Julian John Chisolm of Charleston, South Carolina, enabled the surgeons to use a far smaller dose of the drug in a much more direct and effective fashion. Traditionally, ether and chloroform were dispensed to the patient in a soaked cloth placed over the nose and mouth until the person became insensible. Fumes from the dissipating liquid sometimes affected the operating team when surgeries were performed indoors. The "Chisolm Inhaler" was a 2½-inch hollow metal box with two small attached metal tubes. The tubes were inserted into the patient's nostrils and chloroform was placed on either wadded cotton or fabric that was inserted into the body of the device or dripped into a perforated area on the top of the metal box. The Chisolm Inhaler was a huge boon to the Southern medics, as it allowed for their stock of anesthesia to last far longer than they had originally anticipated, and it delivered a dosage more directly to the patient.

Despite the drawbacks and risks of using general anesthesia, both Civil War medics and patients found it to be a temporary gift of relief to those suffering from terrible pain.

Before the Civil War, the U.S. Army had purchased medicines on the open market, but during the course of the conflict, the Union began to rely heavily on a few large domestic drug companies for stable prices and inventories.

Fueled by the demand for medicines during the Revolutionary War, a North American pharmaceutical industry had sprung up on the East Coast from Baltimore to Boston, with several firms based in Philadelphia. Many of these businesses were founded by pharmacists and physicians with names like Wyeth, Warner, Upjohn and Dohme. As the Civil War progressed, existing companies including Powers and Weightman and the Pfizer Company increased their production of drugs like iodine, morphine, chloroform, tartaric acid, and camphor.

Dr. Robert D. Hicks assessed the industry development: "Armies both North and South had to innovate to address supply problems, shortages, and medicines or technologies that proved ineffective or insufficient. In the North, to produce pharmaceuticals in quantity, quickly, and to a standard required an innovation in management. Thus, the first government-run drug labs were created." Vaccines appear to be an evolution of an ancient practice known as "variolation," a prophylactic defense against the highly contagious and frequently fatal disease of smallpox. Evidence points to the practice of variolation as early in human history as 8th century India, and the same protective procedure was recorded two centuries later in China. In both cases, pus or scab material from an infected person was inserted in an incision in the skin of a healthy person.

New England's early 18th-century Puritan minister Cotton Mather was the owner of Onesimus, an enslaved man from West Africa who had experienced the procedure as a child in Africa and described the process to Mather. Several years later, the minister supported the theory of variolation during a smallpox epidemic in Boston, where it proved effective in dramatically reducing the number of deaths from the disease. By the end of the 18th century, a successful vaccine for smallpox had been developed.

Smallpox was the only disease for which vaccination existed during the Civil War, and immunization was fairly commonplace as performed by physicians in America since the 1830s. The public perception began to change based on a fear of spreading the disease through inoculated persons during the period they were infectious, and the technique was outlawed in several states including New York and Maryland. The vaccinations did initially reduce the frequency and intensity of smallpox outbreaks, but the procedure became largely illegal, was neglected in many places by the start of the Civil War, and disease rates had begun to rise again.

America did not have public health programs in place to encourage the population to be vaccinated, and the potential side effects and complications were discouraging. It was difficult for the Army dispensaries to produce and maintain a viable supply of the vaccine, and when it was used in hospitals, sometimes additional diseases such as syphilis were spread through the process.

Both the Union and Confederate armies technically required that soldiers be vaccinated against smallpox, although the regulations were largely disregarded as both governments rushed to send men into battle. The collected data indicates that between May 1861 and June 1866, the Union Army reported 12,236 smallpox cases among white troops and 6,716 cases among African American troops.

The Confederacy took aggressive measures to ensure adequate scab material for immunizing the soldiers. Military hospitals had an officer assigned to search the local population for infected children from whom to harvest the scabs or "crusts." The preventive measures and quarantines enforced by both armies managed to avert many outbreaks of smallpox during the war and changed public opinion on the efficacy of the procedure, leading to a larger number of inoculated citizens and a tighter control on the range of the dangerous illness.

Before soldiers set foot on the battlefields, they faced an equally deadly enemy in the form of diseases that ran rampant through the army camps.

During the mid-1860s, Dr. Louis Pasteur, the French chemist and microbiologist, was working on his germ theory of disease, an idea that was not widely known in America. By the end of the war, Pasteur would prove that invisible microorganisms cause disease and fermentation and that they are not spontaneously generated. His discoveries would lead to future methods for preventing the spread of diseases, but would not be accepted in common practice in America until years after the Civil War.

Black soldiers showed proportionately higher rates of disease and mortality. African American troops were diagnosed with anemia twice as frequently as white troops, and among those who had been in slavery in the southeast, there was a high incidence of intestinal worms. Confederate doctor William H. Taylor remembered:

The prevailing diseases were intestinal disorders, though we had a share of almost every malady. Occasionally we suffered seriously from measles. Smallpox was effectively kept in check by vaccination. Intermittent and other malarial fevers at times incapacitated regiments.

Estimates place disease deaths among Union troops at a minimum of 225,000 during the war, although there are no established statistics for those who died after the war from the effects of diseases contracted during the conflict. The Army camps were known for their filthy conditions, contaminated water, and terrible diet and it was commonly said that a Civil War army could be smelled before it was seen.

Little more than 160 years ago, the medical profession in America was unregulated and primitive in practice, as the evidence establishes. Adding the fact that surgeons were frequently operating by candle or torchlight, or, in most cases, initially without much experience, it is astounding that so many of the sick and wounded actually lived on. It is estimated that of the amputees, most of whom likely suffered post-surgical infections, approximately 75 percent survived their injuries and subsequent treatment.

More Civil War soldiers died from disease than from wounds received in battle: half of all Civil War deaths were the result of intestinal disorders such as typhoid fever, diarrhea, and dysentery. These diseases were caused by drinking polluted water and by the lice, fleas, and flies that abounded in the filthy army camp conditions. "Fever" was considered a disease, not a symptom.

Gastrointestinal disorders including diarrhea and dysentery were the most common of all camp diseases, and the mortality rate from them was very high. Records indicate that there were approximately 711 cases per 1,000 soldiers each year. The Union army counted more than 75,000 cases of typhoid fever during the course of the war, likely resulting from exposure to contaminated food and water in addition to flies. Typhoid fever killed 17 percent of affected soldiers at the beginning of the war and 56 percent by 1865. It was the disease that killed President Lincoln's eleven-year-old son, Willie. Union major and surgeon S. C. Gordon, witnessed the terrible effects of diseases on the soldiers.

> The death list from disease was a fearful one in the Department of the Gulf. Fever and diarrhea, the former disabling and the latter killing, were worse foes than bullets, ten to one. It was estimated that at least ten thousand soldiers died and were buried in the Department of the Gulf, from disease of the bowels alone. It was a standing joke in our department that to be a good soldier here bowels are of more consequence than brains.
>
> The slang phrase in regard to the soldier who was discharged, was "He hasn't got the guts to stand it." The marches were long, the water poor, the weather torrid, and the rations oftentimes of poor quality. Fatigue duty under such circumstances was deadly. The bones of the best young men of New England lie in unknown graves all over Louisiana.

Most of 1860s America was rural and farmers made up almost half of the Union army. Young soldiers from the sparsely populated countryside had never been exposed to the common contagious diseases that spread rapidly through the crowded military encampments. Thousands of men were felled by measles, chicken pox, mumps, and whooping cough. Colonel Daniel Hand, M.D. of the U.S. Army, continually observed surprising events and statistics among the suffering men.

> While in our winter quarters we had many cases of measles. It was astonishing to find so many grownup men who had never had measles, and we found the number of such candidates was

much greater in the country regiments than in those raised in cities.

In many other ways we found the city-raised soldiers had an early advantage over their country comrades. They had caught everything that was going while children, they were used to being up and out late at night, and they were prompt to take care of themselves, while the lads from the country had been coddled by their mothers, kept out of harm's way, and were slow to act.

Measles outbreaks were common in the camps: extremely contagious and highly lethal, the disease affected at least 67,000 Union soldiers resulting in more than 4,000 deaths among white troops and a mortality rate almost twice as high in African American soldiers. Doctors recorded that the measles deaths were primarily caused by the involvement of respiratory and brain function.

At the time of the Civil War, the concept of contagion, of diseases being spread from one person to another, was somewhat uncertain. If a disease was perceived as contagious, quarantine was usually recommended. The question of quarantine, and its interference with personal liberties, became a political issue among the civilian population. Business was affected, as enforced quarantines would interfere with commerce, and the business community sometimes protested the classifications of diseases as contagious.

Disease made its way into the civilian population. Thousands died from yellow fever and malaria, considered the tropical diseases, which had several shared symptoms: chills, fevers, and nausea. The symptoms could last for many hours and then returned periodically, possibly afflicting the victim on a daily basis. Physicians believed these diseases were caused by the vapors given off by swamps. The term "malaria" was derived from the Italian "mala aria," meaning bad air. The medical community of the time did not connect malaria to mosquitos, although working by canals or sleeping outdoors were conditions known to increase risk. They were aware that locating army camps a significant distance away from stagnant water and having sleeping quarters that were elevated above the ground reduced the chance of contracting malaria. The disease was not usually fatal, but it was capable of debilitating entire camps. Colonel and Surgeon Daniel Hand faced thousands of cases of malaria in the troops.

> We had two large convalescent hospitals at the sea-shore, on Beaufort harbor, and in summer sent most of the sick who could travel. This no doubt saved the lives of many poor fellows broken down by malarial poison. This poison in many districts was almost certainly fatal to those exposed to it after nightfall. Again and again, we had sentinels struck down insensible and dying while on duty. So often did this happen in 1863, we provided for it by having surgeons sit up all night and keep hot water ready, so as to put such men immediately in a hot bath.
>
> This course saved many lives, but so powerful an effect did these congestive chills have on the brain, we could for weeks after such an attack recognize a man who had it, and I doubt if these men ever fully recovered.

"Malarial poison" was another name for the swamp vapors that were believed to cause malaria. While a hot bath wouldn't have cured the disease, bathing the patient probably had other positive effects, such as discouraging the fleas that carried typhus and the flies that carried typhoid fever. During the Battle of Shiloh, Tennessee, in April 1862, troops on both sides were ravaged by malarial diseases. By May, Union General William Tecumseh Sherman's troops were diminished by half, as sickness had affected 50 percent of the men.

Fortunately for the sufferers of the disease, it was well known that quinine was proven to ease its symptoms. The drug did not cure the disease, but it suppressed the symptoms strongly enough to keep soldiers functioning.

It was used as a prophylactic measure and, mixed with whiskey, it was regularly distributed to troops. U.S. Surgeon John Shaw Billings endorsed the use of quinine.

> Quinine was always and everywhere prescribed with a confidence and freedom which left all other medicines far in the rear. Making all due allowances for exaggerations, that drug was unquestionably the popular dose with doctors.

Due to its popularity, quinine was frequently in short supply, however, and the Confederate Army was forced to substitute turpentine in many cases, although its effectiveness was not comparable. Quinine remained a primary treatment for malaria for many years. The disease was caused by the parasite *Plasmodium*, but the parasite's carrier, the mosquito, would not be clearly identified until the end of the century.

Epidemics of yellow fever have appeared throughout American history, thought to have arrived in the Western hemisphere during the African slave trade. An epidemic was reported in the Yucatan in 1648, and periodic outbreaks occurred for the next two hundred years in Europe and North American coastal cities and tropical areas. The epidemics occurred mostly in summer and autumn months and the illness was termed the "stranger's disease" as newcomers to a given area were the likeliest victims. During the Civil War yellow fever struck more than ten thousand people in the South, with more outbreaks in Texas than anywhere else in the country. Those who survived seemed to have gained a lifetime immunity to the disease.

As Union troops invaded the Confederacy in 1862, Northern soldiers became prey to the multiple tropical diseases common to the bayous and swamps of the coastal regions of the South. The wartime yellow fever epidemics also had a deadly effect on refugees as thousands of African Americans died from the overcrowding and contagion in contraband camps.

In New Orleans, it was noted that outbreaks often occurred after the arrival of ships from Caribbean ports, inspiring a radical plan of action. All ships were quarantined seventy miles below the city for forty days, a prudent decision that eventually almost completely eliminated yellow fever in New Orleans.

Venereal diseases were very common among mid-19th-century troops. It had been known for hundreds of years that syphilis and gonorrhea were transmitted by sexual contact, although the term "gonorrhea" was applied to all forms of urethral discharge during the Civil War. As the devastating complications frequently don't appear for many years, it's impossible to estimate the number of postwar deaths that can be attributed to these diseases. Between 1861 and 1865, 102,893 soldiers were diagnosed with gonorrhea during the war and 79,589 with syphilis, but very few wartime deaths were listed as a direct result of these diseases. The military created some successful public health programs in its efforts to rid camp areas of diseased prostitutes. The women were rounded up, inspected, treated, and released when their symptoms receded.

The dental problems of soldiers presented separate health care issues to which Union and Confederacy would have strongly differing approaches.

Humans have practiced early forms of dentistry for many thousands of years, but it was not until 1840 that the first independent dental school in America opened in Baltimore, which may have occurred as a result of the medical department of the University of Maryland's refusal of a request by students for the inclusion of dental education in its curriculum. Most dental practitioners were likely trained through apprenticeships under experienced "preceptors," or were simply self-ordained, but the trend toward the formal practice of dentistry was demonstrated the following year by Alabama's enactment of the first dental practice act. It was a field of medicine that was beginning to be taken seriously in the country, and by 1859, the American Dental Association was organized in Niagara Falls, New York. Although there was great growth in the field, none of the dental schools in the country were incorporated into medical schools by the Civil War's end.

At the start of the war in 1861, there were about 5,500 dental practitioners in the country, but only about 400 had been graduated from the existing American dental schools. The schools awarded a Doctorate of Dental Surgery, the first degree of its kind in the United States.

The average soldier was not likely to take care of his teeth, did not brush them, and likely had a poor diet. Teeth were, however, important tools on the battlefield as it was normal practice to bite off the end of powder cartridges for the muzzle-loading rifles. If recruits lacked half a dozen opposing upper and lower front teeth, they were frequently turned away from the army.

The Union Army had no dental corps, had strongly resisted forming one for at least ten years, and did not emphasize the importance of dental hygiene to its wartime soldiers. Any dental procedures that were completely necessary were performed by surgeons or hospital stewards, except in instances where practicing dentists had enlisted as surgeons. The most common treatments offered were lancing boils on the gums or the pulling of teeth.

Dentist Dr. William B. Roberts, editor of the *New York Dental Journal*, published in an 1862 article:

> the army surgeon is generally not only utterly incompetent
> to the proper care of teeth, but he is also entire averse to it . . .
> If the soldier could only take reasonable care of his teeth
> himself, he would get on much better, but a toothbrush is an
> article not in the regulations.

Dr. Roberts also decried the lack of appropriate dental instruments allocated to Army surgeons: "attached to the encumbrances of the surgeon are: one turnkey, two pairs of straight forceps, one pair of lower molar forceps, one gum lancet, and the occasional stump screw" and that "the

best trained dentist in the world could not perform with these instruments
. . . to any degree of satisfaction."

The American Dental Association and many practicing dentists agreed
with Roberts's stance in advocating for the assignment of one dentist to each
brigade and educating the men on the importance of proper dental care.
They argued that it would save the U.S. War Department a "useless and
ill-regulated expense," although the admonitions were ignored, no military
dental units were formed, and Union soldiers were not provided with dental
care throughout the length of the war.

The Confederate government required every soldier to have a dental
exam. The shortage of men in the South made it clear that no one could
be exempted from military service because of problems with his teeth. The
Confederate Army's high command advocated for and began to appoint
dentists into their army by 1861, remaining supportive of troops' appropriate dental care and prevention throughout the war.

By 1864, Confederate medical corps had professional dentists in most of
their military hospitals and more were appointed to provide care to soldiers
in the field. Both President Jefferson Davis and Surgeon General Samuel
Preston Moore were strong proponents of dental care and for adding dentistry within the structure of the army. They had also become aware that
proper care for dental ailments frequently allowed a more rapid recovery
for the soldier and his faster return to the battlefield.

In addition to other medical supply shortages caused by the war, the
South had only a single supplier for dental needs—Brown and Hape in
Atlanta—but they began to assemble all available supplies and tools and added
to their regulations that tooth-extracting kits must be issued and included
with medical supplies. The Confederacy also became aware that most
soldiers could not afford professional dental services, and they began to
contract civilian dentists to supply them. In 1861, Dr. J. B. Deadman from
North Carolina was the first civilian dentist to be appointed and employed,
followed by a more formal draft and conscription of dental practitioners.

The 1864 Conscription Act was not welcomed by all Southern dentists, and some were able to obtain exemptions under "special circumstances," but the result of the draft was that the Confederacy gained a significant number of dentists who could also be assigned to work as regimental surgeons.

An additional upside to the increased dental services provided by the Confederate Army was that the practitioners gained skills and advanced the technology of their field. A great deal of work was done in new procedures like endodontic treatment for root canal and maxillofacial surgery to correct or prevent dental or facial deformity. Many soldiers who may not have been considered fit for service were able to rejoin the active troops after skilled dental treatment.

The Confederacy also strongly promoted the importance of dental hygiene and the necessity of possessing, carrying, and using a toothbrush. By the end of the war, most Confederate hospitals had at least one dentist on staff and the government was considering the establishment of a Bureau of Dental Surgery.

Throughout man's history with animals, disease has been the driving force behind the development of veterinary medicine. Animals have been a major part of wars and food supplies for centuries, and Europe was long familiar with disease outbreaks in animal populations that had severely affected both. France established a school of veterinary medicine in Lyon in 1762, created in part because of a disease epidemic and also due to concerns about the need for animals in warfare.

The United States had thus far escaped any epidemic diseases of livestock, and not many people in the country saw the need for formal veterinary education. The density of livestock was not particularly large, leaving few opportunities for any diseases to become widespread. Those who worked with animals gained their experience onsite and firsthand; farriers—craftsmen who trim and shoe horses' hooves—dealt with horses and "cow leeches" worked with cows and other livestock. The care of animals was left largely to their owners and there did not seem to be a call for or pressing need of formal veterinary education in America. As they had been in the Revolutionary War, farriers were considered to be those most knowledgeable about the care of horses and they provided the first veterinary services to the U.S. Army. Although they had no formal education in equine treatment, they possessed the most practical expertise about the animals and were respected by the Army.

By the 1850s, the U.S. Army saw some necessity for establishing an institution that would instruct Army veterinarians, and there were dozens of attempts to start veterinary schools, but most of them failed in the early stages. The American civilian population's farmers and ranchers had begun to express a need for experts in animal health for their communities and some medical colleges began to add lectures on veterinary treatments. An appeal to Congress was made in 1853 by Quartermaster General Thomas Jesup for the establishment of an Army veterinary corps and school, but the request was denied. The U.S. Army, while resisting the institution of a veterinary corps, still pursued experiments in targeting ideal mammals for the military's use. An 1855 experiment in replacing the usual horses or mules as pack animals tested camels as replacements, receiving an initially positive response from the men working with the creatures. The then U.S. secretary of war, Jefferson Davis, headed the camel experiment, which was permanently derailed by the start of the Civil War and Davis's subsequent alignment with the Southern states.

When the Civil War began, there were about 7.5 million horses in America and possibly 50 trained veterinarians in the country, all of them Europeans who had studied abroad. Any soldiers working with animals in the U.S. Army tended to be untrained. No set qualifications yet existed for the position of "veterinary sergeant," and neither Union nor Confederate armies had a formal veterinary corps, although after the first several months of the war the U.S. Army did form a veterinary service. At this point a position was created for "veterinary sergeants," each of whom received the pay and benefits of a noncommissioned officer consisting of fuel, rations, quarters, a horse, and $17 a month (equal to about $570 in today's dollars). The veterinary sergeants were each responsible for three battalions of horses, and despite their lack of formal training or the availability of adequate medications, they faced difficult equine diseases including distemper, "blind staggers," and the highly contagious upper-respiratory ailment "glanders."

An increasing scarcity of food for horses, wounds received in battle, overwork, and terrible neglect by the ignorance of those tasked with their care led to the deaths of many thousands of animals. More than 1.2 million mules and horses died in the Civil War, the loss totaling approximately 20 percent of all the horses in the country.

After the war ended, the government originally allowed the scavenging of horse remains and the selling of the bones. Secretary of War Edwin Stanton contacted the quartermaster general asking that farmers be granted the right to dig up the bones of fallen military horses and mules to be used as fertilizer for crops. The quartermaster refused the request, stating that they were animals who had died in service to their country and consequently their remains deserved honor. An 1865 letter from the quartermaster's office included the statement, "Having died in service he thinks they [the horses] ought to rest in peace."

CHAPTER TWO

WHAT MADE THIS WAR
SO DEADLY?

Both Union and Confederacy were completely unprepared to deal with the medical crises presented by the first "modern war": modern in the sense that this conflict employed high-velocity bullets and cannonballs and relied upon fast-moving railroads that could quickly mobilize tens of thousands of troops. Advances in technology made possible the mass production of weapons, the rifling of gun barrels, and manufacturing of the new repeating guns as they came into use. Communication was greatly enhanced by the 1844 invention of the telegraph and improvements in printing that made multiple copies of publications and pictures more widely available to the public. Transportation on land and combat on the sea were evolving importantly with the appearance of streetcars, submarines, and ironclad warships, but some of the most stunning and memorable advances were in the killing and maiming power of weapons.

Black powder or gunpowder was originally invented in the East for medicinal purposes by practitioners of the Taoist religion and philosophy. Its large-scale production and use in warfare can be traced to 10th-century China when the predecessor of modern guns, the "fire lance," first appeared: an incendiary device composed of a metal tube fastened to the end of a spear, filled with black powder, and lit with a slow match of pinewood soaked in sulfur. Small packages of the combustible substance were also wrapped in paper, attached to arrows, and ignited with a fuse. Military engineers of the Song dynasty (960–1279) used gunpowder as a highly effective weapon in siege warfare and utilized it in the development of the first bombs, mines, cannons, and rockets.

As the trade in weapons increased, the manufacture of more advanced arms appeared in Central Europe, France, Spain, Italy, and the British Isles, where the development of guns was further improved and refined. The 18th century saw large migrations to America, where early colonization required gun-based survival and encouraged the many technological weapons enhancements that were made in the New World.

The Civil War marked a revolutionary leap in warfare: deadly new ammunition, the rifling of gun barrels for greater accuracy, speed, and velocity, and the development of the repeating gun—the direct ancestor of today's automatic and semiautomatic weapons and great-grandfather of the AK-47 and AR-15-style assault rifles. This was also a time when new armaments ran directly up against old medicine. Traditional combat strategies employed in the period included the massed infantry attack that utilized facing linear formations of opposing combatants and was responsible for rapid and vast numbers of casualties.

Advances in medicine lagged far behind this recent technology that had radically increased the power of weapons. The new arms were highly efficient and caused extensive damage. The ten-hour Battle of Antietam in Maryland in September 1862 created 23,000 dead and wounded, while the three-day Battle of Gettysburg, Pennsylvania, in July 1863 resulted in another 53,000 casualties. American trauma medicine, in its infancy, was overwhelmed with the savage effects of the fighting and gaping lacks in experience, education, and support. Current estimates suggest that between 620,000 and 750,000 deaths were a result of the extended violence.

The bladed weapons of centuries past were still found on the battlefields, but wounds attributed to them made up less than 2 percent of the human damage as hand-to-hand combat was relatively uncommon in the Civil War. Advancements in small arms and artillery meant that troops rarely came close enough to fight with bayonets or to club one another with the butt end of their muskets. Swords were carried by officers and served more as a badge of rank than a weapon. Mounted troops frequently carried the formidable sabers, but the cavalry eventually found that firearms were preferable to the edged weapons.

The majority of Civil War wounds were caused by the new ammunition: specifically, the Minié ball. This evolved projectile, developed in France, was a hollow ellipse of soft lead with rifling at its base. The bullet was easily deformed and notorious for passing through two or three bodies in one shot. The Minié ball and its accompanying advances changed the face of combat.

The familiar smoothbore musket, somewhat infamous for its loading difficulty and firing inaccuracies, was giving way to the new guns with rifled barrels and to advanced cannons, which were superior to all the Western weapons of the past. The lines of facing troops in the massed infantry attack were now killing one another far more efficiently with their vastly improved weapons and enhanced ammunition performance.

The long gun with a smoothbore barrel known as a "musket" first appeared in the early 16th century. Its name may have come from the French word "mousquette," for a male sparrowhawk, as firearms were frequently named after animals, or an alternate theory suggests that it may be a derivation of the Italian "moschetto," the bolt of a crossbow. A weapon capable of penetrating heavy armor, the musket's name endured and was assigned to virtually any handheld long gun until the mid-1800s. The American Civil War version was a shoulder gun carried by infantry, usually a large-caliber muzzle-loading smoothbore. The musket was phased out of use with the advent of newer long guns with rifled barrels.

Musket balls, a form of ammunition dating back to the 15th century, were one of the earliest types of bullets ever designed to be fired from a gun. Although stone musket balls have been found, traditional musket balls were usually cast from molten lead in a mold, cooled, and trimmed, and sometimes in desperate circumstances, even manufactured directly on the field of battle. Most musket balls were approximately .7 inches in diameter and weighed about .9 ounces, the size used in American guns up to and throughout the 1846–1848 Mexican-American War. They were fired from muzzle-loading smoothbore long guns and they caused heavy damage at close range. Musket balls were loosely accurate to about 100 yards.

Loading the weapons required the pouring of gunpowder into the musket barrel followed by the insertion of the round ball projectiles, wrapped in a fabric patch, being pushed down the barrel on top of the powder charge with a long, slim tool known as a "ramrod." If the ball was not wrapped in the fabric patch, it could bounce from side to side within the musket barrel, resulting in an unpredictable trajectory. It was also difficult to standardize the amount of gunpowder used, so firing results could be erratic. Musket balls made of lead would expand inside a human body and leave a huge exit wound. Most could be compared to .30–.75 caliber ammunition, but even weightier balls were manufactured for the large-bore pistols that were also in use at the time.

As the Civil War continued, smoothbore muskets began to be phased out by both armies and replaced by rifled muskets. The Northern factories were better equipped to manufacture the new arms compared to the lesser industrialization of the South. The North's manufacturing advantage can largely be credited to advanced mass production techniques developed by Eli Whitney, known primarily as the inventor of the cotton gin. Rifled gun barrels had begun to appear in the years before the Civil War, issued to both Northern and Southern troops, and their use, coupled with a new bullet known as the Minié ball, changed the universe of combat.

French army officer Claude-Étienne Minié, born in 1804, had served in a number of African campaigns, achieving the rank of captain. In 1849 he improved upon several earlier efforts by military men and resolved the reliability problem of muzzle-loading guns by designing a new bullet that would replace the long-used globe-shaped musket ammunition. It would become known as the Minié ball.

The Minié ball, despite its name, was a cylindrical, bullet-shaped lead projectile with a conical point. It had a hollow in its base that expanded when fired, and the rifled skirting at the base of the bullet fit tightly against the spiraling grooves in a gun barrel, which stabilized and spun the ball as it exited the barrel. The bullet's velocity was maximized and the accuracy and effective range of the weapon was increased from 100 yards to 300 yards. The ball weighed about 1½ ounces and was frequently wrapped in paper, dipped in tallow, and then slid smoothly into a gun barrel. The new bullet was accurate at long range and frighteningly effective. Civil War doctors described the damage done by Minié balls as a shattering of the bones and "pulpifying" of the muscles.

The new conical bullets, owing to their higher velocity and greater mass, were anathema to the human body. They could go through the bodies of two or three soldiers in one single shot, rarely remaining lodged within the bodies, and they created massive exit wounds. The damage to limbs, including shattered bones and compound fractures, was so severe that amputation was usually necessary in order to save a life. Major blood vessels impacted by the ball frequently had deadly outcomes. The older musket ball retained the possibility of being deflected by a large bone and avoiding serious or permanent injury, but the Minié ball's shape and soft lead composition tended to distort and flatten when it impacted the body, which increased the potential for grave damage as its velocity and weight allowed it to continue traveling through multiple bodies despite its deformation. These powerful bullets fired by small arms were not always immediately or imminently fatal, and field hospital records note many examples of soldiers shot through the head who only died after lingering for hours or days.

The tradition of frontal assaults by cavalry and infantry was ending. The new weapons and ammunition could be fired accurately from a long distance and take down attackers before they got too close. The increased range of the defensive forces was responsible for a revolution in combat and the killing power of the individual soldier was multiplied exponentially.

The Minié ball was enthusiastically adopted by the armies of Europe and the United States and was the most-used ammunition throughout the American Civil War, where it has been estimated that 90 percent of deaths on the battlefield were attributed to the combination of the rifled gun barrel and the Minié ball.

Claude Minié retired with the rank of colonel in 1858 and was rewarded by the French government with an appointment to the staff of a military school and 20,000 francs (more than $250,000 in today's dollars). He later served as a manager for the Remington Arms Company in the United States. Minié's technology had changed Western warfare and medicine by creating the majority of the catastrophic gunshot wounds of the American Civil War.

The Minié ball was the ammunition used by one of the most well-known, requested and lethally effective infantry weapons of the Civil War, the Springfield Model 1861 rifle. It was the Union Army's standard-issue arm, the most widely used shoulder weapon, and was popular in the Confederate Army as well for its accuracy, range, and reliability on the battlefield. The "Springfield" was used throughout the war, had an effective firing range of 200 to 400 yards, and could fire two to three rounds per minute.

The rifle was originally manufactured by the Springfield Armory in the city of Springfield, Massachusetts (formally known as the United States Armory and Arsenal at Springfield), which produced military firearms for the United States from 1777 to 1968.

Due to the weapons shortage at the start of the war, the federal government contracted for almost one million Model 1861–type rifles from about twenty different private companies during the conflict, making it the first rifle ever to be produced on such a large scale.

The Springfield variants of the Model 1861 included the Models 1863 and 1864, but the Model 1861 remained the principal weapon of the Civil War. It was a muzzle-loading percussion rifle that was designed to use the new and deadly Minié ball ammunition. Its manufacturing cost per unit in 1861 was $14.93 ($482.20 in 2021 U.S. dollars) and the pressing need for quantities of the weapon necessitated expanding its manufacture outside of the United States to Manton in England and firms in Germany.

The Springfield was a handsomely designed and produced gun and many Union soldiers, despite being aware of its inferiority to the repeating guns, expressed great pride in its appearance and performance. In a paean of praise to the visual elegance of the weapon, a corporal in the Fifty-Second Massachusetts Volunteers wrote, "dark black—walnut stock, well oiled, so that the beauty of the wood is brought out, hollowed at the base, and smoothly fitted with steel, to correspond exactly to the curve of the shoulder."

The soldiers' pride in their beautiful weapons sometimes led to the reveal of a menacing downside. Although the Enfield muskets that were also used throughout the war usually had blued or browned barrels, the shiny Springfields were frequently kept so clean and well-polished that the reflective nature of their surfaces made it difficult to conceal troops' location. It was reported by some soldiers that their positions were made clear to the Confederates by the moon's reflection on the Union's muskets at the Battle of Fredericksburg, and the guns were said to have glittered in the dust at the Second Battle of Bull Run and the Battle of Petersburg, exposing the motion of the federal troops to the opposing army.

An array of other rifles were used in the Civil War, including the Whitworth rifle, the Smith, Tarpley, and Burnside carbines, the Lorenz rifle, the

Colt revolving rifle, and one of the most revolutionary of the new guns: the Spencer repeating rifle.

The horrors of war inevitably spur human creativity in both the offensive and defensive stances. Weapons technology is refined and honed, then medicine works to advance itself in response to the damage caused by that new technology. Brilliant inventors with vision and philosophical perspectives are inspired to unleash their plans and dreams. Christopher Miner Spencer was an inventor with remarkable ideas, excellent engineering skills, and the tenacity to follow through the lengthy patent and manufacturing processes.

Born in 1833 and growing up on his parents' farm in Manchester, Connecticut, Spencer stayed close to home, spending the bulk of his life and raising his family just a few miles away in the town of Windsor, the first English settlement in the state. He was known as a man fascinated by seeking or inventing solutions to technical problems, and also as a person who was kind, friendly, and possessed of a generous spirit.

At the age of eleven, Christopher was sent to live with his ninety-year-old maternal grandfather, Josiah Hollister, whose encouragement may have laid the foundation for Spencer's future work. Hollister was a gunsmith and veteran of the American Revolution, and the two shared a love of machinery and firearms. Josiah had a foot-operated lathe, which he allowed the boy to use, and also an old Revolutionary War musket that Christopher modified by sawing off the barrel to make it more convenient for hunting.

When the young boy was fourteen, he began working at a silk mill in Manchester, where he wrote later that he "first became imbued with the idea of becoming a mechanic." The mill was owned by brothers Charles and Rush Cheney, with whom Spencer remained close partners for many years. After one year of his vocational training, the Cheneys endorsed Christopher's opportunity for an advanced yearlong apprenticeship with machinist Samuel Loomis in Manchester Center, after which the boy returned to the silk mill. It was during this second apprenticeship that Spencer attended his apparently singular school experience—Wesleyan Academy—for twelve weeks. Over the next several years, as his skills blossomed, the Cheneys gave Spencer the opportunity to experiment with creating machinery for their mill. His first patent, for an automatic silk-winding machine, was earned in 1855 as he became the superintendent of their machine shop.

Over his lifetime, Christopher Spencer would obtain forty-two patents and create the first successful breech-loading repeating rifle. The Cheney brothers continued to encourage his efforts and allowed him to use their machinery in the development of his first repeating weapon, for which he obtained a patent in 1860.

The new gun was designed to allow for ammunition to be loaded into a chamber at the rear of the barrel rather than inserted at the muzzle. The rifle held seven metallic cartridges that were fired by moving the lever back and forth in order to eject a spent cartridge and load a new one. It was necessary to manually cock the hammer before pulling the trigger. It was a very reliable weapon under combat conditions and could fire twenty or more rounds per minute, although it did create a great deal of smoke, which some complained made it hard to target the enemy. Smoke was a common side effect of muzzle-loading guns as well, and under intensive firing conditions was said to produce a thick fog that could blind whole regiments. The Spencer rifle fired metallic ammunition that did not require the usual paper cartridge or fabric patch, and the bullets were lauded for being hardy and waterproof. The Spencer carbine was a shorter-barreled version of the gun that was designed for use by the cavalry.

The new repeating rifle provided stiff opposition for the South's slower muzzle loaders. Capturing the Union's Spencer weapons was a virtually fruitless endeavor for the Confederate troops as the guns fired specific and unique cartridges that were not manufactured or available for sale in the South.

Union President Abraham Lincoln was passionately curious about science and technology, and hopeful inventors frequently brought their creations to him. Fascinated by all things mechanical, he was particularly interested in the engineering of guns. A voracious reader, Lincoln kept abreast of recent innovations in the *New York Times* and *Scientific American* and devoured a journal called the *Annual of Scientific Discovery or Year-Book of Facts in Science and Art.*

His friends and colleagues were used to Lincoln's penetrating examinations of machines and ordnance. His longtime law partner, William Herndon, commented that whenever presented with an unfamiliar or new creation, Lincoln would examine it "inside and outside, upside and downside." Another colleague, attorney Henry Clay Whitney, recounted that when the two men traveled together and stopped by local farms for dinner, Lincoln would invariably become fascinated by

> some machine or tool, and he would carefully examine it all over, first generally and then critically; he would "sight" it to determine if it was straight or warped, if he could make a practical test of it, he would do that, he would turn it over or around and stoop down, or lie down, if necessary, to look under it.

Lincoln's interest, coupled with his urgent desire to equip the Union's soldiers with the best possible weaponry, led him to personally test the new arms that were replacing muskets, although the District of Columbia then had a distinct standing order against the firing of weapons in the city.

In August of 1863, Christopher Miner Spencer of Connecticut brought his lever-action repeating rifle to the White House. President Lincoln, Spencer, and a naval aide walked to a small nearby park and set up a makeshift pine board target so that the President could test the new rifle himself. Hitting the mark over and over again, Lincoln was impressed with the accuracy and repeating capabilities of the weapon, and upon their return to the White House presented Spencer with a fragment of the crude pine target they had used. Lincoln immediately recommended the rifle for a formal evaluation by the U.S. Army and Navy and soon tens of thousands of Spencer rifles were being delivered to Union troops.

Gettysburg, Pennsylvania, in 1863 was the first major battle in which the new Spencer rifles made their debut, having been recently issued to the Thirteenth Pennsylvania Reserves. The Spencers appeared prominently again at the Battle of Chickamauga, Tennessee, in that same year, and became widely used in the Western armies by 1864. The repeating rifles were carried by many Union cavalry and infantry regiments, maintaining a strong advantage over the Confederates' weapons.

Lincoln's aggressive sponsorship of the excellent Spencer gun certainly helped to give it the serious attention it warranted and contributed to its rise in popularity and widespread use. A Spencer gun would appear again, strangely, at Lincoln's death. The president was killed by assassin John Wilkes Booth, then armed with a .44 caliber Derringer pistol, but a few days later, when Booth was captured and shot in a barn on Garrett's farm in Virginia, he was in possession of a Spencer carbine.

The massive rapid-fire gun patented in 1862 by American inventor Richard Gatling again raised the bar on the killing power of weapons. It sparked the creation of repeating magazine rifles and manually operated machine guns, and its DNA remains in every contemporary automatic and semiautomatic gun.

In a stunning twist of fate and choice, one of the most advanced and deadliest weapons created during the Civil War—a weapon that caused untold thousands of deaths and losses of limbs and opened the door to an ever-evolving field of assault rifles and machine guns—this weapon was invented by a trained medical doctor.

Richard Jordan Gatling, M.D., was born in North Carolina in 1818 and early in his life demonstrated a great gift for inventions and technology. He created a screw propeller for steamboats (although another inventor patented his own first), a rice-sowing machine, and a wheat drill for use in planting wheat. Gatling's inventions helped to revolutionize the country's agriculture system and earned him a small fortune.

At the age of twenty-seven in 1845, Richard Gatling contracted smallpox while on a business trip. He recovered, but the experience inspired him to seek a medical education. The Ohio Medical College awarded his M.D. in 1850, although he then decided not to practice medicine, but to return to creating and patenting his own inventions. Over the course of his life, Gatling would create or redefine devices for improving bicycles, toilets, pneumatic power, steam cleaning, and tractors, but his concept for an advanced weapon would forever change the present and future of combat and warfare.

Gatling's inspired creativity was stirred by the outbreak of the Civil War. Although he was born in the South, he was a strong supporter of the Union. He had witnessed the soldiers' devastating wounds from muskets and bayonets. He knew of the terrible raging diseases that claimed so many of their lives and he began to think about a way to curtail the trail of death and disease. After the war, he described his original intentions in a letter to a friend:

> It occurred to me that if I could invent a machine—a gun—which could by rapidity of fire, enable one man to do as much battle duty as a hundred, that it would, to a great extent, supersede the necessity of large armies, and consequently, exposure to battle and disease [would] be greatly diminished.

Richard Gatling hoped to discourage large-scale battles with the huge and terrible power of his new weapon and he devoted his energy to improving and perfecting the device. He invented the first Gatling gun in 1861, received the patent for it on November 4, 1862, and founded the Gatling Gun Company in Indianapolis, Indiana, that same year. The gun would become the first successful and widely used machine gun.

The Gatling gun was based on six metal gun barrels mounted in a rotating circular design on a wheeled cart. It was operated by a hand crank and could fire up to two hundred rounds per minute. The weapon used gunpowder and .58-caliber bullets that were loaded into paper cartridges. As the crank was turned by the operator, gravity-fed bullets from a magazine entered each barrel and then advanced to the firing position. The barrel continued to revolve after each bullet was fired and was reloaded with a new bullet.

Inventors since the 1700s had maintained visions of a grouped-barrel concept for guns, but previous designs and engineering had been unsuccessful. Gatling's gun was unique in featuring an independent firing mechanism for each barrel and simultaneous actions of some of its smaller moving parts.

The U.S. Army officially adopted Gatling's patented "Battery Gun" invention on August 21, 1866. It was the first successful iteration of a rapid-fire repeating gun and was superior to all other rapid-fire guns of the time.

Gatling kept improving upon his invention in later years, and when brass cartridges were introduced, he was able to create a version that could fire up to four hundred rounds per minute. The spent casing would be ejected out of the bottom of the device, and the empty barrel would have a few seconds to cool before it rotated back to the top position, allowing higher rates of fire without serious overheating of the barrels of the gun. It was the ancestor of the electric motor-driven rotary cannon and introduced a new field of rapid-fire weapons.

In the four decades following the American Civil War, the Gatling gun was utilized by many world powers. It was frequently mounted on ships and employed during military conflicts including the Boshin War (or Japanese Revolution), the Indian Wars, the Great Railroad Strike of 1877 in America, the Anglo-Zulu War, the Spanish-American War, Philippine-American War, and the Boxer Rebellion in China.

Dr. Richard Gatling's contributions were acknowledged and commemorated during World War II by the U.S. Navy when the Fletcher-class destroyer DD-671 was christened the U.S.S. *Gatling*.

One of the most effective and deadliest large weapons of the American Civil War was the Model 1857 twelve-pounder "Napoleon" cannon, the most popular and widely used of the smoothbore cannons available during the war. The gun was named after Louis-Napoléon Bonaparte, the French president and emperor and the nephew of Napoleon Bonaparte, and had been developed in 1853 in France, where it was known as the "Canon de L'Empereur." Its outstanding performance and versatility led to its replacing many of the earlier field guns. The cast-bronze weapon defined a revolution in artillery by combining the functions of a cannon, which was designed to fire ordnance in a flat trajectory, and a howitzer, which was usually a shorter gun that could fire shells on high-arcing trajectories. The Napoleon was light enough to be pulled easily by a team of horses, was reliable, accurate, and capable of firing balls, shells, canisters, and grapeshot. The versatility of its combined functions allowed it to destroy fortifications a half-mile away and also to reach close-range targets in trenches or behind cover. It remains somewhat unclear as to the gun's original design but it is frequently attributed to Louis-Napoléon, who had been educated as a military engineer while serving in the Swiss Army and was regarded as a notable gunner.

Jefferson Finis Davis was a Democratic American politician representing Mississippi in the U.S. Senate and House of Representatives, later serving as United States secretary of war under President Franklin Pierce from 1853 to 1857. He subsequently became president of the Confederate States of America from 1861 to 1865. As U.S. secretary of war, Davis kept himself aware of artillery developments being made in Europe and in 1854 sent a three-man commission to observe European armies and the Crimean War operations. The commission was impressed with the new French cannon and recommended it for America's military.

The U.S. Army adopted the French design in 1857 and adapted it as the "light 12-pounder M1857." Five of the bronze guns were originally cast with some modifications but there remained only a few in service until 1861, when the weapons went into serious production. By the time of the Battle of Gettysburg, Pennsylvania, in 1863, the Napoleon cannons were the most popular smoothbores in use by both armies. The cannon became a universal piece of artillery as captured guns could be easily used by both sides. It created massive wounds that presented mostly insurmountable challenges for the surgeons. Dr. Samuel D. Gross of the Jefferson Medical College described the damage.

> Cannon balls often do immense mischief by striking the surface of the body obliquely, pulpifying the soft structures, crushing the bones, lacerating the large vessels and nerves, and tearing open the joints.

The weapon's refined simplicity of design allowed for easy replication, and wartime foundries in the North produced about 1,100 Napoleon cannons; Southern manufacture numbered about 600. The effectiveness of the gun compared to other available weapons was so outstanding that in 1863, Confederate general Robert E. Lee had all older "six-pounder" cannons in the Army of Northern Virginia melted down and recast as Napoleon twelve-pounders. In the same year, the Union Army near Chattanooga, Tennessee, seized the Ducktown copper mines, effectively blocking the Confederate supply of copper for making bronze, so later Confederate models of the Napoleon cannon were cast in iron.

The American version of the Napoleon was reasonably accurate up to 1,700 yards, but most effective at about 250 yards. The barrel weighed 1,220 pounds (550 kilograms) and had a bore of 4.62 inches (117 millimeters). The solid spherical projectiles for it weighed approximately 12.30 pounds (5.58 kilograms) with a maximum effective range of about 1,620 yards. When it was mounted on its gun carriage, the cannon's total weight was 2,445 pounds (1,100 kilograms) and required a team of six horses to pull it. The average gun crew numbered six men.

No accurate statistics exist, but it is extremely likely that the cannons and their munitions of shells, grapeshot, and canister were responsible for a huge percentage of promptly fatal battlefield wounds. The Civil War artillery was designed to be effective at a distance in order to smash through fortifications and various structures, but at close range against massed troops, the twelve-pound iron balls created crushing and usually terminal injuries. Shells fired by the cannons tended to kill rather than wound as the jagged metal fragments from the exploding shells quickly sliced through bone and tissue, causing lethal damage. Twelve percent of all wounds treated at field hospitals during the war were attributed to shell fragments. Grapeshot and canister rounds accounted for 1 percent of the field hospital treatment total, as few men survived long enough to reach a hospital. "Grapeshot," a primarily antipersonnel weapon, consisted of small iron or lead balls held in clusters by iron rings and combined with iron plates and a central connecting rod, reminiscent of a cluster of grapes. "Canister" was a tin can filled with musket balls and, when fired, it sprayed the balls over a wide area along with shards of metal from the can. Men caught by canister blast usually received multiple wounds in a single shot and sometimes their bodies were basically obliterated by the onslaught, leaving little to identify them.

Union soldier Colonel St. Clair Mulholland, Congressional Medal of Honor winner of the 116th Pennsylvania Regiment, never forgot the hideous rain of destruction at the Battle of Gettysburg.

> No tongue or pen can find language strong enough to convey
> an idea of its awfulness. Streams of screaming projectiles poured
> through the hot sir, falling and bursting everywhere. Men and
> horses were torn limb from limb, caissons exploded one after
> another in rapid succession, blowing the gunners to pieces. No
> spot within our lines was free from this frightful iron rain. The
> infantry hugged close to the earth and sought every slight shelter.

It was literally a storm of shot and shell. That awful, rushing sound of the flying missiles is everywhere.

The Minié ball holds the distinction of causing the greatest number of Civil War wounds, and the Gatling repeating gun is credited as one of the most lethal weapons to be employed in the war. Lesser arms included the bladed weapons, which were far less common than in earlier wars, but the grenade, a centuries-old concept, was still a prominent factor in several Civil War battles. A grenade is a small chemical or gas bomb that is used at short range, causing shockwaves and spreading fragments of its metal casing at high speeds.

The 8th century had introduced incendiary hand-thrown weapons—jars filled with "Greek Fire," a combustible compound—and lobbed at enemy soldiers. These devices apparently first appeared in the Byzantine Empire, one of the world's leading early civilizations, a huge territory encompassing most of the land around the Mediterranean Sea. Over the next few centuries the technology spread through the Islamic world and across the Far East, where early advancements by the Chinese included transitioning to a hollow metal casing and filling the shell with gunpowder.

By the 15th century, grenades were used in Europe, their name deriving from the French word for "pomegranate"—"grenade"—as the early weapons visually resembled the fruit and also because as it ripens, a growing pomegranate tends to explode and spread its seeds over a wide area.

By the 16th century in Europe, grenades were in widespread use with the military: hollow iron balls were filled with gunpowder and ignited by a fuse, each weighing from 2½ to 6 pounds. European armies of the 17th century created specialized divisions of soldiers who were trained to throw grenades, and called "grenadiers."

By the mid–19th century, the grenades used in the Civil War either resembled a cast-iron ball or a slim dart with stabilizing fins of cardboard. The nose of the weapon was backed by a percussion cap. The limiting factor of the device was that it had to land on its nose in order to detonate. In one 1863 failed Union grenade attack in Port Hudson, Louisiana, Confederate soldiers caught the unexploded grenades in blankets and hurled them back at their enemies.

Grenades were widely used in the 1861 siege at Fort Sumter and were common in land warfare by both armies afterward: in 1862 the Union claimed that civilians in Winchester, Virginia, threw grenades from their houses, wounding and killing their soldiers.

Northern and Southern armies frequently included grenades in their arsenals, as did the U.S. Navy throughout 1863 and until the end of the Civil War. Current versions are vastly enhanced by modern technology and grenades remain an integral part of offensive and defensive combat and warfare.

The Civil War term "torpedo" was assigned primarily to an explosive device later termed a "mine" and it also referred to a wide range of bombs, booby traps, and "sub-terra shells." The use of torpedoes—a name inspired by the torpedo fish, a creature that gives powerful electric shocks—by both the Confederate and Union armies raised new questions of ethics regarding "weapons that wait."

Confederate General Gabriel J. Rains, chief of the Confederate Torpedo Service, appears to have sown the seeds of modern land mine usage—he sought to delay the Union's pursuit of retreating Southern forces by burying artillery shells with pressure fuses in the road, tactics that the Union generals strongly protested. Recorded in the memoirs of Union general William Tecumseh Sherman is Sherman's furious response to the practice:

> On the 8th, [of December 1864] as I rode along, I found the column turned out of the main road, marching through the fields. Close by, in the corner of a fence, was a group of men standing around a handsome young officer, whose foot had been blown to pieces by a torpedo planted in the road. He was waiting

for a surgeon to amputate his leg, and told me that he was riding along with the rest of his brigade-staff of the Seventeenth Corps, when a torpedo trodden on by his horse had exploded, killing the horse and literally blowing off all the flesh from one of his legs. I saw the terrible wound, and made full inquiry into the facts. There had been no resistance at that point, nothing to give warning of danger, and the rebels had planted eight-inch shells in the road, with friction-matches to explode them by being trodden on. This was not war, but murder, and it made me very angry.

Torpedoes were used by both armies, on land and on the sea, where the Confederates found their use particularly appealing owing to the South's significantly smaller navy. General Rains lauded the device for use at sea, stating, "Ironclads are said to master the world, but torpedoes master the ironclads!" The Southern army made serious use of the weapons on the water with what is referred to today as a "contact mine"—floating on or below the water surface by means of an air-filled flotation device or otherwise being bottom-moored. The torpedoes detonated when struck by a ship, but could behave unreliably, although not enough to dissuade the combatants from a torpedo arms race.

The technology existed to allow torpedoes to be detonated electrically from the shore so that friendly vessels or enemy vessels of low value could bypass them while the shore operator waited for a more valuable target. The chronic shortages in the Confederacy of supplies including copper, platinum, and acid for batteries severely impacted the reliability of their mines, and the new technology of electricity was not understood well enough for predicting the limitations of the voltages.

Despite the moral considerations of the use of torpedoes and the Union's practice of ordering Confederate prisoners to clear mines from designated areas, their use proliferated and their design was refined. Confederate General Rains voiced the dilemma of using these weapons in warfare:

Each new invention of war has been assailed and denounced as barbarous and anti-Christian, yet each in its turn notwithstanding has taken its position by the universal consent of nations according to its efficiency in human slaughter.

The debate over "weapons that wait" did not end with the Civil War in 1865 and the argument over the ethics of the use of landmines continues to this day.

Army officers have been considered the military's elite for centuries. Many officers of past generations came from nobility, were often mounted on horseback, and were armed with swords that marked them as a breed apart, compared to the bows or long thrusting spears called "pikes" that were carried by the infantry. When pistols came into use, the small guns seemed like a more convenient and chivalrous arm for officers to use as a close-quarters weapon. Conferred with a measure of related status, pistols remained a traditional officers' sidearm for many years.

Pistols used in the American Civil War were multi-shot weapons usually carried by officers and cavalry; Northern men used the U.S. Army Model 1860; the Confederates received the .36 caliber Navy revolver. They were not standard issue in either army, and although an infantryman was permitted to carry and use a pistol, he had to purchase it with his own money. Some regular soldiers who acquired pistols decided over the span of the war not to continue carrying them but to simply stick with their long-range rifles, as hand-to-hand combat had become less and less common. They liked the multiple shot aspects of the pistols, but the guns were slow and difficult to reload, had a very limited range of about fifty paces compared to that of rifles, and were somewhat burdensome to use and carry.

The Colt revolver revolutionized combat when it was introduced in 1836. The gun could fire six bullets without a pause to reload and used percussion caps, which allowed it to operate reliably in wet weather. Inventor Samuel Colt's new weapon and its related designs became an important part of the

United States' arsenal for most of the 19th century. The Colt Army Model 1860 was a .44-caliber revolver that came into use just before the beginning of the Civil War. It met with enthusiastic reception from North and South, and 2,200 were contracted for the Confederacy and 130,000 guns built for the Union alone. The evolution of firearms was again demonstrated with the Colt Single Action Army and the invention of metallic cartridges that eliminated the need for carrying a separate powder container, ramrod, and percussion caps. The gun saw action in every American military campaign and war until 1905 and was familiarly dubbed "The Peacemaker."

Colt's revolver not only changed armed conflict, it revolutionized U.S. manufacturing, triggering the industrial revolution and hugely impacting the settlement of the American West. The revolver, also known as a "six-shooter," became an iconic weapon in the West, gaining great and legendary popularity and was in such demand that people there were willing to pay up to $500 (more than $16,000 in today's dollars) for the gun, which was available in the East for $25 (now $826).

The Colt weapons remained the most popular small arms during the Civil War, but their chief competitor, E. Remington and Sons in Ilion, New York, one of the oldest gun makers in the United States, also provided thousands of revolvers to the U.S. Navy and Army. Remington offered its revolvers to the U.S. at a lower price than that charged by Colt, and in 1863, 64,900 .44 caliber revolvers (with all appendages except bullet molds) were contracted for $12 each, which was $2 less than Colt's price. Remingtons remained popular with the U.S. Navy during the war and the revolvers were carried on many Union vessels.

The federal forces were supplied with additional revolvers in more limited numbers by a variety of firms including Smith and Wesson, Allen and Thurber, and Savage-North as well as a variety of European makers including the French LeFaucheux, which armed many Union troops in the Western theater. The LeMat weapon familiarly called the "Grape Shot Revolver" invented by Jean Alexandre LeMat of France was popular with the Confederate forces, as was the LeFaucheux "pin-fire," which took a special .45-caliber cartridge and was a favorite of Confederate Generals J.E.B. Stuart and Pierre Beauregard.

The Confederacy did manufacture some of its own revolvers, although in far fewer numbers than the North. The South's access to some materials necessary for production, including steel, brass, and copper, was extremely limited or nonexistent during the war. The firm of Griswold and Gunnison was the most successful of the Confederate revolver makers, producing their .36-caliber "Griswolds." They were supplemented with weapons produced by smaller Southern firms like Spiller and Burr and Leech & Rigdon.

By the end of the Civil War, small arms were actually widely available in both armies. The North's manufacturing capabilities and a massive four-year importation of guns by both sides created a surplus of small arms that lasted into the next century.

CHAPTER THREE

THE DOCTORS

The U.S. Army was caught unprepared for full-scale war on April 12, 1861, when Fort Sumter near Charleston, South Carolina, was bombarded by the South Carolina militia. No military leaders, including then U.S. Surgeon General Thomas Lawson, had any plans in place for dealing with a huge and lengthy war, or with hundreds of thousands of casualties, and the rudimentary existing U.S. Army Medical Department was severely understaffed.

The American Civil War retains the unfortunate distinction in medical and military history as the last large-scale conflict fought without the medical community's knowledge and incorporation of the work on germs and disease by Dr. Louis Pasteur of France or of Dr. Joseph Lister's work in Scotland on the terrible problem of infection.

The people who wrestled with the wartime injuries and diseases of 1861–1865 were a unique and diverse collection of healers. At the start of the war, the Union Army had 113 doctors and more than 16,000 troops. When the hostilities began, twenty-four of the U.S. doctors left for their Southern homes and three were dismissed for reasons of "loyalty." By the end of the war in 1865, there were in excess of 12,000 doctors in the Union Army and more than 3,000 in the Confederate Army. The victims of Civil War violence were treated by doctors ranging in age from their very early twenties to grandfathers in their late sixties. The physicians came from everywhere in the country; some were commissioned by their armies, some were volunteer or contracted; they came from rural practices and city offices. Volunteer and commissioned surgeons were sometimes only medical students with one year's worth of classes and no clinical experience, and some wartime physicians were originally trained as dentists, although they served as surgeons during the conflict. American doctors generally attended two years of medical school, although many of those who could afford it also studied in Europe, where medical education was far more intensive and encompassed four years of study. The U.S. was markedly behind—Harvard Medical School did not own any microscopes or stethoscopes until after the Civil War, and at the time of the war, many states still prohibited human anatomical dissection for medical education. Confederate doctor William H. Taylor reflected on the extremely limited availability of medical equipment and supplies during the war.

> In reviewing my acquirements during my three years and a half
> of service in the field, I find that I gained an excellent working
> knowledge of the art of practicing medicine without medicines
> and surgery without surgical appliances.

Two men who did not formally serve in the Civil War, but whose works likely impacted many of the wartime physicians were Dr. Samuel David Gross and Sir Thomas Longmore. Their publications probably formed the foundation of much of the treatment that was given to the wounded and sick soldiers in the American war. The handbooks they authored were the mainstay of the surgical training for a large proportion of the young doctors whose formal educations and experience had not included techniques used in surgical operations.

Samuel David Gross was born on a Pennsylvania farm in 1805 and grew up speaking Pennsylvania Dutch, a dialect of German, only learning English as a teenager. He had expressed a desire to become a physician from the time he was a child, and by age seventeen was seeking apprenticeships in medicine. Gross pursued his goal through tutoring, followed by a return to preparatory schools, and finally enrolled in the newly founded Jefferson Medical College in Philadelphia, where he received his degree in 1828 after a two-year course of study.

Dr. Gross was appointed demonstrator of anatomy at the Medical College of Ohio, later becoming a professor of pathological anatomy and chair of the department at the Cincinnati Medical College. He published his famous groundbreaking work *Elements of Pathological Anatomy*, which remained the leading reference work in its field for more than twenty-five years. After filling prestigious positions at medical schools in Kentucky and New York, Gross returned to his alma mater, Jefferson Medical College in Philadelphia, and remained there for the rest of his life. A prolific author, he published a hugely successful two-volume work called *A System of Surgery: Pathological, Diagnostic, Therapeutic and Operative*, which was translated into multiple languages and appeared in six editions between 1859 and 1882.

Training in military medicine was not a part of the curriculum in American medical schools, and at the start of the Civil War a number of books on surgery were rushed into publication, with a particular emphasis on treating gunshot wounds. Dr. Gross was especially concerned with adding to the educations of the wave of new young doctors and, in 1861, published his treatise *Manual of Military Surgery or Hints on the Emergencies of Field, Camp and Hospital Practice*. For many of the newly minted wartime surgeons, it was their first introduction to trauma surgery and surgical techniques.

Dr. Samuel David Gross was a skilled and innovative surgeon, a widely admired teacher, and an influential author. He pioneered many advancements in surgery and taught the United States' first systematic approach to surgical operations. He was immortalized in the huge 1875 painting by Thomas Eakins titled *The Gross Clinic*. The wall-sized composition is a celebrated and graphic depiction of Dr. Gross's removal of a tumor from the thigh of a patient as he is observed by an audience of students in the medical amphitheater of the Jefferson Medical College. The artwork resides in the collection of the Philadelphia Museum of Art.

The doctors of both Union and Confederate Armies benefited from an extremely useful handbook by the British surgeon general Sir Thomas Longmore, a doctor who had also served as inspector general of the British Army. Originally an essay on gunshot wounds based on his experiences in the Crimean War, Longmore's *Treatise on Gunshot Wounds* was reprinted in the United States in 1862 by J.B. Lippincott & Company and provided one of the major textbooks for the American Civil War physicians. The book covered a wide range of the aspects of gunshot wounds including shock, hemorrhage, amputation, gangrene, and the use of chloroform as an anesthetic.

Longmore brought a distinguished career along with his expertise and experience. Born in 1816, the son of a surgeon who had been a member of the Royal Navy, the younger Longmore also served the military in a wide range of locations including the Ionian Islands west of Greece, the West Indies, and Canada. As an Army doctor and surgeon, he was present at every major engagement of the Crimean War, despite suffering from frostbite.

Longmore wrote extensively on medical subjects including battlefield ambulances, ophthalmology, and gunshot wounds. His writings had a profound influence on the knowledge and skill of the young, inexperienced Civil War surgeons as they faced thousands of casualties. Having witnessed firsthand the plight of the wounded in battle, he felt strongly that there should be international rules for the treatment of wounded men and their caretakers during armed conflict and he represented Britain at the 1864 conference that ignited the force that became the original Geneva Convention.

Knighted by Queen Victoria and lauded for his invaluable work, Sir Thomas Longmore, K.C.B., Surgeon-General, A.M.D., and honorary Physician to the Queen, created a legacy of skill, knowledge, and humanitarian aid that was shared with the inexperienced young Civil War doctors.

The posts of surgeon general in the Union and Confederacy both cycled through more than one man leading up to and throughout the Civil War, but the two most influential and dynamic were Samuel Preston Moore of the Confederacy and William Alexander Hammond of the Union. These powerful leaders were quite disparate in age—Moore was forty-eight when he accepted the post while Hammond was only thirty-four—but they shared many interests, concepts, and a strong drive for positive change.

Both men had history in the United States military, educated and experienced backgrounds in medicine, and a deep interest in botany. Although Hammond's brash personality would prove to be his downfall in the office, both he and Moore valued excellence and organization in medical practice. They would each transform their armies' medical divisions, keep careful records, and institute updated and increasingly hygienic procedures.

Dr. Samuel Preston Moore, born in 1813, served as the Confederacy's surgeon general throughout most of the American Civil War. A native of Charleston, South Carolina, Moore graduated in 1834 from the Medical College of the State of South Carolina and became an assistant surgeon in the Medical Corps of the United States Army during the Mexican-American War. While he was stationed in Texas, Moore met Jefferson Davis, the future president of the Confederate States of America, and strongly impressed Davis with his medical and organizational abilities. Moore was promoted to surgeon in 1849 and remained at that rank with the Army through the 1850s, although when his home state of South Carolina seceded from the Union in 1860, he resigned his U.S. Army post and moved to Arkansas, planning to go into private practice. He was intent on avoiding doing battle against a country to which he had devoted much of his life.

Jefferson Davis began to contact Moore, imploring him to join the Confederate Army, describing the lack of qualified physicians and the army's desperate medical and military conditions. He finally persuaded the forty-eight-year-old Moore to accept the position of Confederate surgeon general in 1861, replacing the acting surgeon general, Charles H. Smith.

Early in the war the Confederate Army was already facing a dire medical crisis including extreme shortages of medicines, equipment, and relevant supplies. Crippled by the Union's naval blockade of Southern ports and without enough trained surgeons, Moore created solutions or salves for a staggering array of problems. His resourcefulness was unparalleled, and some of the systems he created would reverberate through the field of medicine for many years.

Under immense pressure to improve the army's terrible conditions and facing thousands of wounded and sick men, Moore turned out to be a brilliant visionary and knowledgeable creative who reimagined the entire Confederate Medical Department. In order to weed out any unqualified men who applied to work as physicians, he instituted an examining board for surgeons and assistant surgeons and introduced new methods to improve the education of army doctors. He created an effective army hospital and field ambulance corps and under his guidance treatment protocols were improved throughout the army. To combat the shortages caused by the blockade and other Northern offensives, Moore established factories across the Confederacy to manufacture drugs, surgical instruments, and hospital supplies; he created laboratories to prepare alternative medicines made from indigenous Southern plants. He commissioned two important volumes as resources to support the army: Dr. Julian Chisolm's *Manual of Military Surgery* and surgeon and botanist Dr. Francis Peyre Porcher's *Resources of the Southern Fields and Forests*.

Among Dr. Moore's many achievements was the forming of a professional organization, the Association of Army and Navy Surgeons of the Confederate States, and founding a notable medical publication titled *Confederate States Medical and Surgical Journal.*

Samuel Preston Moore's revolutionary changes transformed the medical corps of the Confederate States of America into one of the most well organized and effective departments of the Confederate military—changes that undoubtedly saved the lives of thousands of Southern soldiers.

The Union actually cycled through four surgeons general through the length of the Civil War. At the time the first shots of the war were being fired, Surgeon General Dr. Thomas Lawson had held the post for more than twenty-four years. He was in somewhat poor health at age seventy-two and died unexpectedly on May 15, 1861. In a surprise move by the incoming political party and the newly elected Republican president Abraham Lincoln, Dr. Clement Alexander Finley, a graduate of the University of Pennsylvania, was named the tenth surgeon general of the United States Army.

Surgeon General Finley appears to have had a discordant relationship with Secretary of War Edwin Stanton, and was "retired on his own application" in April 1862; Assistant Surgeon General Robert C. Wood served temporarily in the post. Probably causing Secretary Stanton additional angst, President Lincoln chose to name the brilliant and brash young Dr. William Hammond to the post with the rank of brigadier general against Stanton's recommendations and advice.

Despite what would be the brevity of his service, Hammond's powerful vision and strong personality fostered many positive and forward-thinking reforms. During his tenure he effectively redesigned and vastly improved the Union medical corps. He was also a volatile and emotional personality whose removal from office was effective in September 1863. Edwin Stanton's friend and personal physician Joseph K. Barnes became the twelfth surgeon general of the United States Army, serving throughout the rest of the Civil War and until 1882.

William Alexander Hammond, born in 1828 and surgeon general for the United States Army from 1862–1864, grew up largely in Pennsylvania, the son of a successful doctor whom the young boy greatly admired and wished to emulate. From an early age, Hammond's appearance, brilliance, and achievements all seemed larger than life—at sixteen he began his medical education and earned his M.D. from the University of the City of New York at age twenty in 1848. After some months in practice, he joined the U.S. Army in 1849 as an assistant surgeon and shortly thereafter was named Medical Director of Fort Riley in Kansas, remaining in the service for the next eleven years.

Hammond left the Army in 1860, accepting an offer to become the chair of anatomy and physiology at the medical school of the University of Maryland, but his resignation would be short-lived. He rejoined the service in May 1861, and less than a year later became the eleventh surgeon general of the United States Army, still a young man at age thirty-four.

Hammond's prior army experience and superb organizational abilities helped him to tackle the woefully inadequate and lax Union hospital network. He began a system-wide reorganization, upgrade, and expansion. Like Surgeon General Samuel Moore in the South, he instituted demanding medical examinations to weed out unqualified doctors and ordered strict inspections of existing hospitals and medical facilities for cleanliness and adequate ventilation. He directed new hospitals to be built, supplied them with modern equipment, updated age-old protocols, and authorized Major Jonathan Letterman's creation of an ambulance corps for the Army. He collected reports from the hospitals and medics that were later published in the revolutionary and invaluable six-volume *Medical and Surgical History of the War of the Rebellion*, and in 1863 wrote *A Treatise on Hygiene: With Special Reference to the Military Service.*

Although Hammond's changes to the Union medical system vastly improved the quality of care and lowered the mortality rate, his outsize personality and opinionated rhetoric caused personality clashes with other physicians and with Lincoln's secretary of war, Edwin Stanton. He was dismissed from the service by court martial in 1864, although he petitioned for a reconsideration and was reinstated as a brigadier general in 1878.

Despite difficulties resulting from his brash personality, Hammond's genius and powerful energy enabled him to help found the Army Medical Museum (now the National Museum of Health and Medicine), the American Neurological Association, and to set new and higher standards for military medical care.

The Civil War retained the rare distinction of its combatants having friends and family on both sides of the divided nation. Many doctors of the period had gone to school together or originally served at the same time in the U.S. Army before the country was sundered. Dr. Hunter Holmes McGuire became a prominent Confederate physician who typified the connections to both North and South. Born in 1835 in Winchester, Virginia, his medical education began in Philadelphia, Pennsylvania, at the Jefferson Medical College. By the late 1850s, developing national hostilities had begun to affect the medical community in the city, enrollment of Southern students in Northern medical schools had started to decline, and when news of abolitionist John Brown's raid on Harpers Ferry, West Virginia, in October of 1859 reached Philadelphia, medical student Hunter McGuire led an exodus of Southern students from the city. He would later complete his education at the Medical College of Virginia and begin a distinguished career as not only surgeon, but as teacher, orator, and soldier.

McGuire would go on to teach at Winchester Medical Academy in Virginia, Tulane University in New Orleans, and the University of Pennsylvania in Philadelphia, but at the onset of the Civil War he returned to the South to join the Second Virginia Regiment. McGuire was prepared to fight as a foot soldier, but the lack of trained doctors in the Confederacy meant he was sorely needed as a medical officer. In 1861 he was detached as a brigade surgeon to General Thomas J. "Stonewall" Jackson, known as a bold and powerful commander with a reputation for terrorizing Northern forces. Although Jackson initially denigrated McGuire's youth, they soon became close friends, and Dr. McGuire treated General Jackson after the First Battle of Manassas, the place where Jackson acquired the nickname "Stonewall" when he rushed his troops to close a gap in their line against an attack by Union forces.

McGuire was promoted to chief surgeon of Jackson's corps and was present at all of the battles of the Army of Northern Virginia. General Jackson was impressed with McGuire's ideas about reforms to the Confederate Army's medical service and championed many of them to positive effect. At McGuire's urging, Jackson allowed Union prisoners who were doctors to be paroled in order to attend to casualties. Both North and South would adopt the practice, which was later endorsed and incorporated by the American Red Cross.

The deepening friendship of mutual respect and admiration between Jackson and McGuire reached a tragic conclusion at the Battle of Chancellorsville, Virginia, in May of 1863. As they returned from an attack, Jackson and his soldiers were fired on by their own troops, who mistook them for Union soldiers. The general was hit in the left arm by two bullets and developed pneumonia shortly after, although his friend tried desperately to save his life. A devastated McGuire amputated Jackson's arm as the wounds were too severe to repair, and cared for him around the clock in the following days as the thirty-nine-year-old Jackson succumbed to what may have been either pneumonia or a pulmonary embolism. McGuire served as a pallbearer in General Jackson's funeral and always revered the friend with whom he had shared such intensive and dramatic service. He remained with the Army of Northern Virginia after Jackson's death and for the rest of his life maintained his commander's image and reputation. He wrote biographical briefs about the general and gave speeches about his life and achievements.

Dr. McGuire lost several close friends, companions, and his brother Hugh to the war, and his home in the Shenandoah Valley was destroyed by a devastating fire. He moved to Richmond, Virginia, after the war, where he became chair of surgery at the Medical College of Virginia, married Mary Stuart, and fathered ten children, some of whom would grow up to follow in his footsteps in medicine.

Hunter McGuire created a tradition of leadership in medical progress not only in Virginia, but nationally. He founded Virginia's St. Luke's Hospital and Training School for Nurses and helped establish the Medical Society of Virginia. Among his many achievements and contributions to the field of medicine are educational institutions, his prolific writings, and the memory of his compassionate treatment of patients. In 1893 Dr. McGuire initiated the College of Physicians and Surgeons in Virginia (later University College of Medicine) and later served as president of the American Medical Association. He has been immortalized in name by many medical facilities in Virginia; his statue is prominent on the grounds of the Virginia State Capitol and written accolades to the excellence of his performance as soldier, surgeon, teacher, orator, and author are numerous and glowing.

An international bequest by Dr. Hunter Holmes McGuire was his contribution to the First Geneva Convention. During McGuire's military service in the Civil War, General Jackson's army captured Winchester, Virginia, in May 1862, including seven prisoners who were U.S. Army surgeons. McGuire believed that medical personnel should be classed as noncombatants and he encouraged General Jackson to release the captured doctors. The ensuing agreement signed by the Union physicians was known as the "Winchester Accord" and called for "the unconditional release of all medical officers taken prisoners of war hereafter." On June 6, 1862, the United States immediately and unconditionally released all of the Confederate doctors then being held as prisoners of war.

McGuire joined European advocates of the classification of medical personnel as noncombatants, a movement that revolutionized battlefield medicine. The concept became part of the Geneva Conventions, and both the American Red Cross and the International Committee of the Red Cross upheld the motion as a foundational principle. Upon Dr. McGuire's death in 1900, the *Boston Medical Journal* stated in his obituary that he had "humanized war."

The hard-won medical lessons of the Civil War were written first in blood on the nation's battlefields, and a second time in print in the libraries that conserved and preserved the information that had been traded for American lives.

One of the less well-known doctors of the Civil War was one of the most important shepherds of the written records of American medicine. John Shaw Billings was a surgeon, librarian, and building designer, all at the highest levels of innovative excellence. Dr. Billings modernized the Surgeon General's Library, which was at the time the nation's first comprehensive collection of materials on medicine; he was a major player in the both the physical building and the curriculum design of the medical school for Johns Hopkins University Hospital, and he served as the first director of the New York Public Library.

John Shaw Billings was born in 1838 in a sparsely settled Indiana region to a family that had immigrated to America in the mid–17th century. His early life was spent on his family's farm and he attended country schools, demonstrating an exceptional memory and a passionate love of reading. The young boy was also tutored in Latin, Greek, and geometry by a clergyman, Mr. Bonham, who was extremely impressed with his proficiency and mastery of the subject matter. At age fourteen, John Billings passed the entrance exam and was admitted to Miami University in Oxford, Ohio, graduating second in his class in 1857. He was admitted to the Medical College of Ohio in Cincinnati the following year, graduating as doctor of medicine in 1860 and immediately appointed demonstrator of anatomy at the school. His treatise, "The Surgical Examination of Epilepsy," was published in the journal *Cincinnati Lancet and Observer* of 1861.

At the outbreak of the Civil War, young Dr. Billings offered his services to the Union Army. He was commissioned first lieutenant and assistant surgeon, serving for more than a year in military hospitals in Washington and Philadelphia. In 1863 he was transferred to field service with the Fifth Corps of the Army of the Potomac.

The Battle of Chancellorsville, Virginia, fought over a week in the spring of 1863, yielded tens of thousands of casualties on both sides. Billings's exceptional skills as both surgeon and executive officer were apparent. He followed the Army north to the bloodbath at Gettysburg and was present at the trail of devastation and destruction that led to the siege of Richmond, Virginia. As a battleground surgeon, Billings organized the movement of entire field hospitals, kept statistics on injuries, and honed the working of the Union Army's ambulance corps. He was appalled by the treatment of wounded soldiers, felt that amputation was overly performed, and objected to the technique used for surgical bullet removal, believing it could lead to additional infection. He was a remarkably skilled surgeon, and many of the most difficult operations were referred to him.

In August of 1864 Billings was assigned to the office of the medical director of the Army of the Potomac in Washington, where he assembled the field reports that would eventually form a part of the *Medical and Surgical History of the War of the Rebellion*. He was transferred in December of that year to the office of the surgeon general where he spent the next thirty years, there accomplishing what is viewed as the most important work of his life: incorporating his expertise in military and public hygiene, hospital construction and sanitary engineering, vital and medical statistics, medical bibliography and history, the advancement of medical education and the condition of medicine in the United States, and as a civil administrator of outstanding ability.

After the war, Billings planned and designed institutions including the Barnes Hospital at the Soldiers' Home, the Army Medical Museum in Washington, D.C., the William Pepper Laboratory of Clinical Medicine in Philadelphia, and the Peter Bent Brigham Hospital in Boston. He proposed that medical statistics should be included in the United States Census of 1880 and personally took part in drawing up the vital statistics for the tenth, eleventh, and twelfth census.

In a longtime dedicated role, Dr. John Shaw Billings developed and modernized the Surgeon General's Library and created the Medical Index Catalogue, as he believed strongly in the need for a great reference work for the use of researchers and writers on medical subjects. By the year 1876 he had collected 40,000 volumes and as many pamphlets and begun the publication of the first series of the catalogue.

Billings aided the U.S. secretary of the treasury in the reorganization of military hospitals, oversaw work for treating yellow fever patients, and served as Johns Hopkins University Hospital's medical advisor. His immense contributions to the hospital included the architecture, infrastructure, and the curriculum for the medical school.

Upon his retirement from the Army in 1895, he was appointed director for the New York Public Library, a position he held until his death in 1913. This brilliant and multitalented man demonstrated the great truth that not all progress in medicine is restricted to the operating table or in the hospital wards—it is measured in the collection and analysis of data and the preservation and availability of medical information, background, and specifics.

Dr. Billings received honorary degrees from universities including Edinburgh, Oxford, Dublin, Munich, Budapest, Harvard, Yale, and Johns Hopkins and was a member of many medical and scientific societies.

Some of the Civil War doctors brought their international educations and observations to the American conflict. Dr. Moritz Schuppert, born in Marburg, Germany, in 1817 and receiving his degree from the university there, immigrated to New Orleans at age thirty-three, becoming a leading surgeon and an early champion of the use of antiseptic techniques. He was a fierce supporter of the pioneering work on sepsis espoused by Dr. Joseph Lister in Scotland. Schuppert was named city physician of New Orleans in 1854, continuing his work in vascular surgery and pioneering new techniques in orthopedic surgery.

When the war began, he authored a handbook targeted to the inexperienced young surgeons now tasked with performing many rapid lifesaving surgeries. *A Treatise on Gun-Shot Wounds: Written for and Dedicated to the Surgeons of the Confederate States Army* was published in 1861. Dr. Schuppert's heart was with the South and there was a poetic tone to his observations.

> Large armies are rushing to the contest. We may expect to see many a bloody battle, many a hard won field. The soldier is already dreaming of glory and renown, but military tactics leave out of the question the ghastly field, its wounded, and the bed of suffering. There the province of the physician begins, and on the field of the battle itself, his knowledge and skill are put to the severest test. He must be prepared and ready for every emergency; he has no time to consult, no time to read up, he must act; for while he hesitates, the current of life may be ebbing away.

The very first African American man to receive a degree in medicine was unable to gain admittance to a United States college owing to his African and European mixed-race heritage, which classified him as "mulatto." Free-born New Yorker James McCune Smith opted instead to travel to Scotland, where he entered Glasgow University, earning three degrees including a doctorate in medicine. Dr. Smith returned to New York where he served as the doctor at the Colored Orphan Asylum for twenty years, until it was burned down by a violent mob in the New York Draft Riots in 1863. Dr. Smith died of a heart attack two years later at age fifty-two, but he left a legacy of achievement and perseverance. A gifted writer, he published a number of academic works and composed the introduction to social reformer and abolitionist Frederick Douglass's book *My Bondage and My Freedom*.

Thirteen of the first degreed African American doctors served in the Civil War as physicians and surgeons. Many of these doctors had attended medical school in Canada as, with a very few inclusive rarities like Ohio's Oberlin College, American medical schools would not allow them admittance. These pioneers who had to rise above the rampant bigotry of their time, who faced oppression, rejection, distrust, discrimination, and sometimes violence, still blazed a path for millions of people who would follow their lead.

Dr. Alexander Thomas Augusta, whose life exemplified not only the practice of medicine but the breaking of archaic educational and professional barriers, was a lifelong champion of the rights of others. He was born in 1825 to free people of color in Norfolk, Virginia, and had wanted to be a doctor since childhood. Reading and writing were going to be essential skills for him, although education for blacks was illegal in the state of Virginia. The law had originally applied to enslaved people but the state had also restricted the rights of free people of color following the Nat Turner slave rebellion of 1831. Alexander Augusta found it necessary to draw on every discreet opportunity available to him in his dangerous pursuit of learning to read.

He moved to Baltimore, Maryland, as a young man and began to work as a barber while continuing to seek the realization of his dream of a medical education. Although the University of Pennsylvania would not accept him as a student owing to what he described as a "prejudice of color," he would have been unable to fulfill other required prerequisites for entrance due to the existing laws preventing the education of blacks. In a stroke of good fortune, a faculty member from the university took an interest in him and agreed to teach him secretly, and despite every obstacle in his path, Alexander was able to achieve literacy.

He married Mary O. Burgoin (listed in various records as "Native American" or "coloured"), and they apparently enjoyed a strong mutual love and partnership throughout their lives. The Augustas moved to Toronto, Canada in 1850, a city that was pleasantly known for its racial tolerance and its opportunities for educated African Americans to thrive. Alexander was granted acceptance to the Medical College at the University of Toronto and he also opened an apothecary on Yonge Street in the city, working as a druggist and chemist to support the couple and pay for his medical education. He received his M.B. (equivalent to an M.D. in America) from the college six years later. The president of the college described him as one of his most "brilliant students" and the brand new physician established a successful practice in Toronto where he accepted patients regardless of race or income. Dr. Augusta became an active member of the community and was later appointed the head of the Toronto City Hospital, president of the Association for the Education of Colored People of Canada, and was known for speaking out against racial injustices, all of which were opportunities that would not have been available to him in the country of his birth.

The occasion of President Abraham Lincoln's January 1, 1863, signing of the Emancipation Proclamation, which called for the freedom of enslaved people in the Confederate states, was a defining moment for Dr. Augusta. The proclamation also allowed for the Union Army to recruit blacks, and on January 7, owing to his belief that "the coloured people have a duty to perform at this present time," Augusta wrote to President Lincoln and Secretary of War Edwin Stanton. He offered his services to the black regiments, subsequently receiving a presidential commission from Lincoln.

Alexander Augusta was aware of the danger of such an assignment and of taking part in a massive and bloody conflict, but he believed that as an educated person of color in a position of authority, he could give strength to the Army while supporting black soldiers.

The Augustas left Canada and returned to the United States upon his receipt of a confirmed appointment for a military examination. Two days before the examination was due to take place, his invitation to join the Army was canceled, again owing to his classification as a "person of colour" and the accusation that, having lived in "British North America" for ten years, he was technically a British subject. Under the antiquated ruling, he would not be able to serve in the American military.

Dr. Alexander Augusta's hard-won literacy again served him well. He wrote another letter to President Lincoln and to members of the Army's Medical Board:

> I have come nearly a thousand miles at great expense and sacrifice, hoping to be of some use to the country and to my race at this eventful period.

He made additional arguments about the doubly high death rates among black soldiers from illness and disease and recommended an increased medical field staff. A few months later the board reversed its position and in April of 1863, Dr. Alexander Thomas Augusta was commissioned as a surgeon with the rank of major in the Union Army, becoming the first black doctor to hold such a commission. He was appointed surgeon-in-charge at the Contraband Hospital for former slaves and free blacks in Washington, D.C.

Dr. Augusta's next assignment was as regimental surgeon for the Seventh Infantry of the United States Colored Troops in Maryland. Another letter was addressed to President Lincoln, this time signed by several white surgeons who were objecting to a superior officer who was black and referring to the situation as "humiliating."

Again facing racial discrimination that affected his professional advancement and proffered service, Dr. Augusta's next role was at a recruiting station for black troops. At the time, white privates in the Union Army were paid $13 a month (equivalent to $433/month in 2021 dollars); black privates received $7 a month ($233 today). As an Army surgeon with the rank of major, Augusta was entitled to a salary of $169 per month ($5,631 today). In 1864, the Army paymaster, based on the color of Augusta's skin and disregarding his medical qualifications, slashed his pay to $7 a month.

While facing his own personal challenges, Alexander Augusta sparked many positive changes in his lifetime, and this was another opportunity. He wrote a letter describing and decrying the inequity of pay for black soldiers and sent it to Republican senator Henry Wilson of Massachusetts, chairman of the Senate Committee on Military Affairs. The senator championed the restoration of Augusta's salary, although it took slightly longer to change the landscape for the black soldiers, but in June of 1864, Congress established equal pay, regardless of color, for United States soldiers.

Another Republican senator from Massachusetts, Charles Sumner, a well-known abolitionist, was at that time sponsoring a law that would make it illegal for streetcar companies to racially segregate passengers. In an 1864 Washington, D.C., rainy winter day incident, Dr. Augusta, in full military uniform, was physically pushed off of a streetcar for insisting on remaining under the cover of the roof rather than on the outside platform. This time Dr. Augusta's descriptive letter protested segregation on trains and requested the president's protection for other African American soldiers and families. It was sent to his commanding general and found its way to Senator Sumner in D.C., who was enraged by the account. The change was not immediate, but by March of 1865, Congress passed legislation making racial discrimination on streetcars illegal in Washington, D.C.

Augusta left the service in 1866 having earned the respect of much of the military and medical leadership and was awarded the prestigious honorary rank of brevet lieutenant colonel, becoming the highest-ranking African American officer in the United States military. His distinguished service and activism also made him one of the first African Americans to be invited to the White House—Dr. Augusta and his Canadian-born assistant, Dr. Anderson Ruffin Abbott, who was also black, were invited to a reception in February 1865 by President and Mrs. Lincoln, which they attended and enjoyed.

During a full life characterized by courage and the pursuit of justice and equality and despite huge obstacles owing to his race, Dr. Alexander Thomas Augusta achieved a remarkable number of "firsts": first African American physician commissioned as an officer in the Union Army; first black hospital administrator in United States history; first African American to serve on the faculty of a medical school (Howard University), and, upon his death in 1890, he became the first African American officer to be interred in Arlington National Cemetery.

More than 12,000 doctors served in the Union Army during the Civil War: thirteen of them were African American. These men, most of whom had overcome impressive odds to attain their educations, were the front-runners of a new era in medicine and community.

William Peter Powell Jr., freeborn in New Bedford, Massachusetts, in 1834, was one of the first African American physicians to be contracted as a United States Army surgeon. Powell's mother, Mercy Haskins, was Native American; his father, William Powell Sr., was African American and a staunch abolitionist. Powell Sr. operated several boarding houses that catered to African American seamen and former and fugitive slaves in New York City and in New Bedford, which was part of the Underground Rail-road that aided escaped slaves in finding their way to freedom in Canada.

With a wife and seven children of color, Powell Sr. became increasingly concerned about the possibilities raised by the Fugitive Slave Act of 1850. Superseding the earlier 18th-century law, the revised compromise was designed to deter early calls for Southern secession. The new law demanded that citizens were to participate in the capture of runaway slaves, that slaves were denied the right to a jury trial, and that federal commissioners were offered a form of bounty for returning suspected runaways. Horrible instances occurred when freeborn Northern blacks were captured and accused of being runaway slaves, and many abolitionists doubled their efforts to assist fleeing enslaved people. William P. Powell Sr. wrote a letter to the *National Anti-Slavery Standard*, an abolitionist newspaper and the first official weekly publication of the American Anti-Slavery Society, describing the law as a declaration of war against the "free coloured population," and in 1851, he decided to move his family to England to escape the danger posed by the laws.

When the family settled in Liverpool, England, a story in Dublin's *Freeman's Journal* of February 1851 focused on William Powell Sr., known as a "militant champion of black seamen." "He had come to this country to procure for his children that education and means of supporting themselves denied them in Boston on account of their colour." A letter from Powell Sr. in England to a white friend in Boston, Maria Chapman, stated, "I came to this country a poor despised outcast—outlawed American negro—driven from my native country for no 'color of crime' but for the 'crime of color.'"

The younger Powell had grown up largely in New York where, as a teenager, he found a job with an apothecary, sparking his early interest in becoming a doctor. When the family settled in England, he helped his father run a hotel for black sailors and fugitive slaves, but his interest in medicine grew. It is believed that he applied to and was accepted for training by the College of Physicians and Surgeons in London. Although records of his degree are uncertain, it appears that he had qualified in 1857–58 in Dublin. He was employed at St. Anne's District Hospital, Liverpool, as a house surgeon, and also worked on a temporary basis at the Liverpool South Hospital. When the Powell family returned to New York in 1861, Dr. William P. Powell Jr. began practicing medicine in his native country.

Three of the Powell sons served in the Union Army: Edward, Sylvester, and Isaiah. Their brother, Dr. William, applied to become a contract assistant surgeon with the Union Army in 1863 and was assigned to the Contraband Hospital (later called the Freedmen's Hospital) in Washington, D.C., a hospital that took care of black soldiers and fugitive slaves. Dr. Powell worked under the direction of Major Dr. Alexander T. Augusta, the first African American medical officer and the first surgeon-in-chief at the hospital. Powell was later appointed to head the hospital when Dr. Augusta left for his regiment, the Seventh U.S. Colored Infantry. Powell ushered in a new era by hiring several African American nurses who received regular wages. He also made requests for camp improvements such as protective perimeter fencing.

Serving as head of the hospital camp, Dr. Powell noted that it was common for the camp to receive five or six new smallpox patients each day and that many patients and staff were sickened by the poor quality of the drinking water. Dr. Augusta had campaigned to improve the fresh water supply, but his efforts were declined by the Medical Department. During Dr. Powell's tenure at the hospital, one of his fellow surgeons remarked that as other staff members caught the highly contagious smallpox or were sickened by the foul water, Powell labored around the clock to ease the situation.

After the war, Dr. Powell returned to his medical practice until poor health forced his retirement in 1881. He petitioned the U.S. government for an Army pension, which was repeatedly denied on the grounds of lack of medical proof of disability and the fact that he served as a contract surgeon, not a military officer. He eventually returned to England to care for his gravely ill younger brother and remained there for the rest of his life. Dr. William P. Powell continued to petition the U.S. government for twenty-four years to approve his pension application, citing his disability and his Army service. He wrote to presidents William McKinley and Theodore Roosevelt without success.

Dr. Powell's death was recorded in Liverpool, England, in 1915, age eighty-one. He was never able to secure a pension, and ended his life in impoverished circumstances. His name, however, has been permanently engraved on the annals of American history as a man and a doctor who, despite facing terrible societal obstacles, became a respected professional, a healer, and a leader who holds a distinct place in the Civil War as one of thirteen unusually brave and dedicated physicians.

Eleven additional men faced daunting obstacles to attain their educations and earn their degrees in medicine. Their names constitute a list of courage and resolute devotion even before stepping onto a battlefield. They are: Dr. Anderson R. Abbott (Canadian, Toronto School of Medicine, Toronto, Canada); Dr. Benjamin A. Boseman (Dartmouth Medical School, Hanover, New Hampshire, Medical School of Maine, Brunswick, Maine);

Dr. Cortlandt Van Rensselaer Creed (Yale University, New Haven, Connecticut, first African American to be graduated from Yale Medical School); Dr. John Van Surly DeGrasse (Medical School of Maine, commissioned as surgeon in U.S. Army); Dr. William Baldwin Ellis (Dartmouth Medical College, Hanover, New Hampshire); Dr. Joseph Dennis Harris (Western Reserve College, Hudson, Ohio, later College of Physicians and Surgeons, Keokuk, Iowa); Dr. Charles Burleigh Purvis (Oberlin College, Oberlin, Ohio, then Case Western Reserve University, Cleveland, Ohio); Dr. John H. Rapier Jr. (Iowa College of Physicians and Surgeons in Keokuk, Iowa, first African American west of the Mississippi River to graduate in medicine); Dr. Willis R. Revels (Medical College of Louisiana, New Orleans). Although time has obscured their affiliated educational institutions, Dr. Charles H. Taylor and Dr. Alpheus W. Rucker also served honorably throughout the Civil War.

Almost all mid-19th-century American medical schools barred admission to women, but 200–300 diplomas in medicine may have belonged to some of the country's first female physicians. It is also likely that a considerable number of women possessed serious medical knowledge as a result of working with their physician husbands or fathers, gaining useful skills and experience that they brought to treating and nursing the wartime ill and injured.

The Female Medical College of Pennsylvania (later Woman's Medical College of Pennsylvania), founded in 1850, was one of the only institutions to provide a medical education for qualified women students. Dr. Chloe Annette Buckel, an 1858 graduate of the school, opened her first medical practice in Chicago and later worked with the pioneering physicians Dr. Elizabeth Blackwell and Dr. Emily Blackwell at the New York Infirmary in New York City. In 1863 at the request of General Ulysses S. Grant, she left the Infirmary to organize field hospitals for the Union Army. While on location in Tennessee she set up six field hospitals in warehouses and stores and was later appointed to consult on the selection of female nurses. Although Dr. Buckel possessed a diploma in medicine, she was addressed as "Miss Buckel" throughout her service, and, affectionately, as "The Little Major."

The first woman to graduate from an American medical school was British-born Elizabeth Blackwell, followed by her sister, Emily Blackwell. The Blackwell family had moved from Bristol, England, to New York in 1832, when Elizabeth was eleven years old. Their father, Samuel, was active in the abolitionist movement and encouraged his nine children's wide-ranging social and political awareness. They were certainly cognizant of the fact that American culture of the time fostered the opinion that a woman's place was in the home, unless she chose to teach.

Samuel Blackwell died when Elizabeth was seventeen, leaving few monetary assets to support his children. With two of her sisters, Elizabeth opened a small school, which helped them survive financially for the next four years, and she began to contemplate an almost unthinkable new chapter for herself. She decided to study medicine and began to pursue the avenues that would lead her to that goal, spending a year studying and living with two physician friends while she continued teaching in order to afford her medical education. Although it seems that she was initially repelled by the laboratory examination of tissue—she was very uncomfortable when a teacher presented the eye of a bull for study—she seems to have overcome her distaste and continued forcefully in pursuit of a medical degree. The clinical aspect of her career was eventually just a portion of her enormous influence on women and on the medical field.

> My mind is fully made up. I have not the slightest hesitation on the subject; the thorough study of medicine, I am quite resolved to go through with. The horrors and disgusts I have no doubt of vanquishing. I have overcome stronger distastes than any that now remain, and feel fully equal to the contest.

Demonstrating remarkable determination in a country and time that did not endorse higher education for women, let alone for scientific studies, Elizabeth Blackwell set out to overcome a monolith of refusal from medical schools. She was rejected from every established medical school to which she applied, including all of those in New York and Philadelphia, followed by a dozen smaller colleges, as her gender was perceived to characterize her as intellectually inferior. There was apparently even some discussion of disguising herself as a man in order to gain admittance. Her single acceptance came from Geneva Medical College (presently known as State University of New York Upstate Medical University) in New York in 1847, where the 150 male students voted unanimously for her admission. She attended her courses in New York and during the summer worked at an almshouse in Philadelphia, gaining valuable experience and gathering research for a thesis on typhus.

Elizabeth Blackwell, M.D., graduated from Geneva Medical College in 1849. It was reported that at the graduation ceremony, when her degree was conferred by Dr. Charles Lee, the dean, he stood and bowed to her.

She became the first woman in America to earn a formal medical degree. After her graduation, the thesis she had written on typhoid fever was published in the *Buffalo Medical Journal*: the first medical article to be published by a female medical student in the United States. The article conveyed her sensitivity to suffering and her knowledge and advocacy for social and economic justice—a perspective that was labeled as "feminine" by the medical community. That perception and labelling was actually more insightful than offensive—Elizabeth was a lifelong active and outspoken champion of women, their care, their opportunities, and their right to medical educations.

She met with resistance at every turn of her education and career. After graduating with her medical degree, she spent two years working in London and Paris, where, in order to be able to gain practical experience, she was permitted to work at the Maternity Hospital in Paris only under the condition that she would be considered a student midwife.

In 1851 Elizabeth returned to New York, opening a practice and dispensary with her sister, Dr. Emily Blackwell, an effort that again was met with negativity and opposition, describing it as "a blank wall of social and professional antagonism."

Perhaps prepared in childhood by her father's acceptance and endorsement of progressive ideas and organizations, Dr. Blackwell displayed an impressive strength and ability to quietly crash through society's gender discrimination, prejudice, and additional hurdles. She began to focus her work on the promotion of hygiene and preventative medicine with an emphasis on advocating for medical education and opportunities for female physicians, finally finding the arena where she could fully devote her heart.

> My whole life is devoted unreservedly to the service of my sex.
> The study and practice of medicine is in my thought but one
> means to a great end . . . the true ennoblement of woman.

Dr. Blackwell championed the cause of women entering the medical field, and also the medical care and treatment of women and children. Elizabeth and Emily Blackwell jointly founded the New York Infirmary for Indigent Women and Children in 1857, which later became New York University Downtown Hospital. The Infirmary, which also served as a training facility for nurses, was extraordinary in having women physicians, women on the board of trustees, and women on the executive committee.

Elizabeth returned to England in 1859 as a medical doctor advocating for women to pursue medical educations. She would become the first woman admitted to the British Medical Register and was then legally enabled to practice medicine in both the U.K. and the U.S.A.

During the American Civil War, as an abolitionist, Dr. Blackwell was a strong Union supporter and wanted to assist in the war effort. She helped to standardize the hygienic practices in which she believed so strongly, and trained nurses in a coordinated effort designed to give them skills for working on the chaotic and horrifying battlefields.

Blackwell's forceful personality created some additional barriers for her wartime participation. She played an instrumental role in the development of the United States Sanitary Commission, but her clashes with the new and emerging leaders of the organization led to Elizabeth's not receiving an offer for a formal role in the U.S.S.C. Blackwell's response was to align with another private relief agency, the Woman's Central Association of Relief (W.C.A.R.) that raised millions of dollars in funds and supplies for support of the Union troops. The W.C.A.R. was eventually absorbed by the Sanitary Commission. She also managed to work at training nurses for the Union effort with the notoriously difficult superintendent of nurses, Dorothea Dix, at Blackwell's New York Infirmary.

Moving away from clinical medical practice after the war, she worked on strengthening her positions in public health advocacy, women's rights, and the abolitionist movement. With some colleagues she established the Woman's Medical College of the New York Infirmary, beginning with an enrollment of fifteen students in 1868.

Returning to Britain in 1869, Blackwell amplified her efforts in social reform. In 1871 she cofounded the National Health Society, whose motto "Prevention is better than Cure" remains a fundamental truth in medicine. She worked with a number of progressive movements including moral reform, preventive medicine, sanitation, family planning, and medical ethics. She did not believe in the effectiveness of vaccines, feeling that it was a dangerous practice, and she disavowed bacteria as a singular cause of disease.

England's first medical school for women, London School of Medicine for Women, was created in 1874 by a small group that included Blackwell, her sister Emily and her friend, the renowned British nurse, Florence Nightingale. Elizabeth lectured at the London School and published many pamphlets and books, beginning with *The Laws of Life with Special Reference to the Physical Education of Girls* and leading to her 1895 autobiography, *Pioneer Work in Opening the Medical Profession to Women*.

When Dr. Elizabeth Blackwell passed away at age eighty-nine, she had changed the world, blazing important new roads for empowering women in medicine and society. Her work is reflected in numerous honors: the American Medical Women's Association has, since 1949, annually awarded the Elizabeth Blackwell Medal to a female physician, and the Elizabeth Blackwell Award to women who have shown "outstanding service to humankind" is presented each year by Hobart and William Smith Colleges.

As unrest and violence cast the dark shadow of the encroaching Civil War, only one African American woman in the United States held a formal medical degree. Her life was filled with extraordinary circumstances and important "firsts" and her mere existence would spark an incredible legacy for her gender, her race, and the field of medicine.

Physician, nurse, and author Rebecca Davis Lee Crumpler was born in Christiana, Delaware, in 1831 and raised largely in Pennsylvania by an aunt who ministered to the local ill and infirm. There were no formal schools of nursing in the United States until 1873, so, drawn to the field of nursing, Rebecca moved to Boston in her twenties and acquired much of her education while on the job, spending eight years working as a nurse. Her physician employers, impressed with the young woman's intellect, skills, and work ethic, gave her letters of recommendation to the West Newton English and Classical School in West Newton, Massachusetts.

She was accepted as a "special student in mathematics" at this unusual institution, also known as the "Allen School." The school, founded in 1854 by progressive and liberal educator Nathaniel Topliff Allen, with the encouragement of American educational reformer Horace Mann, was unique at the time. The school welcomed a racially integrated coeducational student body and a diverse curriculum. During its fifty years in existence, more than five thousand students, many of them international, graduated and pursued impressive careers in education, medicine, law, and government.

In her next unique endeavor, Rebecca continued her medical education at one of the world's first medical schools for women, Boston's New

England Female Medical College (NEFMC). The school grew from a women's medical training association called the Female Education Society that had been founded with twelve students in 1848, although it was not able to grant medical degrees at that time. The Society was reorganized as the NEFMC in 1856 with the ability to confer degrees. Crumpler won a tuition award from the Wade Scholarship Fund, established by a bequest from a local businessman. There were initial questions about the wisdom of admitting this African American woman to the college, and fears that it was an action that might provoke anger from the South, but she was finally accepted and received her medical degree in 1864.

> It may be well to state here that, having been reared by a kind aunt in Pennsylvania, whose usefulness with the sick was continually sought, I early conceived a liking for, and sought every opportunity to relieve the sufferings of others. Later in life I devoted my time, when best I could, to nursing as a business, serving under different doctors for a period of eight years (from 1852 to 1860); most of the time at my adopted home in Charlestown, Middlesex County, Massachusetts. From these doctors I received letters commending me to the faculty of the New England Female Medical College, whence, four years afterward, I received the degree of doctress of medicine.

The original graduates of the Female Medical College were titled "Doctress," and it would be another twelve years before they were officially accorded degrees of "Doctor of Medicine." In an open display of gender discrimination, most of the white women graduates were initially denied training or jobs in established hospitals. Rebecca remained the lone African American graduate during the existence of the school and continued to break new ground as she traveled to postwar Richmond, Virginia, where more than ten thousand freed slaves lived in deplorable conditions in tent cities on the outskirts of Richmond. Working under the Freedmen's Bureau, she and other black physicians, nurses, and volunteers took responsibility for these people who otherwise would have had no access to medical care. She set up a tent hospital and convinced her medical school to send medicines and bandages to Richmond by train, as local pharmacies refused to sell supplies to her and local hospitals would not admit her patients. For more than four years the freshly anointed doctor, suffering bouts of both typhoid and malaria in the process, as well as the intense and vicious racism of the postbellum South, ministered to these thousands of people caught in the frightening transition from slavery to freedom and indigence. Despite the devastating circumstances, her devotion remained strong. She felt that Richmond would be

> a proper field for real missionary work, and one that would present ample opportunities to become acquainted with the diseases of women and children. During my stay there nearly every hour was improved in that sphere of labor. The last quarter of the year 1866, I was enabled . . . to have access each day to a very large number of the indigent, and others of different classes, in a population of over 30,000 colored.

As a medical student, Rebecca had been widowed by the death of her first husband, Wyatt Lee, after ten years of marriage. She married a second time to Arthur Crumpler and had one daughter, Lizzie Sinclair Crumpler. After her postwar work in Richmond, Dr. Crumpler returned to Boston, resumed some of her private medical practice there, and began to write a book based on notes she had kept during her combined years in medical practice. In 1883, she became one of the first African Americans to publish a medical textbook. It focused on medical advice geared to women and children. Her *Book of Medical Discourses in Two Parts* was published by Cashman, Keating and Co. of Boston. She dedicated the book to "mothers, nurses and all who may desire to mitigate the afflictions of the human race."

Although few photographs of Dr. Crumpler have survived, her strong and relentless forward progress through vicious discrimination against her race and her gender remain a singular beacon of light that has guided many African American women aspiring to careers in medicine.

Esther Jane Hill, a white woman born in 1833 in Hooksett, New Hampshire, completed an academic education in public school and at an academy in Kingston, New Hampshire, then began her career as a teacher and a strong supporter of abolition. In 1854 she met and married Dr. John Milton Hawks, surgeon, avid abolitionist, and passionate advocate for assistance to freed blacks and black soldiers.

Esther was fascinated by her new husband's medical books and began to study them, eventually deciding that she wanted to attend medical school. Despite his progressive thinking, her husband was clear in his desire that her focus remain on tending to his comfort, but she persevered, finally receiving her M.D. degree in 1857 from the New England Female Medical College in Boston. Dr. Esther Hill Hawks had become one of the first female physicians in America.

Esther's husband, Dr. John Hawks, joined the United States Colored Troops as a physician in order to care for former slaves, receiving an appointment as acting assistant surgeon in Beaufort, South Carolina, on the mainland near Hilton Head Island. In November 1861, Hilton Head Island was captured and occupied by 13,000 Union troops, rapidly becoming a sanctuary for freed and escaped slaves. Hilton Head was a safe harbor, territory where the new residents were free to go to school, buy land, and begin new lives. Their numbers burgeoned to more than 600 by February 1862.

Dr. Esther Hawks's medical degree was frequently overshadowed by her gender. Refused entrance to serve as an army surgeon, she applied to Superintendent of Army Nurses Dorothea Dix to work as a nurse and was rejected on the basis of her youth and appearance. Dix was intent that her nurses would not be exploited by the Army doctors and therefore restricted her hiring on the bases of age and lack of physical beauty in order to avoid the possibility of her nurses attracting the eye of any ill-intentioned medic.

Intent on supporting the war effort, Esther finally applied for a teaching position with the National Freedmen's Relief Association in Beaufort, South Carolina, a job that allowed her to join her husband and work at educating the soldiers of the First Regiment of South Carolina Volunteers. The regiment was the first official unit of the Union Army to be composed of escaped slaves. The men of the regiment were so eager to learn to read that as a condition of their enlistment, the Army made teachers available to them.

The federal government built a hospital on Hilton Head Island for African American soldiers. It was called General Hospital Number 10 and Esther Hawks was able to work there unofficially as her husband's assistant and nurse while continuing to teach. When Dr. John Hawks was sent on a remote assignment and no other army surgeon was available to take on his duties, Dr. Esther Hawks had the highly unusual experience of taking charge of the hospital and finally being able to utilize her medical skills and training.

> I am left manager of not only the affairs of the hospital, but have to attend surgeon's call for the 2nd (South Carolina Volunteers), so every morning at 9 o'clock the disabled are marched down to the hospital in charge of a Sergeant and I hold surgeon's call for hospital and Regt. And with great success, on the back piazza, sending some to duty and taking into the hospital such as need extra care.
>
> So for three weeks I performed the duties of hospital and Regimental Surgeon, doing work so well that the neglect to supply a regular officer was not discovered at headquarters.

The Fifty-Fourth Massachusetts Volunteer Infantry Regiment of African Americans led an assault on Fort Wagner, South Carolina, in July 1863. The fort was a valuable target, as it guarded the Charleston, South Carolina, harbor entrance. Despite the incredible valor of 600 men, the Fifty-Fourth was not able to seize the fort and almost 300 of them were killed, captured, or wounded. Their sad and heroic story was further immortalized in the 1989 feature film *Glory*, directed by Edward Zwick and nominated for five Academy Awards. The real-life survivors of the mid-19th-century battle were carried to General Hospital Number 10 and treated by the two Dr. Hawks, who worked without rest to attend every patient.

> The only thing that sustained us was the patient endurance of those stricken heroes lying before us, with their ghastly wounds, cheerful and courageous.

Several months later, in February 1864, the Hawks traveled to Jacksonville to care for Union wounded from their loss at the Battle of Olustee, the largest battle to be fought in Florida during the Civil War. The Confederacy would remain in control of the interior of Florida until the end of the conflict.

After the war doctors Esther and John Hawks moved to Port Orange, Florida, where the Homestead Act of 1866 allowed freedmen to purchase government lands in Florida, as well as in Louisiana, Alabama, Mississippi, and Arkansas. The Florida settlement quickly attracted more than 1,500 former slaves and a community began to form. Esther became a teacher with the Freedmen's Aid Society and established a school where both black and white children were welcomed and classes were offered for black adults. It was most likely the first integrated school in the state of Florida.

Her school appeared to be flourishing for the next two years, but in January 1869 it was torched in an arson fire. The doctor returned to Massachusetts, where she was legally permitted to practice medicine, although her husband appears to have remained in Port Orange for the rest of his life. She became active in multiple charities and served as an officer of the Women's Rights or Suffrage Club. Although Dr. Esther Hill Hawks had been denied the right to work as an Army surgeon during the Civil War, she was elected an honorary member of the New Hampshire Association of Military Surgeons in 1899.

In the field of medicine, dentistry is one of the oldest professions, with evidence indicating its existence as early as 7000 B.C.E. in South Asia's northwestern Indus Valley Civilization. America's first dental college opened in Baltimore in 1840, followed by Alabama's dental practice act the next year. By 1860 the American Dental Association had been formed and two years after the end of the Civil War, in 1867, Harvard University Dental School was founded.

The Civil War would reveal another divide between the armies—the Confederate states had about five hundred dentists then practicing, and President Jefferson Davis was a strong proponent for a dentistry corps in the army. When Davis served as United States secretary of state under President Franklin Pierce, he had lobbied unsuccessfully to establish a dentistry corps for the U.S. Army. At the onset of the Civil War, the Confederate Army established a dental program and in 1864 began conscripting dentists into the army. With fewer men available to fight in the South, the army could not allow dental problems to sideline their soldiers.

Dentists in the Confederate Army usually held the rank of hospital steward, and under some conditions they could also be full surgeons complete with surgeon's pay and benefits. The Union remained unmoved as to establishing a dental corps, but the army did accept many dentists as assistant surgeons and surgeons. Both armies were grateful for their trained dentists, whether or not they were ranked as such—they were invaluable in dealing with potentially fatal fractures and gunshot wounds to the jaw at a time before tube feeding and intravenous drips existed. Some army dentists performed daring maxillofacial surgery that prevented deformities and disfigurement. The dentists had also introduced anesthesia to the medical profession and brought it into common use during the war.

One of anesthesia's strongest early champions was American dentist and physician William Thomas Green Morton, born in 1819 in a farmhouse in the village of Charlton, Worcester County, Massachusetts. His childhood wish was to become a physician, although his father, a farmer of Scottish descent, was not wealthy. William attained a New England common school education and at seventeen went to work in various businesses in Boston as a salesman or a clerk. Unfulfilled by these labors, and without the funding to attend medical school, he moved to Baltimore, Maryland, and enrolled in the College of Dental Surgery in 1840.

Morton returned to New England in 1842 and opened a dental office in Farmington, Connecticut, where he met dentist Horace Wells, a practitioner who was interested in anesthesia and was experimenting with nitrous oxide gas. The two men went into practice together in Boston, but found the partnership unprofitable and soon dissolved it, although Morton remained in the city. He also fell in love with Elizabeth Whitman of Farmington, the niece of former congressman Lemuel Whitman. Elizabeth's parents had hoped for a more prestigious and moneyed match for their daughter, and they also objected to Morton's dental profession. They gave permission for the couple to marry in 1843, but only after he promised to study medicine.

Morton entered Harvard Medical School in 1844 to study for his medical degree, but due to mounting financial pressures he was forced to leave before graduating. In his short time at Harvard, he attended chemistry lectures given by Dr. Charles Thomas Jackson, an American scientist and physician with strong interests in chemistry, medicine, and minerology. In Morton's brief enrollment at the school, Jackson introduced him to ether and its anesthetic properties. (Although Morton was not financially able to complete Harvard's degree requirements, several years later he was nonetheless awarded an M.D. degree "honoris causa"—a degree conferred as a mark of esteem without examination—in 1852 by the Washington University of Medicine, later called the College of Physicians and Surgeons of Baltimore.)

Dr. Jackson's Harvard chemistry class demonstrations of the loss of consciousness from the inhalation of sulfuric ether were fascinating to William Morton, who had continued his work in dentistry while enrolled in medical school in order to be able to pay for the education. He had become particularly interested in the manufacture of artificial teeth and was concerned about lessening the pain caused to the patient by tooth extractions. He had experimented with various intoxicants including opium, but found none satisfactory until he tried the inhalation of sulfuric ether on himself, and, impressed with the result, proceeded to anesthetize a goldfish, a hen, and his pet spaniel, all of whom recovered successfully.

William Morton became convinced of the safety and effectiveness of ether as an anesthetic agent, and in September of 1846 he administered ether to a patient and then performed the extraction of an ulcerated tooth while clearly causing no pain to the patient. The procedure was written up in the *Boston Daily Journal* newspaper a day later and deeply impressed a young Boston surgeon named Henry J. Bigelow, who was associated with Massachusetts General Hospital. The hospital's surgical chief, Dr. John Collins Warren, invited Morton to demonstrate his discovery by anesthetizing a young male patient named Gilbert Abbott for a procedure to remove a vascular tumor of his neck, just below his jaw. The success of the operation in removing the tumor while the patient remained unconscious was reported around the world, and Dr. Bigelow wrote about Morton's discovery in the *Boston Medical and Surgical Journal* in November of that year. It was an event that signaled the end of the fear of pain during surgery and opened the field of surgical operations in a revolutionary way, conferring what is widely regarded as a blessing to the human race.

Morton's world began to crash down after he patented his discovery in the United States and England in 1846, expecting to be financially compensated and lauded as the discoverer of anesthesia, but instead he received competition for years from other doctors who had also experimented with various forms of anesthesia, including his former partner Horace Wells and his professor Charles Jackson. Although Morton had received a patent, the government simply appropriated his discovery for its own use and disregarded any ownership or claim. Morton became angry, depressed, and litigiously combative over his losses.

In 1862 Dr. William Morton joined the Army of the Potomac as a volunteer surgeon and specialized in administering ether to thousands of wounded soldiers during Virginia battles including Fredericksburg, Chancellorsville, and the Wilderness. He was known to go out over the fields after a battle and dispense anesthesia to wounded men awaiting rescue and hospital transport, giving them a window of respite from their pain.

Morton remained obsessed with the controversy over the discovery and use of inhalation anesthesia and failed to receive financial compensation for his work although he was granted some honors. The last twenty years of his life were embroiled with his legal battle for Congressional approval of his discovery and patent, and he dedicated himself to the pursuit while neglecting his practice, accumulating legal bills and being eventually reduced to frustration and poverty. He suffered a sudden major stroke in New York City at the age of forty-eight and died shortly after. Morton was rushed to St. Luke's hospital, where his wife reported that when the chief surgeon saw the new patient and recognized him, he made the following comment to his students: "Young gentlemen, you see lying before you a man who has done more for humanity and for the relief of suffering than any man who has ever lived."

Dr. William Thomas Green Morton was buried in Mt. Auburn Cemetery near Boston, with many prominent physicians in attendance at the ceremony. A monument was erected over his grave by the citizens of Boston with an inscription written by Dr. Bigelow:

William T.G. Morton,
Inventor and Revealer of Anesthetic Inhalation.
Before whom in all time surgery was agony.
By whom pain in surgery was averted and annulled.
Since whom, science has control of pain.

Dr. Morton's life and work were further immortalized in the book *Triumph Over Pain* by René Fülöp-Miller and the 1944 film from Paramount Pictures *The Great Moment*, starring Joel McCrea and Betty Field.

Dr. Joseph Janvier Woodward Jr. achieved the dubious distinction of attending two U.S. presidents after their assassination attempts.

He was born in Philadelphia in 1833 and appears to have excelled in his academic work. Woodward attended Philadelphia's Central High School, the first high school in Pennsylvania, known as "the worthy apex to a noble pyramid," earned a degree and graduated as his class valedictorian. He began to study medicine privately with Professor George B. Wood while attending lectures at the University of Pennsylvania, which awarded his M.D. in 1853.

The microscope was a lifelong passion of Woodward's, and he gave private instruction in its use in addition to working as a demonstrator in operative surgery at the university and managing the surgical clinic. He had begun to experiment with photomicrography, the science of taking photographs through a microscope, but when the Civil War began, he offered his services to the U.S. government and became an assistant surgeon in the army.

In 1862 Dr. Woodward was assigned to the surgeon general's office in Washington, D.C., an office where he served for the rest of his life. His duties were to collect materials for the planned multivolume series of books about a medical/surgical history of the war, later realized as the impressive six-part *The Medical and Surgical History of the War of the Rebellion*, and for a planned Military Medical Museum.

During the war Woodward wrote and produced several publications on war-related diseases, and also authored handbooks at the suggestion of

Surgeon General William Hammond, writing *The Hospital Steward's Manual*, designed for use in the military hospitals. The manual gave explicit instructions for duties of hospital attendants including stewards, nurses, and ward masters. The book included recipes that had been developed during the Crimean War for use in hospital cooking. His *Outlines of the Chief Camp Diseases of the United States Armies: As Observed During the Present War* was published in 1863. He worked on planning the museum with a colleague in the office, Dr. William Thomson, finding that the two exceptionally gifted and dedicated young physicians shared an interest in photomicrography and its uses in pathology. They both made significant contributions to the development of the Army Medical Museum and its reputation for excellence in the field of pathology.

Woodward is renowned as a pioneer in applying photomicrography to pathology, even developing improvements in the photomicrographic camera. Becoming known worldwide, he was one of the first pathologists to explore the field and devised new methods for the work, revolutionizing the science and use of photomicrography and opening the groundwork for the study of modern surgical pathology.

In 1881, Dr. Woodward assisted in the care of President James A. Garfield after the president was shot and wounded in an assassination attempt, and he later recorded Garfield's autopsy. Woodward had had some similar prior tragic experience, having been one of two physicians who performed the head-only autopsy on President Abraham Lincoln in 1865. He also carried out the autopsy on Lincoln's assassin, John Wilkes Booth, and wrote the autopsy reports on both.

Army Assistant Surgeon Dr. Edward Curtis worked with Woodward to perform the autopsy on the president.

> Dr. Woodward and I proceeded to open the head and remove the brain down to the track of the ball. The latter had entered a little to the left of the median line at the back of the head, had passed almost directly forwards through the center of the brain and lodged.

After the procedure was completed, Woodward reported on the president's autopsy to the surgeon general.

April 15, 1865,
Brigadier General J.K. Barnes,
Surgeon General, U.S.A.

General:

I have the honor to report that in obedience to your orders and aided by Assistant Surgeon E. Curtis, U.S.A., I made in your presence at 12 o'clock this morning an autopsy on the body of President Abraham Lincoln, with the following results: the eyelids and surrounding parts of the face were greatly ecchymosed and the eyes somewhat protuberant from effusion of blood into the orbits.

The wound in the occipital bone was quite smooth, circular in shape, with beveled edges. The track of the ball was full of clotted blood and contained several little fragments of bone with small pieces of the ball near its external orifice. The brain around the track was pultaceous and livid from capillary hemorrhage into its substance. The ventricles of the brain were full of clotted blood. A thick clot beneath the dura matter coated the right cerebral lobe.

There was a smaller clot under the dura matter of the left side. But little blood was found at the base of the brain. Both the orbital plates of the frontal bone were fractured and the fragments pushed upwards toward the brain. The dura matter over these fractures was uninjured. The orbits were gorged with blood. I have the honor of being very respectfully your obedient servant,

J.J. Woodward, Assistant Surgeon, U.S.A.

What does Lincoln's death say about Civil War medicine? The president of the United States was treated by doctors who weren't unskilled or unsophisticated; they were competent physicians, some of them prominent and respected men. They gave the best care they knew how to give, but Abraham Lincoln's assassination still stands as the tragic moment that illustrates how far medicine had *not* come.

In 1865, people weren't expected to survive penetrating head wounds. Lincoln was unusual in that he had a head wound and didn't die quickly. No one then understood brain function: the surgeons kept him alive by keeping the wound open to allow for brain swelling as it had been understood for centuries that excess pressure in the cranium was deadly.

The most important man in the United States got the best medical care of his time from physicians working with minimal knowledge. All their skills could only serve to make their patient as comfortable as possible.

Lincoln stands as an icon of Civil War medicine, illustrating both its strength and its weaknesses. His death marked the end of the war and was shortly followed by a gigantic leap forward into new areas of medicine: medicine with the understanding of sterilization and the germ theory of disease.

The scientific advances that were made during the Civil War couldn't save the president, but his influence was felt in the organizational and clinical progress that rescued countless lives in future generations. These gains increased our understanding of the workings of the human body and mind and they have eased the suffering of untold numbers of the sick and wounded.

The tenacity, persistence, courage, and daring of these wartime medics led to some effective solutions for centuries-old problems. Faced with outbreaks of deadly contagious diseases that included yellow fever, measles, chicken pox, and mumps, they saw that quarantining patients with transmissible diseases led to containing that disease to a limited population. Yellow fever, dreaded for generations, was virtually eliminated by the practice of quarantine.

Despite their limited training and experience and lack of supplies, sleep, tools, and facilities, Civil War doctors managed to save a higher percentage of the lives of the sick and wounded than physicians in any previous American or European war.

Peter J. D'Onofrio, Ph.D., president emeritus, Society of Civil War Surgeons, founded the prestigious group that has studied, written, and published results and observations on the phenomenon for many years. His reminder cautions that "we must not forget that the medical professionals of the Civil War era were some of the best trained doctors of their time, given the standards of care and knowledge that existed during the most turbulent time in American history."

CHAPTER FOUR

THE EMERGENCE OF WOMEN AND THE EVOLUTION OF SKILLED NURSING

The 1850s and 1860s in America saw the rise of the "sentimental domestic idea." Women were held up as examples of purity, piety, and submissiveness. They were not seen unaccompanied in public, pregnant women isolated themselves at home, and the forming of friendships with men was considered inappropriate.

In the American antebellum period, precise and strict rules were recommended for women's socially acceptable and appropriate behavior. A popular etiquette guide for ladies, published in 1860, offered some advice to clarify the expectations of "polite" women's manners and behavior:

> In the street a lady takes the arm of a relative, her affianced lover, or husband, but of no other gentleman, unless the streets are slippery, or in the evening.
>
> . . . every lady will endeavor to become, not only well educated, but accomplished. It is not, as some will assert, a waste of time or money.

Paintings and illustrations of the period frequently depict the fact that a woman getting formally dressed required an additional set of hands for tightening her "laces" or adjusting her voluminous skirts. The most common and popular silhouette of the period featured a closely fitted bodice and a wide, floor-length skirt. The skirts were typically made of fabric with sewn channels that acted as casings for materials that held the skirt stiffly out from the body. The channels in the skirts and bodices held whalebone or steel strips that maintained the fullness of the skirt or the form-fitting silhouette of the bodice. The outer garments were worn over a tight corset, chemise, and drawers. It was a confining combination of clothing and frequently precluded a wide range of motion. The glamorous wealthy belles of the South modeled traditional Victorian hoop skirts and boned bodices that were adorned with ribbons and bows. It was a style depicting status and wealth, and its restrictive nature only emphasized its detachment from physical work.

The Civil War would change the social, economic, and political landscape for women from every walk of American life. Women demonstrated a remarkable adaptability in the savagely altered wartime world, responding to the great need of the nation while acquiring and utilizing skills to ease the pain of the country. Women's new wartime assertiveness would give them tremendous gains in opportunity and stature.

Dr. Robert D. Hicks of the College of Physicians of Philadelphia explained: "At the beginning of the war, a 'nurse' meant a soldier recovering in hospital from a wound or injury, untrained in healing, who aided doctors with miscellaneous duties. The idea of women handling the bodies of men not related by family was unthinkable. By the end of the war, the term meant women who, as para-professional volunteers or paid employees of the government, aided doctors by cleaning and feeding patients and occasionally assisting doctors in their surgeries and treatments."

Nurses in America had usually been men. When the Civil War began, there was not a single school in America devoted to nursing, although internationally, there was an exciting hint of new doors opening. Inspiring news about the British Florence Nightingale's nursing and training work in the Crimean War of the 1850s had reached Europe and America.

The history of nursing can be traced to many early civilizations as most cultures included nursing as a religion-based service. The beginnings of both Christianity and Islam included dedicated nurses as an integral part of their belief systems. The Sanskrit text *Charaka Samhita* from approximately 100 B.C.E. in ancient India states that a nurse was required to be knowledgeable and skilled at working with and preparing formulas and dosages, to be sympathetic to all people, and was expected to be clean. Early Christianity offers the record of the woman emissary Phoebe being sent to Rome by St. Paul. As a wealthy member of a religious community, there is speculation that it was also intended that she would work there as a nurse or healer. Rufaidah bint Sa'ad, a 7th-century contemporary of Muhammad, is described as the first Muslim nurse, a woman who dared to lead a group of women to treat injured warriors on the battlefield.

Both men and women are recorded to have served as nurses throughout our early history, but by the mid–19th century in America, it was no longer considered to be a job for a woman. The founding of modern professional nursing in the West can be said to begin with Florence Nightingale, whose influence on nursing during the American Civil War was profound and revolutionary.

A young woman from a very wealthy British family, Florence was given a lavish and liberal education including literature, mathematics, history, philosophy, and Italian, and she displayed a remarkable talent for collecting and analyzing data. She was thought to be an interesting but eccentric character from an early age, and, at seventeen years old, had a series of experiences that she believed were messages from God inspiring her to devote her life to service.

The social conventions of the upper-class British precluded nursing work—caring for and intimately working to heal strangers, whether in their homes or in hospitals, was not seen as a respectable activity for young ladies of wealth and tradition. It was acceptable to perform these acts for family members or close friends, but pursuing nursing as a profession or a calling was considered to be extremely inappropriate behavior for a woman.

Florence Nightingale was an exception to many of the social expectations of her time. Despite the opposition of her family, she believed that a career in nursing was a valid opportunity to provide intellectual and social freedom for women, who otherwise had few options for professional work. At age thirty she visited a Lutheran religious community in Germany and observed the pastor and deaconesses caring for the sick and indigent. It was a period of time that would be the basis for changing her life path in a passionate and dedicated way. She published her findings anonymously, and underwent four months of medical training at the German facility. Two years later she became the superintendent at the Institute for the Care of Sick Gentlewomen in London.

Britain's Crimean War, beginning in 1854, was the flashpoint of change and the beginning of defined, professional nursing for the Western world. Florence Nightingale arrived in Crimea in 1855, began to visit and care for the wounded, and trained a group of women as nurses, sharing with them her knowledge, skills, and vision.

The British hospital in Constantinople was in horrifying condition—filthy and overrun with rodents, excrement, and trash. Supplies including food, medicine, blankets, and water were limited or nonexistent. Florence Nightingale's moment had arrived, and she seized the opportunity, leading a massive cleaning effort and bringing her experience, beliefs, and theories into play. She believed that cleanliness decreased the spread of infection, and that measures such as handwashing were desirable hygienic procedures. She ordered that nourishing food be prepared and served to the patients, that windows be opened for ventilation, and that medications were to be administered on a schedule. Within weeks, the death rate at the hospital had plummeted and even the public had heard about the "Lady with the Lamp" and her nightly rounds to comfort the patients.

The news of Florence Nightingale's transformation of health care facilities, practices, and training spread throughout Europe and America, providing a foundation for radical change in hospitals and treatments. By 1860 she had set up a training school for nurses at St. Thomas' Hospital in London and the Western world was beginning to see and incorporate some of the dramatic changes she had wrought. By the start of the 20th century, educated, skilled nurses would be a mainstay in every hospital and health care facility.

When the American Civil War began, although no trained nurses yet existed in the country, women came out of the parlors and kitchens in force. They traveled to the battlefields and the hospitals and took charge of running businesses. By the tens of thousands, they sought to comfort and heal the sick and wounded and they trained other female volunteers to administer much-needed aid.

For the first time in America, female personnel held responsible positions in a traditionally male military environment and some were even paid or salaried for their work. Thousands of women, Northern and Southern, volunteered their service as nurses in the hospitals and at the fronts. Many "Angels of the Battlefield" served throughout the war; laywomen as well as Catholic nuns from many orders across the country. Nuns who served as nurses were known for their dedicated work ethic and their willingness to treat patients suffering from known dangerously communicable diseases like smallpox and yellow fever. A Sister of Charity from Maryland remembered the patients' surprise.

> Our small-pox patients appeared to think that the Sisters were not like other human beings, or they would not attend such loathsome contagious diseases, which everyone else shunned. One day I was advising an application to a man's face—and I told him this remedy had cured a Sister. The man looked at me in perfect astonishment. "A Sister!" He exclaimed. I answered

"Yes," "Why!" said he, "I didn't know the Sisters ever got anything like that." I told him "To be sure they did. They are liable to take disease as well as any one else." "To be sure NOT!" he said, "For the boys often say they must be different from other people, for they do for us what no other person would do. They are not afraid of fevers, small-pox or anything else."

During a period of anti-Catholic sentiment in America, when Catholics made up only 5 percent of the population, when rioters in Boston burned down a convent belonging to Roman Catholic Ursuline nuns in the 1830s and when Catholic churches in Philadelphia had been torched in 1855, the largest organized group of women in the country with any concentrated medical training was Catholic nuns. In an atmosphere of hatred for them, when many Sisters chose not to wear their habits outside of the convents, the vilified nuns nevertheless became somewhat more acceptable to Protestants across the country, as they were openly supported by the Protestant Union surgeon general William Hammond. Sisters from twelve orders including the Daughters of Charity, Sisters of St. Joseph, Sisters of the Holy Cross, and Sisters of Mercy dedicated themselves to serving the sick and wounded of the Civil War. It is estimated that between 600 and 700 nuns served as nurses in Union and Confederate hospitals: as many as 20 percent of all nuns in the United States.

In medieval and early-modern Europe, the role of a nun was a prestigious one as the convents were funded by the generous dowries of enrolled daughters from wealthy families. Providing nursing and health care for the poor was considered to be a part of the calling of the Sisters and for many centuries, European religious had visited and cared for the sick in their homes.

When the American Civil War erupted, the governments of the divided country had not prepared for a lengthy and epic combat situation and its resulting casualties. Arrangements had not been made for transporting or treating tens of thousands of wounded and sickened men. Both North and

South were hesitant to call for female nurses, but officials on both sides, including President Abraham Lincoln, eventually requested aid from the Catholic sisterhood. It was an especially difficult decision for the Confederacy, as Southern tradition in particular found the intimate physical contact of nursing to be highly inappropriate for women.

In the mid–19th century, with waves of immigrants coming to America, some European Sisters were included, nuns who had actually assisted and learned from Florence Nightingale in her pioneering nursing efforts in the Crimean War. Their knowledge and experience would benefit the American nuns and secular nurses.

Despite the existing religious prejudice, and fulfilling an important service with both militaries, the Sisters were lauded for their willingness to risk their health and lives to care for all patients regardless of religious affiliation, including victims of known contagious diseases such as yellow fever and smallpox. They were invaluable for their dedicated service in hospitals, hospital ships, and directly on the battlefields; known to work long hours and to require little for themselves. As Christianity encouraged practical charity and the tending of the sick, hundreds of religious women followed these edicts into uncertainty and unknown dangers. They created and solidified new roles for America's women in the changing and evolving country.

The newly created parameters for women combined with the advancement of technology brought aid to the battlefield wounded more rapidly than ever before. The first medical teams to arrive at the Battle of Shiloh were Sisters of Charity, who appeared at the scene via steamboat. The U.S.S. *Red Rover*, a captured Confederate vessel that became a U.S. Navy hospital ship, was the first to be staffed by women nurses—nuns from the Sisters of the Holy Cross from Notre Dame, Indiana, who boarded the vessel on Christmas Eve 1862. This voyage would become naval history's forerunner of the United States Navy Nurse Corps.

Throughout the duration of the Civil War nuns were sent to administer hospitals, to serve on hospital ships, to teach other workers about establishing guidelines for the cleanliness they believed in so strongly for combating infection, to visit prisoners of war, and to continue to treat and comfort the wounded and the dying.

After the war, most of the surviving nuns returned to their communities, where they continued to assist in the country's recovery by nursing, teaching, and caring for the widows, orphans, and sick and aging veterans of the war. They quietly helped to ease prejudice for their faith and their gender and played a large role in making nursing a respectable and desirable profession for women.

In a 1924 commemoration of the service of the many women's religious orders that served in the Civil War, Catholic leaders, with the blessing of Congress, unveiled the *Nuns of the Battlefield* monument in Washington, D.C., outside of St. Matthew's Cathedral. The monument is inscribed with these words:

> *They comforted the dying, nursed the wounded, carried hope to the imprisoned, gave in His name a drink of water to the thirsty—To the memory and in honor of the various orders of Sisters who gave their services as nurses on battlefields and in hospitals during the Civil War.*

Cornelia King, chief of reference and curator of Women's History of The Library Company of Philadelphia, pointed out that women were "learning nursing on the ground. They were acquiring leadership skills and getting larger roles in important arenas. They were acquiring confidence and connections. The war created an opportunity for many women to develop leadership skills within a large-scale organization."

For upper- and middle-class white women, this socially sanctioned game changer came from a long tradition of women being engaged in philanthropy as volunteers. They were accustomed to "helping the poor" and had an inherited sisterhood in charity work and fundraising. During the war they held prominent roles in organizing fundraising fairs and writing letters to the newspapers, letting the public know what conditions were like for the soldiers.

White teenage girls of Southern "society" would have normally been planning for elaborate parties, gowns, and hairstyles for their traditional social debuts, but instead, they found themselves thrust into the terrible swirling melee of the war's shortages and the desperate needs of its victims. The privileged and sheltered sixteen-year-old Louise Wigfall and her younger sister volunteered for the cause of relief and were swept into service on a Confederate hospital train from Atlanta to Macon. Packed beyond capacity with no space for any person to lie down, the train was

> filled with wounded, sick and dying soldiers in all imaginable stages of disease and suffering . . . I never imagined what a hideous, cruel thing War was until I was brought into direct contact with these poor victims of "Man's inhumanity to man."

Although devotion and dedication to the cause of relief transcended social class and race to some degree, there was still inequality among women. Huge contributions to the effort included many unsung African American women, former slaves, contrabands, and freeborn, who also risked their lives on the battlefields and helped to staff hospitals and hospital ships.

Harriet Tubman, born into slavery, is primarily known for her roles as a courageous conductor on the Underground Railroad, a Union spy, and scout. She is less remembered for her influential role in nursing during the Civil War.

In childhood and adolescence Harriet endured vicious and violent treatment from various "masters," including suffering a serious head injury that plagued her with seizures for the rest of her life. In 1849, she made the daring and successful attempt to escape slavery and the South via the Underground Railroad into Pennsylvania. After reaching safety in Philadelphia, she again risked her life to guide family members and many others to the freedom to be found in the Northern states and Canada. Her final rescue mission was in November 1861. It is estimated that in eleven years, Harriet Tubman rescued more than seventy slaves from Maryland, and as many as fifty or sixty others who survived the journey to the Canadian border. Harriet's then-husband, John Tubman, elected to spend his life in Maryland rather than attempt the escape to the North.

When the Civil War cast its ugly shadow over the country, she offered her services to the Union Army and traveled to South Carolina to provide desperately needed nursing care to black soldiers and newly freed slaves. She also began scouting and spying missions behind the Confederate lines, supplying valuable intelligence. She was lauded by the press for an 1863 mission that she carried out with Colonel James Montgomery along the Combahee River in an assault that rescued more than 700 slaves from plantations there.

Tubman was a gifted and compassionate nurse who reportedly cared for thousands of wounded soldiers both black and white. She was highly skilled in the use of healing herbal medicine and her ability to cure the dangerous dysentery was legendary.

From an 1886 biography called *Harriet: The Moses of Her People* by Sarah H. Bradford:

> She nursed our soldiers in the hospitals, and knew how, when they were dying by numbers of some malignant disease, with cunning skill to extract from roots and herbs, which grew near the source of the disease, the healing draught, which allayed the fever and restored numbers to health.

In 1865 Harriet Tubman was appointed matron of a hospital for sick and wounded black soldiers in Fort Monroe, Virginia. Four years later, in Auburn, New York, she married Civil War veteran Nelson Davis. Her passion for the abolition movement transitioned to the cause of women's suffrage, for which she worked tirelessly. She and her husband resided in Auburn until his death in 1888.

It was many years after the war and thirty-four years after Harriet Tubman's first application when at age seventy-nine she was finally able to secure a pension from the government for her wartime work. The Dependent and Disability Pension Act of 1890 made her eligible for a widow's pension from her marriage to Nelson Davis. New York congressman Sereno E. Payne introduced a bill in 1897 to grant Tubman a monthly pension for her wartime nursing service, but some members of Congress objected to a woman being paid the full amount of a soldier's pension. In 1899 she was awarded an additional compromise amount of $20 per month. Her work as a spy and scout was never compensated.

In 2003 the U.S. Congress approved an additional posthumous pension of $11,750 that was intended to make up for the lack of appropriate payments made during her lifetime. The compensatory funds were allocated to the maintenance of her historical sites.

Harriet Tubman was reported to have been surrounded by family and friends when she died on March 10, 1913. She was buried at Fort Hill Cemetery in Auburn with military honors and her bequest of observations, wisdom, and compassion live on:

> Every great dream begins with a dreamer. Always remember,
> you have within you the strength, the patience, and the passion
> to reach for the stars to change the world.

Susannah Baker King Taylor, raised as an enslaved person from her birth on the Valentine Grest plantation in Midway, Liberty County, Georgia, in 1848, created an extraordinary life as teacher, nurse, and author.

The state had harsh orders forbidding education for African Americans under the slave edicts of Georgia, which were cruelly limiting and specific. Under "Crimes of Masters and White Persons Regarding Slaves" it was declared that teaching slaves to read was illegal. The law was originally enacted in 1770 and reenacted in 1829 to include free persons of color.

Defying the restrictive decrees and in dangerous territory, young Susie secretly sought lessons and tutoring sessions. She was apparently originally taught to read by her plantation mistress, attended two clandestine schools operated by African American women, and received tutoring from two white youths, becoming a skilled reader and writer. At the age of seven, she moved to Savannah to live with her grandmother for several years and attended additional illegal underground schools. This perilous activity in criminalized education was overseen by Mother Mathilda Beasley, Savannah, Georgia's first known African American Catholic nun.

The young girl was eventually sent back to live with her mother on the plantation where she had been born shortly before Union forces attacked nearby Fort Pulaski. Susie's freedom came in 1862 when she and her uncle daringly enacted a successful escape from slavery. With a small group of African Americans, they fled by boat in the Jones River and sailed into St. Catherine's Sound and the Atlantic Ocean. They were rescued by a federal gunboat from waters close to Fort Pulaski and reached nearby Union-occupied St. Simons Island off Georgia's southern coast. She first worked there as a regimental laundress, and at the age of fourteen, impressing the commanding officers with her literacy, Susie became a teacher to other formerly enslaved refugees. During the day on the island, Susie taught reading and writing to almost forty children, and after school, her class filled with adults.

> [They] came to me nights, all of them so eager to learn to read,
> to read above anything else.

While serving as an instructor at the school on St. Simons Island, Susie met and married Sergeant Edward King of Darien, Georgia, a literate black noncommissioned officer in the First Carolina Volunteers of African Descent (later known as the Thirty-Third United States Colored Infantry).

She moved with her husband's regiment for the next "four years and three months without receiving a dollar," serving as laundress and teacher, cleaning muskets, cooking for the troops, and nursing wounded soldiers. She also worked as a nurse in Beaumont, South Carolina, at a hospital for African American soldiers, where she met and served with relief worker Clara Barton.

After the war, she strove to continue her career and calling as a teacher and opened a private school in Savannah for the children of freedmen, followed by at least two more serious efforts at establishing schools. Widowed in 1866, Susie moved to Boston several years later and remarried to Russell Taylor in 1879. For much of the rest of her life, in addition to her service with civic and patriotic groups, she worked with an organization created for female Civil War veterans, the Women's Relief Corps.

Susie King Taylor was instrumental in helping to educate and elevate many others out of slavery. She was the first African American woman to write and then self-publish a memoir of her wartime experiences, *Reminiscences of My Life in Camp with the 33d United States Colored Troops, Late 1st S.C. Volunteers*, and she was the only woman of her time to have written about the perspective from inside a Civil War regiment.

Susie never stopped championing causes for equal rights and justice. She supported the creation of the Army Nurse Pension Act, but based on her initial enlistment title, she was denied a pension. Susannah Baker King Taylor died in Boston in 1912, having created a legacy of devoted compassion, support for patriotic and civil causes, and the vital importance and advancement of literacy.

The desperate situations created by the war prompted many women, Northern and Southern, to break long-held traditions and social mores in order to move aggressively to the forefront of the war and assist in healing the terrible damage caused by the fighting. Women stood up to years of preconceived ideas about their strength and tenacity, assuming support and leadership roles in arenas where they had never been invited or admitted.

The war was bringing out the iron backbones and passionate contributions of many people whose passivity had always been encouraged, expected, and demanded.

Captain Sally Louisa Tompkins, also known as the "Angel of the Confederacy" became, at the age of twenty-eight, the first woman to be commissioned into the Confederate Army; also the first woman in American history to be formally inducted into the military. Her commission was unique as the first known case of a women being openly commissioned as a female. (A number that may never be known is that of commissions thought to have unwittingly been given to a small number of courageous women who disguised themselves as men in order to serve as soldiers.)

Sally was the youngest of eight children of a wealthy Virginia family. In 1842, when she was nine years old, three of her four older sisters died within a few weeks of one another, followed a few months later by the loss of her mother. For the next several years, Sally may have worked through her grief by her thoughtful nursing of the community's sick, free or slave, an aptitude and affinity that she had exhibited since childhood. When the Civil War began she was living in Richmond, Virginia, which became the capital city of the Confederacy.

The first major hand-to-hand combat of the war occurred in Virginia at the First Battle of Bull Run, also known as the First Battle of Manassas, in July 1861. Although the Confederacy emerged victorious, hundreds of its men were wounded and were sent to Richmond for treatment via the Virginia Central Railroad. It would be one of the actions defining the first "modern" war—the transport of large numbers of troops and casualties by powerful trains.

The city of Richmond was suddenly inundated with hundreds of wounded men; the capacity of existing hospitals was overrun, and citizens began to open their homes, factories, and churches to care for the wounded. Suddenly the war was literally in everyone's parlor.

Sally's natural compassion and empathy were dramatically affected by this exposure to the evidence of the devastating effects of war. She decided to dedicate her life and her inheritance to the care of the wounded and sick.

Circuit Court Judge John Robertson of Richmond had moved his family to the countryside in hopes of maintaining their safety in the face of impending war. Having known Sally for some years, as both were members of the Saint James Episcopal Church, he arranged to donate the use of his Richmond home and entrusted the young woman to utilize his house at Third and Main Streets as a hospital for as long as needed. Sally contributed her own funds to help transpose the house to a hospital. More of the ladies of Saint James's Church joined the effort and organized, opened, and operated the home as "The Robertson Hospital." With a capacity of twenty-two patients, it was among the largest wartime hospitals in the South at the time.

The medical practices of the private Robertson Hospital reflected Sally Tompkins's compassionate and meticulous dedication to cleanliness and care, and its reputation began to spread. It was said that wounded soldiers in Richmond would beg for admittance to the Robertson hospital and commanders were known to send their most critical cases there.

In order to avoid accusations of malingering and dodging of military service, Confederate president Jefferson Davis issued regulations requiring all hospitals to be under military command and the private hospitals were, for the most part, forced to close. In a stunning move that broke military and social tradition, he allowed Tompkins to continue her work and keep her excellent facility open by commissioning her as a captain in the Confederate States Army. She was then legally able to sustain the hospital's operation and to obtain her medical supplies from military stores. The newly commissioned Captain Tomkins refused payment for her military service, writing on her commission, "I accepted the above commission as Captain in the CSA when it was offered. But, I would not allow my name to be placed upon the pay roll of the army." She seemed always to be conscious of the privilege of her upbringing and throughout her life gave her entire inheritance and additional monies to charities.

Virtually all of the hospitals in the South struggled to obtain supplies as a result of the North's huge naval blockade and were frequently short of everything including blankets, clothing, food, and medicines. The Robertson Hospital was no exception, and Tompkins frequently spent her own money to purchase what was needed and at times hired a blockade runner to obtain supplies.

Sally's patients, who called her "Captain Sally," displayed their gratitude and affection for her with many declarations of love and marriage proposals, all of which she graciously declined. She was said to have commented, "Poor fellows, they are not yet well of their fevers."

Sally Tompkins operated the Robertson Hospital throughout the war, treating 1,334 wounded men with only seventy-three deaths in its forty-five months of existence, a survival rate of 94.5 percent, thought to be the highest of any Confederate military hospital during the war.

After the war, Sally Tompkins continued to use the remainder of her assets for charity work and was considered a local hero in Richmond, hosting a reunion for her patients in 1896. When her fortune was gone, she moved into the Confederate Women's Home in Richmond in 1905 as an honored guest and there spent the remainder of her life. She had deliberately overcome society's limiting traditional attitudes about women and managed to provide invaluable lifesaving care to Confederate troops. Upon her death at age eighty-nine, Captain Sally Tompkins was buried with military honors at Kingston Episcopal Parish Church cemetery in Mathews County, Virginia.

As immigrants from many countries appeared in the great 19th-century melting pot of America, their diversity was reflected in the medical theater of the war. The newly arrived and the first-generation citizens were an integral part of the tapestry of medics and volunteers who worked to staunch the staggering death rate.

Kate Cumming's large family had emigrated from Scotland when she was a small child. They arrived first in Montreal, Canada, and eventually settled in Mobile, Alabama. While Kate's Scottish family ties were strong, she came to love the South, identifying the Confederacy as her home, and she embraced the cause of secession.

In the first year of the Civil War, Kate joined the relief effort, at first working to gather supplies for the hospitals and later finding great inspiration in a talk given by the Reverend Benjamin M. Miller at a local church. Miller was calling for Southern women to accept nursing duties for the sick and wounded at the war front. She was fascinated by news of the work of Florence Nightingale in Crimea, finding the British nurse to be an admirable role model, although the Cumming family was of the opinion that ladies of refined upbringing should not perform the intimate work of nursing male soldiers. Kate declined the first call to head north to the war front, instead assisting other volunteers with their preparations, but eventually defied the preferences of her family and her own lack of medical training by agreeing to join a group of forty local women volunteers heading north by train to the Mississippi-Tennessee border in order to provide aid for the returning soldiers from the Battle of Shiloh. The women were all quite aware that they were entering a new and entirely unfamiliar social and professional arena where there was always the possibility that they would not be welcomed or would be found unfit to serve.

The bloodiest battle of the Civil War up until that time occurred on April 6–7, 1862, at Shiloh, in southwestern Tennessee, where more than 16,000 men were wounded. The Southern ladies presented themselves at a military hospital, and frustratingly but not surprisingly, were turned away. They had not been commissioned by the Confederate government, and the hospital was under no obligation to allow them access to the patients. Cumming wrote in the journal she kept throughout the war, "I only wish that the doctors would let us try and see what we can do!"

The women were then permitted to travel to the Confederate hospitals at Corinth, Mississippi. They were uncertain and unprepared for what they would find, having had by then some glimpses of the wounded returning from Shiloh. The massive battle had left more than 23,000 men killed, wounded, or captured. The fragile and uncoordinated new Confederate medical system seemed nonexistent by the end of the battle and three days later, the wounded were still arriving at the Corinth hospitals, untreated, maimed, sick, and hungry.

The Confederate army camp and hospitals presented a scene of horror unlike anything Kate Cumming had ever seen or imagined. Floors awash in slop consisting of mud, blood, excrement, and trash were populated by a crush of the mutilated bodies of Union and Confederate soldiers, of all ages, some so young that they seemed mere children, all crammed so closely together that she found it almost impossible to walk without stepping on them.

The nurses, armed only with bread, biscuits, coffee, and tea, without plates or utensils, and sometimes lightheaded from kneeling in the stinking filth, handed the slim provisions directly to the patients, making sure that all of the men received some rations and assisting those who were unable to feed themselves.

The hideous conditions had not improved two days later, and only Kate Cumming and one other woman remained onsite to handle the nursing duties. A total lack of organization rendered mostly inaccessible the supplies that were actually available, and the men who were assigned to nursing tasks "knew nothing of caring for the sick," she wrote in her journal, emphasizing that "nursing is a thing that has to be learned."

Later that day, some beds arrived and Cumming was relieved that the most critically wounded would have some comfort, but also that elevating the patients would allow her the clearance to clean the filth of the past three days from the floors.

Many of the Civil War women nurses were only able to serve temporarily or sporadically during the war, but Kate Cumming remained an active nurse throughout the war, gaining experience and confidence. She stayed at Corinth through June, went home to Mobile during the summer, and returned to the hospitals in the autumn, traveling to Chattanooga, Tennessee, to voluntarily serve at Newsome Hospital and remaining there for the next year.

While Kate was working in Chattanooga in September 1862, the Confederate government decreed that hospitals could pay nurses, rather than simply relying on volunteers. This changed her status from volunteer to professional, and the Scottish immigrant was then officially enlisted in the Confederate Army Medical Department. She received the rank of hospital supervisor or matron, staying at work in Chattanooga for almost a year, then traveling with the Army of Tennessee in surgeon Samuel Stout's medical corps, winning his endorsement as "refined, intellectual, self-denying" in demeanor. Moving on to Georgia, she served in many mobile field hospitals that were established there in response to the devastation wrought by the Union troops led by General William Tecumseh Sherman.

Kate Cumming continued her habit of daily journaling and wrote of the scenes she witnessed, her observations, and her emotional responses to the horrors and the dedication she noted. Her journal was published after the war in 1866, titled *A Journal of Hospital Life in the Confederate Army of Tennessee*, and was considered one of the most intensely vivid and accurate accounts of the wartime Southern hospitals. It was one of the only written accounts of the conflict beginning with the Battle of Shiloh and following throughout the war from a woman's experience, giving a rare and colorful perspective from a Southern female nurse. The book was republished in 1890 as a shorter version called *Gleanings from Southland* and is still considered an extremely valuable addition to American and medical history.

Returning to Mobile after the war, she was active in associations including the United Daughters of the Confederacy, supporting herself by teaching school and music. With her father, Kate moved to Birmingham, Alabama, in 1874, where she lived until her death in 1909, and was buried in Magnolia Cemetery in her chosen city of Mobile. In addition to her compassionate kindness, her bequest to her adopted country includes one of the most comprehensive existing firsthand descriptions of the operations of Confederate hospitals during the Civil War.

Prior to the Civil War in America, nursing was not considered to be a job for women. It is, however, estimated from records that between 3,000 and 4,000 women volunteers may have served as nurses in the Union and Confederacy, so many that in the North, Dorothea Dix was hired to manage them as Superintendent of Women Nurses. The numerous African American women who also labored were not included in those numbers and it would be years before they were recognized for their service.

Ann Bradford was born into slavery in Rutherford County, Tennessee, in 1830. Little is known about her early life, although she was apparently not able to read or write until she learned those skills after the Civil War. In 1863 she risked her life to escape the plantation and slavery, making her way to the Cumberland River and hiding there. At some point she was taken aboard the Union ship U.S.S. *Red Rover* (originally a captured Confederate vessel turned hospital ship) and was first classified as "contraband," a term for escaped slaves. The timing of Ann's escape was fortuitous for her, as President Lincoln had recently signed the Emancipation Proclamation, and Ann Bradford's status was upgraded to "free woman." She could legally leave the ship if she wanted to, but instead she chose to stay on board, embracing a new life by formally becoming a volunteer with the Sisters of the Holy Cross of Notre Dame. The governor of Illinois had asked the Sisters to work as nurses on the ship. Ann became the first African American woman to serve on a Union military vessel and was one of the first women ever to openly serve as a nurse in the U.S. Navy. She was one of five African American women—including Alice Kennedy, Sarah Kinno, Ellen Campbell, and Betsy Young—who served on that hospital ship and were assigned the rank of "first-class boy," a term usually applied to very young men who worked as general-duty sailors. The women's new situation was even more novel in that the "first-class boys," male and female, were paid regular wages for their service.

In a very short period of time, Ann Bradford had transitioned from slavery to living as a free, paid worker. She and the other four female former slaves on board performed a wide range of responsible duties, nursing the sick and wounded and also cooking, cleaning, and laundering. They had no formal medical training, so they relied on the folk remedies from the plantations on which they had grown up, and they added their own insights and common sense based on their surprising new experiences. The Holy Cross nuns welcomed the female contrabands, whose familiarity with midwifery gave the Sisters faith in their abilities to face the torrent of blood and death expected aboard the hospital ship as it traveled the Ohio and Mississippi Rivers and their tributaries.

Conditions on the U.S.S. *Red Rover* were made even more horrific owing to the intense heat, humidity, flies, and mosquitoes of the Southern summers. Foul-smelling blood and pus-soaked bandages oozed and stank despite the nurses' unending cleaning and washing. The patients were terribly wounded, ferociously maimed, and many were extremely sick, including with typhoid, malaria, and cholera. The five former slaves spent eighteen months on the ship, caring for almost three thousand patients. When Ann Bradford had to resign from active duty in October 1864, the cause was exhaustion.

After her retirement from the service, Ann married a young African American soldier, Gilbert Stokes, whom she had met on the ship. Unfortunately, Gilbert died just two years later, and, later, Ann remarried to George Bowman and they moved to Belknap, Illinois. In her fifties, despite her inability to read or write, she managed to apply to the Navy in order to receive a pension as a soldier's widow on behalf of her first husband, Gilbert Stokes. The Navy denied her request, but Ann was not deterred. Her health was becoming precarious, but she persevered, learned to read and write, and reapplied to the Navy with a different request. This time, she wanted a pension based on her own military service, rather than her late husband's. When she reapplied she was specific about her health and stated that she had "piles and heart disease."

It was a unique situation and she was persistent. The Navy reviewed her case and verified that she had, indeed, served as a "boy" for eighteen months aboard the *Red Rover*, which entitled her to benefits based on her own military service and she had a pensionable disability as well. In 1890, the United States Navy awarded Ann Bradford Stokes a pension of $12 per month (about $366 in current U.S. dollars), a standard amount for nurses at the time, making her the first American woman not only to apply for but to be granted a pension for her military service.

When Ann passed away in Illinois in 1903, she left a record of extraordinary and courageous "firsts" as one of the earliest and original African American women to have enlisted in the U.S. Navy, and the only one known to have applied for and received a pension. She was one of the first female nurses to serve on a Navy vessel. She had dared to escape slavery and accepted and embraced an entirely new life and profession. Her tenacity, hard work, and willingness to pursue literacy in her later years make a strong and lasting statement from an exceptional person.

One Northern woman who had a tremendous impact on Western nursing and health care was not actually a nurse herself. Superintendent of Union Army nurses during the Civil War, Dorothea Dix was driven to help people who could not help themselves—she worked for many years as an advocate and reformer for prisoners and the mentally ill. Dix fought to improve conditions in prisons and mental asylums in North America and Europe as a longtime champion for the weaker or forgotten members of society.

Dorothea Dix was born into a deeply dysfunctional family in Hampden, Maine, in 1802; her mother suffered from mental illness and her father, a traveling minister who was away from home for weeks at a time, was apparently alcoholic and abusive. At the age of twelve she left the unhappy circumstances and went to live with her grandmother in Boston. When asked about her childhood, it is reported that her common answer was, "I never knew a childhood."

With her grandmother's encouragement, Dorothea attended school in Boston, indulging her passion for education and for tutoring other children. Her health had always been poor, and she struggled with it periodically, although as a teenager and young woman she was still able to work at establishing some schools in Boston and Worcester. When her health became a roadblock to those efforts, she began to write textbooks, including her *Conversations on Common Things, Or Guide to Knowledge*, published when she was twenty-two.

During one of her bouts of ill health, Dorothea's doctor recommended that she plan a trip to Europe and spend some time there. It was on that journey that she met people working with activist and reform groups whose focus was on changing the treatment of the mentally ill. The cause struck a deep chord within her and, upon her return to the United States, she embarked on a mission to tour mental hospitals across the country. She reported on her shocking findings of inhumane conditions to several politicians, remaining a tireless advocate and a persistent reformer, earning some support for the causes. In a time when few women dared to speak their minds passionately in public, she missed no opportunities to seek participation to establish improved hospitals and asylums, and she worked to pass federal legislation to regulate conditions, both in her own country and overseas. Dorothea Dix would transform a field of health care and set in motion a complete reform of medical management for the mentally ill.

Dorothea Dix was among the American women who had traveled to Britain, Turkey, and Crimea to learn from the legendary Florence Nightingale. After the attack on Fort Sumter in 1861, Dix went to New York to meet with Dr. Elizabeth Blackwell.

The American Civil War brought a new need and mission to the fifty-nine-year-old Dix. She would again make a huge impact, this time as a pioneer of modern nursing and patient advocacy. In 1861 a Massachusetts regiment was attacked by a secessionist mob in Baltimore, Maryland. Horrified by the large-scale violence, Dix took a train south to the city in order to assist with caring for the wounded and, upon ascertaining that improvised hospitals were making effective care available, she continued to Washington, D.C., and gained a meeting with the U.S. secretary of war, Simon Cameron. She offered her services as a nurse to the Union Army, but Cameron, impressed with her assertiveness, organizational skills, and tenacious nature, appointed her the superintendent of Union Army nurses instead, a position she held until 1865. It was a title for which Dr. Elizabeth Blackwell had also been considered, although Dr. Blackwell continued to play an important role in the additional selection and training of nurses for service.

Dorothea Dix took on this new responsibility and function with her usual passion and dedication, although her somewhat abrasive personality caused periodic friction. In an environment and a nursing job that had always been male territory, and when many male doctors openly opposed or refused the presence of female nurses, her intentions to hire and instruct women were met with derision and opposition, but she managed to convince military officials that women could be trained to do the job well. Dix powered through a field of resistance and during the course of the war would appoint and arrange for the training of more than three thousand nurses, about 15 percent of all Union Army nurses.

Dorothea Dix was the first woman ever to serve at such a high level in a federally appointed position. She dove into the work, helping to set up field hospitals and aid stations; always quick to learn, she mastered the acquisition and distribution of medical supplies. She was criticized for her aggressive style, for ignoring orders from officials, was frequently considered inflexible in her demands, and was nicknamed "Dragon Dix." She was thought to have impossibly high standards for her nurses, but she continued to advocate for them to receive more formal training and increased work opportunities and responsibilities. She took good care of her nurses, the women who were extremely critical to advancing the role of nursing in the war and in medicine overall. The nurses were working under extremely difficult wartime circumstances, and when needs were high and government stocks perilously low, Dix sometimes labored to acquire supplies from private agencies. She was extremely strict with the women, requiring them to be plain in appearance, at least thirty years old, and to wear dull-colored dresses; they were forbidden to wear hoop skirts, jewelry, or cosmetics. Despite her rigid requirements and the demanding nature of the job, her nurses were respected for being efficient, effective, and reliable.

It would be remembered long after the war that Dorothea Dix and her nurses tended to both Union and Confederate wounded with equal compassion, sometimes providing the only available care in the field to Southern soldiers. In the summer of 1863, after the Confederate retreat from Gettysburg, Pennsylvania, five thousand wounded Southern soldiers were left behind. Many of Dix's nurses provided care for the destitute men. Union nurse Cornelia Hancock served in that terrible time, later writing, "There are no words in the English language to express the suffering I witnessed today."

Despite some serious personality clashes with Army officials, Dix remained in her post until the end of the war, at which point she returned to her advocacy work for prisoners and the mentally ill. Her wartime service was formally recognized by the federal government and she was awarded two national flags for "the Care, Succor, and Relief of the Sick and Wounded Soldiers of the United States on the Battle-Field, in Camps and Hospitals during the recent war." She was elected "President for Life" of the Army Nurses Association, had many parks and hospital wards named for her, and was inducted into the National Women's Hall of Fame.

After the war ended, she traveled throughout the South evaluating the wartime damage to their prisons and asylums and offering consultation on their redesign. She continued in her pursuit for reform for the rest of her life, establishing thirty-two hospitals and influencing the creation of two more in Japan. The life's work of Dorothea Dix had a huge impact on the

19th-century medical field: she transformed the American mental health care system and she helped introduce and revolutionize the field of skilled nursing.

The war took many women to places where they had never expected to go. Phoebe Pember found herself in alien territory when she agreed to accept work as a nurse and hospital administrator—both areas where American business and tradition had never before invited women.

Phoebe Yates Levy was born in 1823 to a prominent Jewish American family from Charleston, South Carolina. Her father, Jacob Clavius Levy, was a successful merchant and the son of Polish immigrants; her mother, Fanny Yates from Liverpool, England, was an acclaimed actress with a successful career in the Charleston theater. The wealth and accomplishments of the popular Levy family seem to have allowed them acceptance among the social elite of the city, despite any anti-Semitism that existed. Phoebe, her five sisters, and one brother may have received some formal education or been privately tutored, as her personal letters, memoirs, and administrative talents reveal a polished intellect and a sharp, sophisticated, and interested thought process.

At the age of thirty-three, Phoebe Levy embarked on a series of new journeys: she married outside of her faith to Thomas Pember, a Christian from Boston, although throughout her life she continued to speak proudly of her Jewish heritage. She moved north with her husband, but shortly after their wedding Thomas developed tuberculosis, and although she nursed him devotedly for the next five years, he succumbed to the disease in 1861. Childless, Phoebe moved back with her parents, who were then living in Marietta, Georgia, but she felt unproductive and confined and her frequent quarrels with her father created an unhappy environment.

Her next chapter came in the form of a very unusual but welcome offer from a good friend—Mary Pope Randolph was the wife of the Confederate secretary of war George W. Randolph, and she had a challenge for Phoebe, who she suggested serve as chief matron for Chimborazo Hospital in Richmond, Virginia. Phoebe felt loyalty to the Confederate soldiers, as a widow she desired to earn an independent living, and she believed that five years of nursing her invalid husband had given her a solid experience in caring for patients. It was an unheard-of position at the time for a woman, and completely foreign territory for the aristocratic Mrs. Pember, but despite her concerns, she accepted the offer and traveled to Richmond, Virginia, in December 1862 to accept her appointment to Hospital No. 2, Chimborazo, then the largest military hospital in the world.

The name Chimborazo comes from that of an Ecuadorian volcano, and the area was thought to have been named by a widely traveled local resident who felt that the Virginia parcel of land resembled the South American site of the famous volcano. The hospital, spread over a large plateau, was one of the largest military hospitals in U.S. history. During the course of the war, more than 76,000 soldiers were treated in its five divisions of 150 wards. No woman had ever been appointed to the hospital staff before, and it was remarkably rare for a female to hold a leadership position in any institution, let alone a military one.

From the time she first stepped foot into Chimborazo, Phoebe Pember encountered stiff internal opposition and resistance to her female presence and continuous efforts by staff to undermine her authority. She was treated with an initial lack of respect by the surgeons and the hospital stewards, and she faced a constant challenge to stop the staff from stealing medical supplies, especially the whiskey that was kept for medicinal purposes. She eventually threatened one thief with a gun she usually kept hidden:

> "You had better leave," I said, "for if one bullet is lost, there are
> five more ready, and the room is too small for even a woman to
> miss six times."

Pember's duties as chief matron of the second division of the hospital included the production and administration of prescribed medications and of special dietary needs. She supervised the hospital workers, house-keeping, and nursing operations, oversaw sanitation procedures and food preparation, and cared for, read to, and wrote letters for an estimated 15,000 men who came under her direct aegis between 1862 and 1865. The initial opposition to her presence eventually turned into the patients' and staff's affection for her charm, dedication to her patients, and her friendly but firm authority. She gained respect for her compassion, her superb management skills, and her personal integrity, later described by journalist, author, and playwright Thomas Cooper De Leon of Richmond as a "brisk and brilliant matron" with a "will of steel under a suave refinement."

Phoebe Pember had a deep affection for the soldiers, finding the enlisted men to be more well-mannered and sincere than the officers or surgeons. She encountered death on a daily basis at Chimborazo, and never stopped making all possible efforts to provide comfort for the dying. One young soldier, gravely wounded in a recent battle and very weak, asked only for "Perry." She wrote:

> On inquiry I found that Perry was the friend and companion who marched by his side in the field and slept next to him in camp, but of whose whereabouts I was ignorant. Armed with a requisition from our surgeon, I sought him among the sick and wounded at all the other hospitals. I found him at Camp Jackson, put him in my ambulance, and on arrival at my own hospital found my patient had dropped asleep. A bed was brought and placed at his side, and Perry, only slightly wounded, laid upon it.

When the young soldier awoke, he was overjoyed and moved to see his good friend and was able to spend the last minutes of his life with the fellow soldier and companion who was most important to him, thanks to the efforts of the indefatigable Mrs. Pember.

After the war, Phoebe traveled extensively in America and Europe and wrote a very well-received memoir, *A Southern Woman's Story: Life in Confederate Richmond*, considered one of the best accounts of Civil War hospital life. The United States Postal Service honored her in 1995 with a stamp featuring her portrait. Phoebe Yates Levy Pember's eighty-nine years were a testament to her strength, dedication, and resilience in proving that a woman was well able to brilliantly and efficiently organize, administer, and manage a huge hospital facility, even in times of war.

Women began to appear more frequently in key administrative and leadership roles. One particularly strong, determined, and colorful woman, Mary Ann Ball Bickerdyke, born in 1817 in Knox County near Mount Vernon, Ohio, was admitted to Oberlin College, one of the only American institutions of higher learning then open to women, to pursue the study of herbal medicine. Mary Ann did not graduate, but instead became a nurse, working as an assistant to physicians in Cincinnati, Ohio, during the cholera epidemic in 1837, later marrying Robert Bickerdyke in 1847 and moving to Galesburg, Illinois. Robert died in 1859 and Mary Ann supported herself and her two sons by working as a nurse and a practicing "botanic Physician."

In the early years of the Civil War, the citizens of Galesburg were moved by a published letter from a young volunteer physician working in the military hospitals in Cairo, Illinois, describing the chaotic and filthy conditions there. The people of Galesburg collected $500 (more than $16,000 in today's dollars) worth of supplies and requested that the dynamic Mrs. Bickerdyke deliver the supplies to Cairo. Bickerdyke, then in her forties, delivered the much-needed supplies and then stayed in Cairo working as an unofficial nurse and an agent of the United States Sanitary Commission.

Spurred by the desperate needs of the sick and wounded, she left her children in the care of friends and followed the path of General Ulysses S. Grant along the Mississippi River. Becoming known variously as "Mother Bickerdyke" or the "Cyclone in Calico," she procured equipment and

130

supplies through the Northwest Branch of the U.S. Sanitary Commission, organized a support staff of "contrabands," and established diet kitchens and laundries for soldiers.

Her remarkable energy, bravery, and dedication to the situation at hand were demonstrated as she organized hospitals, gaining the appreciation of General Ulysses S. Grant. Her enthusiasm and zeal became almost legendary, and Grant sanctioned her efforts, allowing her to move down the Mississippi River with the Army. She became chief of nursing under Grant, set up hospitals wherever there was a need, and earned the admiration of General William T. Sherman, as well, in the process—it was reported that she was the only woman he allowed in his camps.

Bickerdyke also earned some notoriety for denouncing officers who failed to provide adequately for their troops. She became well known for her courage in continuing to search for wounded soldiers even after night fell on the battlefields. She carried a lantern and would enter the high-risk territory between the competing armies to retrieve wounded soldiers for treatment. Her obvious and deep concern for the welfare of the soldiers led them to christen her "Mother to the Boys in Blue."

"Mother" Bickerdyke was constantly in motion, and she engaged in her own fundraising activities for the benefit of the troops. She gave speeches and solicited contributions from the public while continuing her administrative duties as matron of the nine-hundred-patient Gayoso Hospital in Memphis, Tennessee, and overseeing laundry for eleven additional Memphis hospitals. Throughout the war, she was responsible for providing health care and oversight for tens of thousands of men.

General Sherman's staff complained about her outspokenness, insubordination, and failure to regard the Army's red tape and military strictures. Bickerdyke had no patience for complications or inactivity, and no fear of authority. She clashed regularly with some of the doctors at her hospital including one who angrily expressed his wish that she would leave.

I shall stay, doctor, and you'll have to make up your mind to get along with me the best way you can. It's no use for you to try to tie me up with your red tape. There's too much to be done down here to stop for that.

By the end of the war, Mary Ann Bickerdyke had spearheaded the establishment of more than three hundred field hospitals and given aid to the wounded on nineteen battlefields, including Shiloh, Vicksburg, Chattanooga, and the Atlanta Campaign. After the cessation of hostilities, there was a grand review in Washington, D.C., with a parade down Pennsylvania Avenue. General Sherman invited Mary Ann to sit in the reviewing stand as the troops passed by, but she opted instead to accept his offer that she ride at the head of the Fifteenth Corps of the Army of the Tennessee on the triumphant parade route, and afterward she chose to pass out water to the soldiers. It has been reported that she was so loved by the troops that they cheered her as if she were a general.

Bickerdyke's devotion to her soldiers did not end with the Civil War. She worked with the Salvation Army in San Francisco and studied to become an attorney. In her new capacity as a lawyer, she advocated for Union veterans by providing them with legal assistance in applying for government pensions and was instrumental in arranging more than three hundred pensions for women nurses who had served, although she did not receive a pension herself until the 1880s. Moving to Kansas, she assisted veterans in beginning their new lives with help for obtaining tools, supplies, and land. Working with the Chicago, Burlington & Quincy Railroad, she arranged for free rail transportation for veterans planning to settle in Kansas. The rest of her life was devoted to fighting for the rights of veterans and smoothing their journeys in the postwar country.

I have a commission from the Lord God Almighty to do all I can for every miserable creature who comes in my way; he is always sure of two friends, God and me.

Cornelia Hancock of New Jersey became one of the most respected and beloved nurses of the Army of the Potomac during the Civil War. In the summer of 1863, at age twenty-three, Cornelia, born to Quakers of colonial ancestry and educated in Salem County academies, was completely inexperienced in any form of nursing care. At the beginning of July, she heard news of the devastating battle that had just occurred at Gettysburg, Pennsylvania, and resolved to volunteer to help with the huge number of wounded soldiers. Her brother-in-law, Henry T. Child, was a respected Philadelphia physician who was planning to go to the battlefield as a volunteer surgeon and agreed that she could accompany him as a nurse.

Cornelia and a female chaperone joined a group of women seeking to become volunteer nurses and traveled to Philadelphia to meet with the legendary superintendent of nurses, Dorothea Dix. The very pretty Miss Hancock was immediately rejected for nursing service by Dix, whose credo for her nurses included the phrase "mature in years (at least 30), plain almost to homeliness in dress, and by no means liberally endowed with personal attractions."

Cornelia refused to be blocked from service by Dix's rejection, and she quietly boarded the train to Gettysburg anyway, trusting that she would find a way to provide help in what she was aware were terrible circumstances. Upon reaching the scene of the battle on July 6, she knew she had done the right thing and wrote in her journal, "I got into Gettysburg the night of July sixth—where the need was so great that there was no further cavil about age."

Stepping off the train in Gettysburg she was suddenly in the most shocking, horrifying, and alien landscape she had ever seen. Cornelia Hancock went to work immediately upon her arrival in Gettysburg, becoming the first woman to enter the military hospital of the Second Army Corps located at the Jacob Schwartz farm. She was given lodging at the residence of Dr. Charles Horner and stayed at his home on Chambersburg Street until she moved to Camp Letterman later that summer.

The need was immense at the site of the great battle, not only for nurses and doctors, but also for medical supplies. Although she had no formal training, the young woman was quickly up to speed on necessary treatment and care duties, and within three weeks was tending to the lion's share of patients. The lively Miss Hancock became one of the most admired and popular nurses of her day, known for her capable ministrations and her dedication to the soldiers. Cornelia's positive attitude, charm, and encouraging nature made her a very welcome presence among the wounded, and the soldiers named a dance tune for her—"The Hancock Gallop."

In the month after the Gettysburg battle, Cornelia wrote to her mother from Camp Letterman:

I do not read the papers very often now, think I am doing all I can and leave the issue to God. I think war is a hellish way of settling a dispute. Oh, mercy, the suffering! All the worst are dying rapidly. I saw one of my best men die yesterday. He wore away to skin and bone, was anxious to recover but prayed he might find it for the best for him to be taken from his suffering. He was the one who said if there was a heaven I would go to it. I hope he will get there before I do. He was not in my ward now, but I just went over in time to be with him when he died. I hope to keep well enough to stay with the men I am now with until they are all started on their way to heaven or home.

It is very interesting getting them started on crutches. They are so patient, they never bother for anything; they are jolly even, for the most part.

It is great fun to prop yourself up with pillows on a nice little iron bedstead and write letters home. Sergeant Hart has given me one of the best gold pens and it writes so nicely.

From thy daughter, Cornelia Hancock, U.S.A.

The experience of Gettysburg confirmed the direction of the rest of her life for the young Quaker woman She knew that her mission was the dedication of herself to the service of others. When Cornelia left Gettysburg in October, she traveled to Washington, D.C., where thousands of escaped slaves were arriving hungry, injured, and destitute. She volunteered her services on the outskirts of the city at the Contraband Hospital for formerly enslaved people, and worked there through the winter. At Gettysburg she had witnessed the terrible suffering of the physically wounded who had been harmed by military weapons technology, and at the rough Contraband camp and hospital she saw desperation for freedom and the hideous injuries caused by slavery and racism.

> If I were to describe this hospital it would not be believed. North of Washington, in an open muddy mire, are gathered all the people who have been made free by the progress of our Army. Sickness is inevitable. . . . I shall never feel horrified at anything that may happen to me hereafter . . . it seems to me as if all my past life was a myth.

Cornelia reached out to her wealthier Northern friends asking for donations to aid the newly freed people. She was struck by overwhelming compassion for the misery before her and she sought to administer salve with comfort, teaching, healing, and guiding. The experience of the Contraband Hospital stayed with her for the rest of her life.

In 1864, she nursed the wounded from the battles at Wilderness, Fredericksburg, Petersburg, Port Royal, Brandy Station, and White House Landing, becoming almost legendary in the Army of the Potomac. She was one of the first Union nurses to arrive in Richmond, Virginia, directly after its capture by Union forces. Cornelia was never formally associated with any organization, although both the U.S. Sanitary Commission and the U.S. Christian Commission were generous in supporting her requests for supplies. She served in field and evacuating hospitals, the Contraband Camp and Hospital, and, defying the orders of the military, went physically onto some battlefields to give direct aid to soldiers. Her volunteer service to the military lasted from July 6, 1863, to May 23, 1865.

She had loved her work with the emancipated African Americans in Washington, D.C., and was eager to continue, applying for teaching positions. In 1866 she traveled to South Carolina with Laura Towne, who had been one of the first Northern women to work in the South during the Civil War. Laura was part of the federal government's first large-scale initiative to help the former slaves. Cornelia established a school for African Americans in Mount Pleasant, South Carolina. She requested donations and received support from the Freedmen's Bureau and from the Philadelphia Yearly Meeting of the Religious Society of Friends, the central organizing body for Quakers in that area.

After a decade of teaching at the school, she moved to Philadelphia, where she had become aware of the plight of the poor of the city, and helped to found the Children's Aid Society of Pennsylvania, becoming a board member from 1883 to 1895. She served as president of the National Association of Army Nurses of the Civil War and in 1889, she assisted with children who were orphaned after the Johnstown Flood in Pennsylvania, a catastrophe that killed more than 2,200 people.

Cornelia Hancock's memorial is a lifetime of passionate and continuous service to others. This young woman dared to walk into war, was fiercely devoted to the welfare of others, and her heart went out especially to wounded soldiers and black refugees. Ten years after her death in 1927 at age eighty-seven, her Civil War letters, indignant, horrified, humorous, and loving, were published under the title *South After Gettysburg*. To mark its 125th anniversary, the book was rereleased in 2015 by the University of Pennsylvania Press.

The American Civil War turned the tide on the duty of nursing: women finally began to emerge in an area where they had never before been permitted, and the longtime tradition of men being solely tasked with nursing duties was changing. One of the best-known male nurses of the war was the poet, journalist, and essayist Walt Whitman. Considered one of the finest poets ever to write in the English language, Whitman created a brilliant and sensitive body of literary work based on his personal experience, bringing the aura of a Civil War hospital directly to the reader.

When the Civil War began, Whitman was revising a book of his poetry and working as a freelance journalist. As New York City hospitals started to fill with the wounded of the war, he began to visit the injured patients as a volunteer. Whitman's brother, George, had joined the Union Army and sent home disturbingly descriptive letters from the front. Like many civilians, Walt Whitman read the "casualty rosters"—lists of wounded and dead soldiers published in newspapers like the *New-York Tribune*, and noticed the name "First Lieutenant G.W. Whitmore," fearing it was a reference to his brother.

Walt Whitman traveled south to locate his brother George, finally finding him alive with a superficial facial wound. In the process he became profoundly affected by the horribly wounded soldiers, piles of their amputated limbs, and the desolate condition of the hospitals. He knew that he was where he needed to be and that he would not be returning to New York.

Whitman had a friend who helped him get hired to do part-time work in the Army paymaster's office so that he would have time to volunteer as a nurse in the Army hospitals. He wrote an article about his nursing work that was titled "The Great Army of the Sick" and published in the *New York Times* of February 26, 1863.

The overwhelming suffering of the wounded and the fact that there was such a huge and endless stream of them had an overpowering effect on the writer. He sought to console the men by offering emotional support, listening to and writing down their stories, helping to compose letters for them to send home, and giving them small gifts to make them smile. He wrote that his purpose was to give "some trifle for a novelty or change—anything, however trivial, to break the monotony of those hospital hours."

He assisted the physicians and surgeons when they needed him and visited the wounded of both sides, black and white. "The Wound Dresser" from his *Drum Taps* collection of Civil War poems is the verse most specific about his nursing duties; his prose is equally wrenching and eloquent with observations and referenced encounters.

> During my past three years in Hospital, camp or field, I made over 600 visits or tours, and went, as I estimate among from 80,000 to 100,000 of the wounded and sick, a sustainer of spirit and body, in time of need.
>
> I was with many rebel officers and men among our wounded, and tried to cheer them the same as any. Among the black soldiers, wounded or sick, and in the contraband camps I also took my way whenever in their neighborhood, and did what I could for them.
>
> There are many women among the Hospitals, mostly as nurses here in Washington, quite a number of them young ladies acting as volunteers. They are a great help in certain ways, and deserve to be mention'd with praise and respect.

Walt Whitman's writing gave the nation an intensely emotional, heartbroken picture of the victims of the war. He not only grieved the lost, but he created a vivid record of the suffering of the wounded that did not allow them to simply disappear into history.

The 21st-century perception of America's Civil War is shaped and colored by the memories of this gifted writer. Other authors have responded to the profound nature of Whitman's work with the observation that he has been considered the chief mourner on behalf of the nation. If nursing can be said to be based on compassion, the heart and craft of Walter Whitman can be said to embody it.

The evolution and professionalization of nursing in America was spurred and accelerated by the Civil War. Previously, nursing had been the responsibility of family members. The Army had no trained nurses. In military outposts, nursing duties were performed by soldiers' wives or by recuperating troops.

Before the Civil War, most nurses in the country were male. Convalescent soldiers were frequently joined in nursing tasks by volunteers, or by troops called "malingerers," or by men who had proven difficult in the field. Most had no formal training, but some adapted well to the task.

In the United States of 1860, the care of family members who were ill or infirm was typically provided at home, and was considered to be a duty of females. Most women who had garnered any experience in nursing had learned by caring for someone at home. The few women in America who had any serious experience or instruction in nursing were Catholic nuns, usually from a religious order of "nursing sisters," or those nuns who had served in apprenticeships to them. Performing nursing duties outside of the home was frowned upon for wealthy white women, as "working woman" was a derisive term in Victorian America, denoting a person to be pitied or scorned.

When the Civil War began, the armies had no well-organized medical corps or field hospital plans. An officer's wife might accompany her husband to the battlefield, or a mother attend to care for a wounded son or husband, and either might choose to remain and care for the increasing number of wounded. The title of "nurse" was rather all-inclusive in early 1861 and there were no existing schools in America for training nurses.

When the war began, the lack of skilled nursing care became swiftly evident. The number of wounded soldiers multiplied, and epidemic diseases ravaged the troops. Newspaper reports about the lack of medical treatment and supplies in the army camps and hospitals inspired thousands of women to volunteer on the battlefields and hospitals. They began to appear seemingly everywhere, in both cities and remote locations to provide care to wounded or sick soldiers. They were not always welcomed by doctors, and the Union Army in particular was opposed to having women onsite, believing that they were inexperienced, incompetent, and disorganized. It was true that most of the women probably had no prior experience with the kinds of devastating wounds and ailments the men were experiencing, but they were willing to learn and insistent on becoming part of the solution, arguing that the war "was as much a woman's war as it was a man's war."

The women of North and South pressed on in areas that had previously been closed to Victorian ladies, and estimates are that more than 21,000 women served in Union military hospitals and a comparable number in the Confederacy, where 10 percent of the nursing women were African American. More than three thousand women acted as paid nurses and many thousands more worked as unpaid volunteers. The war created a way for women to take an active role in the relief effort from outside of the home and family, assume leadership roles in sanitary commissions, and provide clerical assistance in government and business. It was a new way that women could participate in wartime and feel that their contributions were of value. They demonstrated strength and determination, opening doors to wider professional, social, and political arenas for themselves. Once women overcame the stigma of working in public and felt that they had worthy skills to offer, their self-perception as essential persons in society was forever changed and expanded.

Groups of private citizens and civilian agencies began to offer relief in providing health care to the army. The United States Sanitary Commission, in addition to securing food and medical supplies, began to set standards for nurses who worked under its umbrella and to oversee the work and safety of other women volunteers who were engaged in nursing.

The Union Army's untrained volunteer nurses were gaining the respect of doctors and the trust of patients. In addition to assisting with whatever tasks were requested by the physicians, the nurses comforted patients, read to them, wrote letters, and prayed with them, fed them, and did laundry.

Realizing that the women were providing invaluable services in caring for the soldiers, the Union formalized an arrangement, appointing Dorothea Dix as "Superintendent of Female Nurses of the Army" and more than 3,000 women worked in nursing under her guidance. The emergence and importance of women as nurses during a major health care crisis was undeniable, and was endorsed by Dr. Samuel D. Gross, one of the most revered physicians and professors in the country:

> In order to complete hospital equipments, well-trained nurses should be provided, for good nursing is indispensable.
>
> The question as to whether this duty should be performed by men or women is of no material consequence, provided it be well done. The eligibility of women for this task was thoroughly tested in the Crimea, through the agency of that noble-hearted female, Florence Nightingale; and hundreds of the daughters of our land have already tendered their services to the government for this object. No large and well-regulated hospital can get on without some male nurses.

Dorothea Dix's standards and rules proved too confining and exclusionary for some women, but Northern women found other avenues to gain experience and volunteer as nurses. Some regional aid societies were willing to certify as nurses those who had already served as volunteers, and with the shortage of medical personnel and the vast quantities of sick and wounded, the Union Army permitted surgeons to choose their own nurses. Dr. Gross elaborated on the positive characteristics of a woman nurse:

> The qualities which constitute a good female nurse . . . it will suffice to say that she should be keenly alive to her duties, and perform them, however menial or distasteful, with promptness and alacrity. She must be tidy in her appearance, with a cheerful

countenance, light in her step, noiseless, tender and thoughtful in her manners, perfect mistress of her feelings, healthy, able to bear fatigue, and at least twenty-two years of age. Neither the crinoline nor the silk dress must enter into her wardrobe, the former is too cumbrous, while the latter by its rustling is sure to fret the patient and disturb his sleep.

The Confederate Congress passed a bill in 1862 allowing for the enlistment of women as army nurses. Southern women converged on the battlefields and hospitals. They served as volunteer nurses, provided bandages, food, and clothing, and frequently took the wounded into their own homes to convalesce. As in the North, many society women of the Confederacy traveled great distances to serve their troops. Some of them published memoirs and autobiographies and wrote letters to newspapers and congressmen, bringing public attention to the plight of the sick and wounded. Colonel Buehring H. Jones of the Sixtieth Virginia Infantry expressed his gratitude for the Southern women's unwavering support of their Army.

We had hundreds and thousands of women all over the South, from the East Atlantic to the banks of the Rio Grande, who for four long years, constantly illustrated all the virtues.

They cheerfully yielded their husbands and fathers, their sons and brothers.

They denied themselves comforts and convenience, they toiled and prayed.

Amid the roar of battle, in the crowded and gloomy precincts of the hospital—they were the Angel Ministers of Hope, and Faith, and Charity, and Goodness!

The new female nurses quickly gained skills, becoming more professional and taking on greater responsibilities. They dealt with the management of supplies and the operation of hospital kitchens and laundries. Duties, however, were clearly designated by race and perceived social class. In the South, African American women both free and enslaved were assigned the more physical and less desirable tasks: cooking, cleaning, bedpan duties, and clearing the detritus of the operating areas. The Union had many segregated hospitals to which they assigned black soldiers and contrabands, staffed by African American nurses. In the white Northern hospitals, women who were new immigrants or perceived as lower-class were assigned the more menial and risky jobs.

The hospitals were dangerous places to work and the nurses were exposed to a variety of illnesses and to wounded men with terrible infections. Dr. Louis Pasteur's germ theory of disease had not been fully disseminated among American doctors, so there was no requirement or request for the washing of hands or the wearing of gloves, and sanitizing of surgical instruments was unheard of. Civil War nurses contracted diseases like typhoid, pneumonia, and smallpox in the hospitals and many died from them during the war years.

A huge proportion of the men who served as Civil War physicians and surgeons had little or no clinical experience and had never been in a hospital setting. They were acquiring skills as they went along while learning and adjusting to the military structure, rules, and regulations. Suddenly working in close quarters with women whom they suspected of being undisciplined and untrained created tense situations in the hospitals. Despite their hostile reception and a lack of trust in their abilities and intelligence, the female nurses transformed hospitals with compassionate care and orderly routines. Their competence improved and they learned how to administer treatments and comfort and to encourage patients while supporting the doctors' work. Patient care was exponentially improved by their presence and attentions, and medicine would eventually welcome and value their humanizing of hospital treatment. Trained nurses would become the new and essential health care professionals.

The year before the American Civil War began, 1860, was exceptionally significant for the advent of skilled nursing care, although its benefits would not reach the United States for almost a decade. Florence Nightingale's formal training school for nurses was opened in London.

The British nurse, social reformer, and statistician was the founder of modern nursing and also created the first school for nurses in the English-speaking world. Nightingale's experience in caring for wounded soldiers in the filthy and disorganized hospitals of the Crimean War of the 1850s made it clear to her that major changes in health care were necessary. Her observations led to recommendations for improvements to sanitary conditions and to establishing standards for clean and safe hospitals. She strongly believed that nurses were a necessary and vital part of hospital care, and began to gather and organize her thoughts on the training that would be required to prepare skilled nurses for hospital service.

In 1859, Florence published her book *Notes on Nursing*, which was the first known instruction manual for nurses, and it served as the cornerstone and textbook of the curriculum she was planning for a school. The Nightingale Training School at the newly built St. Thomas' Hospital in London, England, opened in July 1860, with the first formally trained nurses beginning work in May 1865 at the Liverpool Workhouse Infirmary. The school was quickly deemed a success and led to a new public perception of nursing as a professional occupation and one that was worthy of respect. The handbook, *Notes on Nursing*, was a popular publication and actually sold well to the general public. It is still considered by many to be a classic introduction to nursing.

In the United States of the 1860s, the Civil War's thousands of casualties and hundreds of hospitals were making it clear that trained, skilled health care workers were a highly desirable asset and an all-important one. Gender prejudice against women hospital workers was rampant at the beginning of the war, but as violence and diseases proliferated, Army physicians and surgeons became more appreciative of the assistance of female nurses, and many began to see them as indispensable.

During the Civil War and for several years afterward, the clear need for skilled professional nurses became more obvious and led to some hospitals instituting informal training. Students agreed to provide their nursing services to the hospital for free for two or three years and the hospital would offer lectures and clinical instructions to them. It was not a perfect solution and the attaching of nurse training to hospitals rather than schools was a system that allowed and encouraged segregation in the health care system. For years, African American student nurses were refused admission to such schools except those established by African American hospitals.

The first formal schools of nursing in the United States opened in the year 1873. Bellevue Training School in New York City, Boston Training School in Massachusetts, and the Connecticut Training School in Hartford were all based on Florence Nightingale's model for the education of skilled nurses.

Today in the United States, more than eight hundred schools offer degrees in nursing care to men and women of all races.

CHAPTER FIVE

BATTLING SHORTAGES, INEXPERIENCE, AND BLOCKADES: THE SOLUTIONS, REPLACEMENTS, AND INNOVATIONS

The Civil War, a conflict on a gigantic scale never before seen on the continent, tested every reserve of the American population. Organization, management, and maintenance of the massive armies called for a redesign of the mechanisms required to move tens of thousands of men. The social castes and mores of the population were starkly dramatized in a brilliant and harsh new light, bringing into question traditional and popular perspectives on gender and race. A severe lack of medical equipment, supplies, and trained personnel spelled potential disaster for the thousands of victims of the widespread wartime disease and violence.

James G. Mundy Jr., historian of the Union League of Philadelphia, observed that, "As tragic as wars are, wars usually produce shifts in human knowledge because they force us to think of different ways of dealing with problems. As tragic as the Civil War was and still is, it produced a paradigm shift in medicine."

The Union's huge naval blockade effectively stopped the South's access to its accustomed pharmaceuticals from Europe and the Northern states. The Confederacy then made a serious effort to create plant-based therapies to fill the gaping medicinal void. Throughout the war, both armies were plagued with shortages ranging from medicines to food to transport, and both exerted tremendous efforts to replicate, replace, and create solutions to the crippling lacks.

It became necessary to set aside age-old established foundations of acceptable behavior for the sake of preserving lives and, born of desperation, a huge movement of women stormed into the mainstream of a national health crisis. That desperation forced men to accept female presence and assistance in life's most fragile situations. The drafting of African Americans into the armies meant that a new black chain of command and administration must be not simply tolerated, but supported.

Civil War doctors faced the constant threat of medical supply shortages. Early in the war, medical personnel were often forced to obtain provisions by any means possible, even confiscating the supplies of the defeated enemy. As Union and Confederacy revamped their systems and were supported by volunteer organizations, supplies were distributed more efficiently. Southerner Dr. Herbert M. Nash recounted an incident of good fortune for the Confederate medics.

> At the Battle of Seven Pines, May 31, 1862, my command reached the battlefield late in the afternoon. We soon came upon the camp of Casey's division of the Federal army, which had been defeated and driven off in the morning's fighting. The abandoned purveyors' tent, well stored with medicines, liquors, dressings, and other appliances, amazed us, and being fair prey our surgeons soon replenished their depleted supplies.

Sometimes medical supplies were shared by the warring armies, as surgeon Nash experienced at the Battle of the Wilderness, Virginia, in 1864:

> Grant, after the fighting of May 6th, moved off by his left flank. Our cavalry in following came upon one of his large field hospitals with many wounded, and among them not a few Confederates who had been shot down in the charge. My friend, Surgeon C.W.F. Brock, went forward to collect our wounded. The surgeon in charge finding himself and assistants captured, inquired of Brock whether he intended to take away his medical supplies and was informed that the Confederate government did not make war on the sick and wounded, that he only wished to remove his own men. Brock at once paroled the Federal surgeons and men. In return for what he considered such generous treatment he presented Brock with quite a liberal supply of what he most needed.

Supply problems were complicated by changes in treatment and economics. As the dollar fell against foreign currencies, there were shortages of imported drugs and wild price fluctuations, and by 1863 the cost of some pharmaceuticals had risen as much as 500 percent. Stocks of certain medicines were dangerously low. Early in the war, potassium permanganate had been helpful in treating hospital gangrene. The drug hadn't been used much prior to the war, and the new demand was difficult to satisfy.

Southern doctors were particularly hard-pressed to obtain sufficient medical supplies. They tried to procure reserves from Europe, but Union naval blockades, prevalent later in the war, complicated the already desperate situation. Some important drugs were only available to the South through capture or blockade running. The Union declared medical supplies to be contraband in the Confederacy, a ruling heartily protested by many doctors on both sides on humanitarian grounds. Fortunately, the few most important drugs, quinine, morphine, ether, and chloroform, were usually accessible. Dr. William H. Taylor reflected on the South's fluctuating availability of medical supplies:

> Normally, we were scant of medicines, and generally they were of the commoner kinds. At times, however, we were well supplied, and with excellent preparations. These times would be when captures had been made, or medicines of Northern or European manufacture had come through the blockade. The Confederate pharmaceutical laboratories worked industriously, but under great disadvantages, and their output was not surpassingly excellent.
>
> On the battlefield our stock of medical and surgical supplies was particularly condensed. Bandages were plentiful, but we seldom had splints. On one occasion I used a whole fence-rail for a broken arm, being unable to do any better. I had just finished making the rail secure when a turn in affairs forced us to take flight. My patient started to run with the rest, but the distal end of the heavy rail tilted downward, stuck in the ground, and jerked him up short at every step. I do not precisely know what became of him, but unless he had the sagacity to turn round and retreat backward I fear I was instrumental in delivering him into the hands of the enemy.

Even the simplest of medical supplies could be unavailable, and doctors made every attempt to come up with substitutions. Nashville, Tennessee, native Dr. Deering J. Roberts elaborated on the desperation of finding replacements for even the most basic equipment.

> Occasionally, silk for ligatures and sutures was limited; a few times I was forced to use cotton or flax thread of domestic make, and horsehair, boiled, to make it more pliant and soft.

Access to supplies was a major factor in swinging the pendulum of the war. The South was struggling; the North, its larger army bolstered by the vast and well-organized volunteer effort, was able to continue manufacturing and importing.

The medical supply shortages and the large number of sick and wounded men, coupled with limited knowledge, could reduce medical care to its most base level. Sometimes the Confederate regiments received a monthly allotment of one gallon of whiskey, an ounce of quinine, and varying amounts of chloroform. Dr. Taylor revealed that he had often been forced to offer limited and primitive care in the absence of valid pharmaceuticals and other essential supplies.

> Our most valued medicament was the alcoholic liquors, which were furnished to us sometimes in the form of whisky and at other times of apple brandy. These preparations were esteemed as a specific for malaria especially—a condition which was very prevalent.
>
> Early in the morning we had sick-call, when those who claimed to be ill or disabled came up to be passed upon. Diagnosis was rapidly made, usually by intuition, and treatment was with such drugs as we chanced to have in the knap-sack. On the march my own practice was reduced to the lowest terms. In one pocket of my trousers I had a ball of blue mass, in another a ball of opium. All complainants were asked the same question, "How are your bowels?" If they were open, I administered a plug of opium; if they were shut, I gave a plug of blue mass.

Medical supplies were scarce, but even the most basic requirement—food—was often in short supply. The war could not be fought effectively with starving soldiers. Union Army colonel Daniel Hand, M.D., faced desperate situations and difficult decisions throughout his wartime service. He reflected on a nightmarish period in Virginia.

Our scanty supply of food was exhausted, and while trying to hurry up the commissary, Medical Director Hammond called me to one side, and said the bridge across the Chickahominy had been washed away and we could get no provisions that day. He suggested that I have some horses quietly killed.

At once General Sedgwick gave me two cavalry horses and allowed a detail of two butcher-boys from the First Minnesota. We led the horses into a grove near the hospital and in a very short time some beautiful beef was lying on the skins with the edges carefully turned under. Another detail of men carried it to the hospitals, and the cooks were soon making soup and broth. This was served out to the wounded, and no doubt helped many of them to tide over that critical time.

Early in the war, the Union Army had difficulty in getting existing shipments to the troops. The outpouring of donated supplies was tremendous, but there were no efficient systems for delivering them. Without designated transport and distribution, huge quantities of food and hospital supplies were lost, abandoned, or left to spoil. The volunteer United States Sanitary Commission swept in with new guidelines for supply transport and three days after the Battle of Antietam, near Sharpsburg, Maryland, in September 1862, more than forty delegates of the Commission were on the ground extending assistance to eight thousand wounded and sick. Within a week they had brought in ten thousand shirts, underwear, medical supplies, and food, and a huge quantity of materials was delivered to the hospitals caring for the victims.

Union doctor Jonathan Letterman, medical director of the Army of the Potomac, whose ambulance system was a revolutionary advance, was also concerned with the Army's supply systems, or lack of them. He revamped the entire Union Army supply system in 1862, addressing the problems of effective delivery with designated wagons to avoid the huge amounts of supplies that were lost or wasted.

I desired to reduce the waste which took place when a three months' supply was issued to regiments, to have a small quantity given them at one time, and to have it replenished without difficulty; to have a fixed amount of transportation set apart for carrying these supplies, and used for no other purpose. On the 4th of October, 1862, I instituted the system of "brigade supplies."

Creativity and innovation became paramount as the imagination and resourcefulness of leaders and visionaries established new solutions to the myriad problems created by the war. The American Civil War marked the first mass movement of wounded troops. Overwhelming numbers of casualties created the need for new means of transporting wounded men, both from the battlefield to the field hospital, and from the field hospital to general or specialty hospitals.

The first organized wartime transport by ambulance occurred during the campaigns and reign of Napoleon Bonaparte in the late 18th and early 19th centuries. French Army surgeon Dominique Jean Larrey (later baron) followed Napoleon through Egypt, Italy, Germany, Austria, Russia, and Waterloo; in the process he became principal surgeon of the French Army and a baron of the empire. After completing his medical studies, Larrey joined the army in 1792 and was subsequently wounded three times while taking part in sixty battles and approximately four hundred other military engagements. Inspired by the speed of the French artillery and believing that rapid treatment of the wounded was extremely important not only to the injured men, but to the morale of all the troops, he instituted an organized system of vehicles for transport including drivers, stretcher/litter carriers, and corpsmen.

The echoes of Baron Larrey's brilliant and effective system have filtered through more than two centuries of emergency rescue and transport, as have his principles for the training of surgeons, stockpiling supplies and food, reorganizing hospitals, and promoting the importance of sanitation and hygiene, and he is frequently lauded as the true "Father of Military Medicine."

By the mid–19th century, conditions of mass casualties during the American Civil War made it painfully apparent that the need for such systems still existed and were in fact magnified by the size of the massive battles and enhanced weaponry.

Most primary care on the battlefield was given at field hospitals located far behind the front lines. From 1862 on, armies tended to take over a nearby farmhouse, church, or school building for use as a field hospital, although this frequently necessitated moving the wounded miles from where the fighting had taken place. Men, usually those deemed unfit for battle service, were randomly appointed to drive ambulances and carry litters. The wounded who survived the crude emergency efforts were transported to army hospitals in nearby cities or towns, usually by two-wheeled carts or four-wheeled wagons.

The medical corps of the Army of the Potomac was understaffed and disorganized at the beginning of the Civil War, and it exhibited a stunning inability to coordinate a movement of hurt troops from the scene of the battle. At the July 1861 Battle of Bull Run in Prince William County, Virginia, scores of wounded soldiers were left suffering in the hot sun on the battlefield for days, and it was a week before the casualties were completely cleared. Injured men had to make their own way to Washington for medical treatment and were mainly supported by citizens' organizations. Wagons were rarely designated specifically as ambulances, having more use for hauling munitions and other supplies. The United States Army had neglected to budget adequately for medical care and the transport of its wounded.

The Union had no military ambulance corps at the start of the war: the available haphazard ambulance vehicles were driven by civilians or men not able to participate in the fighting. The initial ambulance corps came under the aegis of the quartermaster, and ambulance vehicles were frequently commandeered to deliver supplies and ammunition to the fronts.

Major Jonathan Letterman was born in 1824, the son of a prominent surgeon in the western part of Pennsylvania, and earned his medical degree at Jefferson Medical College in Philadelphia. He applied for an Army commission upon his graduation in 1849 and spent the next thirteen years working throughout North America, caring for sick and injured soldiers in remote locations. Upon his return to the East, Letterman's solid reputation, leadership qualities, organizational abilities, and medical skill led to his appointment as medical director of the Army of the Potomac during the Civil War. Major General George Brinton McClellan recommended the dynamic surgeon as "not quite so thickly incrusted with the habits, forms and traditions of the service."

Horrified by the terrible state of care for the wounded, Major Letterman instituted a plan that was a model of management of medical support, the elements of which are still used today. Calling into play the principles of Baron Larrey, Letterman's design called for transporting the wounded to the hospital and dropping them off with their bedding, picking up new bedding and supplies at the hospital, and returning to the front. The ambulances of a division moved together with specified personnel to collect the wounded from the field, bring them to dressing stations, then to the field hospital. Letterman's plan was implemented in August 1862 when General McClellan issued General Orders No. 147, regulations for the organization of the ambulance corps and the management of ambulance trains. In March 1864, Congress published General Orders No. 106, an act (Public 22) to create an ambulance corps for all the Union armies.

Letterman's ambulance system proved its worth at the Battle of Antietam in Maryland, in September of 1862 when, faced with 23,000 casualties, the new system with its fledgling ambulance corps and medical personnel was able to move all of the wounded from the field in only twenty-four hours. The evolution of those actions can be seen throughout America's wars as the principles of Larrey and Letterman were adopted and echoed by the U.S. Army Medical Corps.

After the Confederacy lost control of most of its major waterways, the Southern states relied heavily on railroads to move their wounded from field hospitals to general hospitals. Trains, introduced to the country in 1830, had never before been used as ambulances in America. The South began to ship supplies in boxcars and return them filled with sick and injured soldiers. The system was plagued with difficulties owing to shortages, raids, and the different track gauges of the various Southern railroad companies.

The American Civil War, also noted as the first "railroad war," marked the initial wartime use of hospital trains in the country. Railroads became the lifelines of the armies—they were used to support combat efforts and strengthen military operations. The trains provided the development of innovative technologies to allow the movement of unprecedented numbers of troops, horses, and supplies. The war saw the introduction of ironclad railcars that were capable of moving big guns and artillery, and it could all be conveyed rapidly to locations where armies were camped.

Most of America's manufacturing was conducted in the more highly industrialized North, which also had constructed about 20,000 miles of railroad track since the introduction of trains, thereby controlling 70 percent of the country's total tracks. The Confederacy was woefully disadvantaged with 9,000 miles of tracks and multiple railroad companies that used different and incompatible gauges.

The beginning of the Civil War signaled a large drop in the production of new railroads, but the use of the existing transportation increased dramatically as the availability and reach of railroads changed the face of the war.

As the number of battle casualties rose frighteningly, the U.S. Army began to explore better methods of medical evacuation and means of transporting wounded men to hospitals. The first rail transports for the sick and injured were empty boxcars returning from delivering supplies to the battlefields. The floors of the boxcars were cushioned with straw, pine branches, or whatever was available to soften the surfaces. There was little or no ventilation in the closed cars and the patients had to bear the pain of the swaying and jolting of the trains. "The worst cases are put inside the covered cars," noted volunteer Katharine Wormeley, "they arrive a festering mass of dead and living together."

There began a move to construct dedicated hospital cars from existing "rolling stock" of passenger cars and to replace seats with bunks. The hospital cars that were used varied from improvised boxcars and passenger cars to purpose-built cars paid for by relief organizations. Soon the hospital cars became part of dedicated trains that sometimes also adapted boxcars as kitchens to provide meals. The designated hospital trains usually numbered between five to ten hospital cars, a passenger car for soldiers who were able to sit, a surgeons' car for medical staff, a kitchen car for preparing food, and a boxcar for supplies, although the cars still provided a rough ride for the patients.

Dr. Elisha Harris of the United States Sanitary Commission, a leading voice in the promotion of sanitation and public health, noted the terrible pain endured by the soldiers in rail transit and designed a special hospital railroad car to be used for the transport of wounded. His plan was approved by Quartermaster General Montgomery C. Meigs, a career United States Army officer and civil engineer. Meigs allowed Dr. Harris the use of several government-owned railcars and persuaded private railway companies to provide additional equipment.

The Harris-designed railcar made it possible for medical attendants to move through the cars and also to go from car to car, attending patients while the train was in motion. It was a novel concept that was not possible in the converted boxcars.

Dr. Harris created a system for hanging patients' stretchers with shock-absorbing rings made of India rubber. The plan also allowed for the same stretcher that carried a wounded man off the battlefield to be used for his transport on the railcar, simplifying the moving of patients. Three tiers of stretchers could be hung in a fifty-foot hospital car. His design was carried out and sponsored by the Philadelphia, Wilmington and Baltimore Railroad in October 1862. The volunteer United States Sanitary Commission purchased a locomotive so that the hospital train could be used exclusively for the transport of the wounded. The design experiment proved successful, and the Sanitary Commission turned over the management of hospital trains to the Army Medical Department.

Dr. Harris's invention of a railway ambulance brought him international acclaim and his design was used during the Franco-Prussian War. He received a bronze medal from the Paris Exposition of 1867, and the Société de Sécours aux Blessés awarded him a silver medal.

It's estimated that during the war, more than 250,000 patients were transported by hospital trains. These trains moved at a slow rate of speed in order to cause the least amount of jostling and pain to their passengers. A yellow flag was frequently flown on the engines and Union trains had large letters reading "U.S. Hospital Train" painted on the outside of the car panels. Some of the Northern trains were distinguished by a bright red smokestack, engine, and tender, and all of the trains carried three red lanterns at night, indicating a need for safe passage. Records indicate that the Confederates never attacked a Union hospital train.

The Battle of Gettysburg, Pennsylvania, in July 1863 marked the railroads' largest evacuation of wounded during the war as almost 12,000 injured soldiers were transported to general hospitals in Philadelphia, Baltimore, and New York City. The removal of mass casualties overwhelmed the intricate railroad system, and additional field hospitals had to be positioned to care for vast numbers of patients awaiting transport. All of the injured had been cleared from the Gettysburg battlefield by July 4, but it took fifteen days and multiple trips to get them moved to general hospitals in the cities. The wounded were evaluated to determine how much travel they could physically handle or if they needed to remain longer at the field hospitals. As soon as a patient was deemed able to survive the trip, he was loaded onto a train bound for a city hospital. Many local Gettysburg residents allowed their homes to be used for temporary hospitals, as the railroads could not keep up. It became clear during the two-week mass process that medical evacuation and transport by railroad were going to be essential elements in winning the war.

The railroads began to run into difficulties, with the Confederacy at a serious disadvantage, especially from the Union naval blockade that had almost entirely shut off its access to supplies. Worn-out parts and equipment were extremely hard to replace for a government that had previously imported its iron from England. Tracks began to wear out and locomotives to fail. Most of the Southern locomotives were wood-fueled, a difficult crop to gather as most of the men were now in the military, with train crews sometimes forced to stop the trains in order to chop wood to keep going.

Normal rail difficulties and minor accidents turned into major stop-pages and catastrophes when coupled with Union sabotage of tracks, tunnels, and bridges and their capture of as much Southern railroad equipment as possible.

Hospital trains have continued to be a part of public health care in numerous countries to the present day. Since 2010, Russia has operated five hospital trains carrying medical staff to remote villages across Siberia; the China Railway operates four eye hospital trains that travel to hard-to reach regions, and India's Lifeline Express is a technologically advanced train providing otherwise unavailable health care to rural areas.

Throughout the history of war, battles fought near large bodies of water have been supported by dedicated vessels for the evacuation and treatment of casualties. The ancient Romans adapted special boats for rescue missions, and once the late-18th-century United States established a maritime branch of its armed forces, it too acknowledged the value of such vessels.

The first floating hospital in America was actually activated two years before the beginning of the Civil War, responding to an epidemic of sailors infected with the highly contagious yellow fever. The existing marine hospital refused to admit them and it was necessary to find a place where they could be secluded and quarantined. New York physician Dr. William

Adison had recently returned from a trip to England where he had observed the H.M.S. *Caledonia*, originally launched in 1808 as a 120-gun ship of the Royal Navy. The *Caledonia* was considered quite a successful ship that had performed well, and after decades of service, she was converted to a hospital ship in 1856, renamed *Dreadnought*, and became a floating hospital for seamen.

In response to the threat posed by the large number of sailors infected with the deadly disease, Dr. Adison suggested adapting a similar vessel for their quarantine and care, and funds were voted by the port authorities to purchase the steamer *Falcon*. Major changes were made to the ship including removing the engines, constructing housing over the deck, and changing her name to *Florence Nightingale*, honoring the British nurse and hospital reformer.

The U.S. Navy's first official hospital ship used in the Civil War was a former Confederate 786-ton sidewheel river steamer named the *Red Rover*. The steamer had been built at Cape Girardeau, Missouri, in 1859 and purchased by the Confederacy in November 1861 as a barracks ship for the crew of the *New Orleans*, a floating battery. Five months after their purchase, the *Red Rover* was captured near Island Number 10 on the Mississippi River by the Union gunboat *Mound City* and quickly put into use as a floating hospital for Northern casualties. Over the course of the summer, the U.S. Army Quartermaster Corps modified the vessel to include bathroom facilities, laundries, operating rooms, and kitchens. The ship was stocked with three months' worth of stores, including 300 tons of ice, for a crew and 200 patients.

The U.S.S. *Red Rover* had a crew of twelve officers, thirty-five men, and a group of thirty surgeons and nurses aboard. In a radical departure from long-held naval tradition, some of the nurses were female. The nuns who came aboard on Christmas Eve of 1862 were later joined by several more sisters and some female African American nurses, a small group who became the seeds of the Navy Nurse Corps.

Newly fitted hospital ships were provided by the volunteer United States Sanitary Commission in 1862 and 1864. All of the major battles in the West took place near large rivers, and the Union was able to evacuate its sick and wounded by ship and transport them to hospitals as far from the front as New York City.

The South used its waterways to convey supplies and troops with barges serving as hospital transports on the James River in Virginia. They were able to move significant numbers of the wounded, but the Union's naval superiority gave the North a strong advantage in conveying supplies and injured men.

In the beginning of the war, the sick and wounded of the U.S. forces were ferried in passenger and cargo vessels, but arrangements were quickly made for more sophisticated means of transporting injured soldiers. By an act of the U.S. legislature on February 28, 1862, Pennsylvania surgeon general H. H. Smith was directed to send a hospital ship to retrieve casualties from Virginia. The steamer *W. Whilldin* was chartered and proceeded to Yorktown, Virginia, carrying surgeons and several Sisters of Charity. The ship returned with scores of men who had been wounded in the Peninsular Campaign, the first of many vessels carrying the human damage of the war.

In 1862, the U.S. Sanitary Commission augmented the government hospital ships with the commission of the *Daniel Webster*. The government provided the ship and the Sanitary Commission furnished the staff and supplies. Many women volunteered to serve aboard these ships, and some from wealthy families documented their firsthand experiences in diaries and autobiographies, and newspapers published many of their letters, giving the public a vivid sense of the conditions aboard a hospital ship. Katharine Wormeley, the daughter of a British rear admiral, grew up in England and moved to the United States when she was eighteen, becoming a devoted volunteer in relief measures for Union soldiers.

The Union's Peninsular Campaign opened in Virginia in 1862 in a low, swampy area where men were ravaged by malaria, and discovered that the federal Medical Department could not support the needs of its army in such difficult territory. When the U.S. Sanitary Commission officials learned this, they applied to Edwin Stanton, U.S. secretary of war, for the use of some large steamships that could be outfitted for the transport of the Army's sick and wounded. The newly assigned *Daniel Webster* shipped 250 severely ill and injured men to New York.

Volunteer Katharine Wormeley sailed on the ship's second voyage from New York to Yorktown and found herself in the unusual position of being a woman with the authority to give orders to men.

> The first vessel, the 'Daniel Webster', was assigned to the Commission April 25, 1862. She reached the York River April 30, being refitted as a hospital on the voyage down. The army was then before Yorktown.
>
> The ship was ready for duty on her arrival; her stores were placed in a warehouse ashore, and the work of relieving the sick in camp and hospital at once began.
>
> Four ladies are attached to the ship. Our duty is to be very much that of a housekeeper. We attend to the beds, the linens, the clothing of the patients; we have a pantry and store-room, and are required to do all the cooking for the sick; we are also to have a general superintendence over the condition of the wards and over the nurses, who are all men.

Conditions on board the hospital ships could erupt into chaos when there were hundreds of wounded men awaiting evacuation and treatment although supplies and attending personnel were severely limited. The largely inexperienced staff faced a hideous vista of men in terrible pain and a lack of material means to make them comfortable. Katharine documented the horrific chaos:

> Captain Sawtelle came on board to say that several hundred wounded men were lying at the landing; that the 'Daniel

Webster No 2' had been taken possession of by the medical officers and was already half full of men, and that the surplus was being carried across her to the 'Vanderbilt', that the confusion was terrible; nor were there any stores or preparation, not even mattresses, on board the 'Vanderbilt'.

We went on board; and such a scene as we entered and lived in for two days I trust never to see again. Men in every condition of horror, shattered and shrieking, were being brought in on stretchers borne by 'contrabands,' who dumped them anywhere. There was no one to direct what ward or what bed they were to go to. Men shattered in the thigh, and even cases of amputation, were shoveled into top berths without thought or mercy. The men had mostly been without food for three days.

We began to do what we could. The first thing wanted by wounded men is something to drink. Fortunately we had plenty of lemons, ice and sherry on board. After that we gave them crackers and milk, or tea and bread. It was hopeless to try to get them into bed; indeed there were no mattresses on the 'Vanderbilt'. All we could do at first was to try to calm the confusion, to stop some agony, to revive the fainting lives, to snatch from immediate death with food and stimulants. Imagine a great river or Sound steamer filled on every deck—every berth and every square inch of room covered with wounded men; even the stairs and gangways filled; while stretcher after stretcher came along, hoping to find an empty place; and then imagine what it was to keep calm ourselves, and make sure that every man on both those boats was properly refreshed and fed. We got through at one A.M.

Later in the war, the Union Army purchased more ships and outfitted them with the most recent innovations in hospital transport, demonstrating revolutionary improvement in the evacuation and conveyance of sick and wounded troops. The *General J.K. Barnes* was called the best vessel of its type—a ship with accommodations for the chief surgeon, his staff, nurses, cooks, and other employees, and wards for 650 patients. The vessel was heated by steam pipes and the berths were arranged to slide up and down so that patients could be placed in them with the least chance of additional discomfort.

Hospital ships continue to provide their compassionate aid all over the globe. Fifty percent of the world's population lives near a coast, so the state-of-the-art medical specialty vessels can bring access to surgeries in these floating hospitals. Modern hospital ships exhibit their protection under the Geneva Convention with the prominent display of the Red Cross or Red Crescent, indicating that they are part of the international humanitarian movements that were founded to "protect human life and health, to ensure respect for all human beings, and to prevent and alleviate human suffering."

When the Confederates had trouble maintaining pharmaceutical manufacturing, they relied on medicines found in their abundant fields and forests. Southern doctors brewed home remedies of herbs and teas, and sometimes a mixture called "old indig" was substituted for quinine. Dogwood, willow, and yellow poplar barks were mashed and used in treatments.

Dr. Samuel Preston Moore, surgeon general of the Confederate States of America, had a lifelong interest in the science of botany and, during his tenure in the Civil War, also had a desperate need for medications for his army. The Union's large and powerful naval blockade prevented the South's accessing their standard pharmaceuticals from Europe and the North. Dr. Robert D. Hicks commented: "The South, lacking drug manufactories and the ability to import from abroad, turned inward by surveying every tree and plant that grew in Southern soil and exploiting whatever had medicinal value as substitutes."

Surgeon General Moore needed an alternative source of medicines, and decided to generate a thorough investigation of the flora of the Confederacy, analyses of the preparation of indigenous botanicals and their uses in healing, with an emphasis on finding a substitute for quinine. It was going to be a massive, meticulous, and complex effort and the man he summoned was uniquely qualified for the task.

Physician and botanist Francis Peyre Porcher, M.D., born in South Carolina's St. John's Berkeley Parish in 1825 to physician and planter William Porcher and his wife, was an outstanding student, excelling in Latin and the Greek classics. Francis graduated with honors from South Carolina College and was accepted to the Medical College of the State of South Carolina in Charleston, where he received his M.D. degree in 1847. Porcher was the valedictorian at his graduation and was also awarded the first prize for his scientific thesis, "A Medico-Botanical Catalogue of the Plants and Ferns of St. John's, Berkeley, South Carolina." His work was published in the *Southern Journal of Medicine and Pharmacy* and he continued to research and compose works on botanicals and medicine.

Dr. Porcher became the coeditor of the *Charleston Medical Journal and Review* in 1849 and an attending physician at the Marine Hospital in Charleston. In the early 1850s he helped to establish the Charleston Preparatory Medical School, and in 1855, working with a colleague, created a hospital for African Americans. He traveled to Europe, visiting many hospitals to refine his knowledge by studying medical procedures and later accepted a post at his alma mater as professor of clinical medicine, *materia medica*, and therapeutics. In 1860 he was awarded a $100 prize from the South Carolina Medical Association for his essay "Illustrations of Disease with the Microscope: Clinical Investigations."

Porcher, as a supporter of secession and a slave owner, volunteered for the Confederate Army in 1861 as a surgeon and remained in the military until the end of the war. He served first at two army hospitals in Virginia, and was approached in 1862 for a project to find substitute medicines for the Confederacy's troops. Surgeon General Moore, aware of impending medical supply shortages and knowing of Porcher's background in medicine and botany, commissioned him to create a work on the botanical resources of the South. Porcher was temporarily excused from field and hospital duty while he worked on the huge and detailed volume, assisted by his mother and his wife, and the following year he published *Resources of the Southern Fields and Forests*, the first detailed listing of regional plant life and its medical uses.

> It is intended as a repertory of scientific and popular knowledge as regards the medicinal, economical, and useful properties of the trees, plants, and shrubs found within the limits of the Confederate States . . . The Regimental Surgeon in the field, the Physician in his private practice, or the Planter on his estate may themselves collect and apply these substances within their reach, which are frequently quite as valuable as others obtained from abroad.

His book, the first of its kind, won praise for its contributions to medicine and to the war effort. It was the only comprehensive study of useful plants indigenous to the South and was the single resource on the subject that was available to the Confederacy. The 600-page compendium was distributed to medical officers; it presented specific directions on how to use local plant life to substitute for commercial pharmaceuticals, including advice on producing homegrown botanicals. The book contained extensive charts and tables listing plants with medical properties, recommended dosages, preparation methods, and administration instructions.

> The mode of action of medicinal plants infinitely varies; these are generally astringent, narcotics, stimulating vegetable oils, cooling, refrigerant acids, bitter tonics, cathartics, etc.

Some of his recommendations met with acceptance, while others did not pass into common usage. No botanical was discovered that produced a valid substitute for chloroform, nor one for quinine. Porcher was an advocate for a smallpox treatment that was known to have been used by Native Americans or First Nations including the Algonquin, Cree, and Iroquois, and that he is reported to have tested on himself. The treatment was made from an infusion of the carnivorous plant *Sarracenia purpurae* (also known as side saddle of fly trap, purple pitcher plant, or turtle socks) and although the reviews were mixed, Porcher claimed that it had widespread use in South Carolina and Georgia and had been found to be effective.

His search for viable anesthetics produced slim results and although twenty-eight plants with narcotic qualities were identified, only a few became useful remedies. There was research on the efficacy of white versus red poppies and an effort was made to cultivate the plant to produce opium and opium byproducts, but the growers' attempts failed. Porcher's research was hampered by the inability to run clinical trials, and he was limited by relying on folklore, tradition, and recommendations from others, but he maintained faith in many properties of plant material including dogwood bark, holly, knotgrass, poplar, and willow bark. Despite his extensive collecting, examining, and experimentation, the search for a substance to replace quinine met with failure.

Chloroform was the favored anesthesia used in the South, and the search for its botanical replacement did not yield impressive results either. Fortunately, Confederate surgeon Dr. Julian Chisolm's wartime invention of an inhaler for chloroform administration provided some relief and leeway for surgical operations. The new metal inhaler required far less of the anesthesia than the older method of using a soaked cloth over the patient's nose and mouth and it allowed Southern surgeons to maximize the use of their limited supplies.

After the war, Porcher revised and reissued his work in 1869 and continued to research and publish valuable medical literature. Botany and medicine remained the devotional attentions of his studies and he returned to South Carolina's City Hospital for the next twenty-one years, making contributions to medicine and science until the end of his life. He had particular interest in yellow fever, heart diseases, the medical and edible properties of plant life, and promoting the understanding and practice of public hygiene.

During his illustrious career, Dr. Francis Peyre Porcher served variously as president of the South Carolina Medical Association, vice president of the American Medical Association, associate fellow of the College of Physicians of Philadelphia, and was one of a few select physicians chosen to represent the United States at international European medical conferences.

Modern medicine and surgery have been moved importantly forward by advances in the sophisticated administration of anesthesia. Anesthesia in the form of opium-based drugs, Indian hemp, and applications made from the mandrake plant appear throughout ancient history as painkillers. In early-19th-century America, opium derivatives and alcohol were the substances most commonly used to induce unconsciousness or to prevent the awareness of pain. Reports list only forty-three anesthesia-related deaths during the war.

The field of dentistry had embraced the use of anesthesia since the 1840s and it was the dental practitioners who would usher in the era of chloroform and ether to surgical practice. Chloroform had a quicker onset than ether, was nonflammable and was generally preferred as an anesthesia. A common technique at the time for rendering a patient "insensible" was to place a chloroform-impregnated cone-shaped cloth over a patient's nose and mouth. It was an erratic solution at best, as much of the chloroform dissipated and evaporated into the air, and frequently the operating surgeons in the crowded hospitals found themselves somewhat affected by it as well. Despite the drastic shortages of medical supplies and many pharmaceuticals, both Union and Confederacy maintained fairly stable stocks of ether and chloroform throughout the war and used it in most of the surgeries that were performed.

The problem of how to adequately and consistently deliver anesthesia to a patient was tackled by Dr. Julian John Chisolm, a native of Charleston,

South Carolina. Born in 1830, the son of a prominent Charleston family, Chisolm served as an "office assistant" to a well-known local physician before beginning his formal education at the Medical College of South Carolina, receiving his M.D. in 1850. He was able to travel in Europe after his graduation and observed the medical care provided to victims of various conflicts abroad. Over the next several years in America, he organized a preparatory school for medical students and a free hospital for slaves. In 1858 he was the youngest doctor to be named professor of surgery at the college where he had earned his degree.

When the Civil War began in 1861, Chisolm was called to duty as an army surgeon for the Confederacy, bringing several years of firsthand knowledge from his practice and travels. He authored a valuable book for use by the Southern surgeons, *A Manual of Military Surgery*, as so few surgical operations had been performed in America before the war. Known for his powerful energy and enthusiasm, he worked to build medical laboratories in the Confederacy, including the creation of a research and drug plant in Columbia, South Carolina, and he began working on a notable invention that would change and refine the administration of anesthesia in a very efficient way.

During the later years of the war, Dr. Chisolm developed a small and simple applicator to deliver anesthesia directly into the nasal passages of the patient. A piece of cotton or wool sprinkled with chloroform was inserted into a small rectangular metal inhaler with twin metallic tubes that were inserted into the patient's nostrils. This method also minimized the danger of the chloroform or the flammable ether being exposed to the flames of torches or operating lamps. The pocket-sized device was only about 2½" in length and its tubes could be stored inside the body of the tool. The new inhaler and technique greatly increased the efficiency and effect of the chloroform and became a much sought-after instrument.

Julian Chisolm's memory and profile are impressive for his many achievements in medical practice and education, publishing more than 100 papers in his lifetime. He became dean of the School of Medicine at the University of Maryland and one of the first American physicians to use cocaine anesthesia for ophthalmic surgery. He remained an important advocate of the use of anesthesia and later devoted himself to diseases of the eye and ear, founding the Presbyterian Eye, Ear and Throat Hospital of Baltimore. He is considered one of the fathers of American ophthalmology. This much-admired pioneer of the medical field died at age seventy-three and is buried in Greenmount Cemetery in Baltimore, Maryland. His invention of the Chisolm Inhaler remains an extremely important turning point in the administration of anesthesia and the cessation of pain.

At the beginning of the Civil War, soldiers who sustained wounds or fractures of the jaw were frequently left without much hope for recovery or even survival. The proliferation of this type of injury from the multiple battles inspired the creation of a lifesaving dental device, and in an almost identical innovation, both Confederate dentist Dr. James Baxter Bean, from Washington County, Tennessee, and Union dentist Dr. Thomas B. Gunning of New York City invented the "interdental splint." During the war, faced with victims of gunshot wounds to the face and mouth, both dentists arrived at very similar devices to stabilize the jaw during healing. It appears that the men were unaware of each other's work, but their intentions created extremely similar tools, both of which strongly advanced the treatment of maxillofacial wounds.

In the North, the prominent dentist Thomas Gunning had been treating jaw fractures for twenty years, including tending to the broken jaw of U.S. Secretary of State William H. Seward. During the war, he worked with Dr. Gurdon Buck, a New York practitioner of "plastic operations," in repairing the facial and dental structures of some severely wounded soldiers. Gunning designed dental appliances to work with and support Buck's surgical repairs.

At the start of the war, the younger James Bean offered his services to the Confederate medical authorities and moved to Atlanta. Dr. Bean had experimented and worked with "plaster and its manipulations," creating customized oral splints and making significant contributions to treating fractured maxillary facial bones. Bean's 1863 "interdental" splint was constructed of vulcanized India rubber with indentations for the teeth and allowed the patient to eat without dislodging the teeth or bones. It was a state-of-the-art technique for handling injuries that could otherwise easily have ended life.

The device was quickly adopted for use in a Richmond hospital. The hard rubber splint was a great success in treating many facial and jaw wounds, and was used in the rehabilitation of Confederate military leaders including General John Brown Gordon. In an Atlanta hospital, a ward was created exclusively for Bean's treatment of jaw fractures. The "Bean Splint" was used in more than 100 cases of gunshot wounds to the jaw and was unanimously adopted and recommended by the Confederate Medical Board in 1865.

After the war, Dr. Bean sought to popularize his splint in the North, discovering that Union dentist Dr. Gunning had independently and successfully invented virtually the same device. Both of these men contributed greatly to the treatment of wounds and injuries that had previously been considered life-threatening. It was a revolutionary advance in dentistry and opened a new window on possibilities for promoting healing that minimized residual dental and facial deformity.

The field known as "rehabilitative medicine" was developed to meet the needs of the huge number of Civil War amputees. Prosthetic limbs had been available for centuries, but the sophistication of the new American and European innovations made them far superior to any that had been produced before. American jurist and legal scholar Oliver Wendell Holmes Jr. fought for three years in the Union Army, observing many of the sad truths of war.

The limbs of our friends and countrymen are a part of the melancholy harvest which war is sweeping. The admirable

HEALING A DIVIDED NATION

contrivances of an American inventor, have risen into the character of great national blessings, while the weapons that have gone from Mr. Colt's armories have been carrying death to friend and foe, the ingenious inventions of Mr. PALMER have been repairing the losses inflicted by war.

It is not two years since the sight of a person who had lost one of his limbs was an infrequent occurrence. Now, alas! That there are few of us who have not a cripple among our friends, if not in our own families. A mechanical art has become a great active branch of industry. War unmakes legs, and human skill must supply their places as it best may.

In 1834 in the village of Meredith, New Hampshire, a ten-year-old boy named Benjamin Franklin Palmer suffered an accident in which one of his legs was crushed. The leg was amputated and the child was provided with a common prosthetic known as a "peg." The artificial limb was so painful and awkward to use that the adolescent Palmer chose to rely on crutches instead.

As a young man, Palmer devoted himself to the development of an artificial limb that could take the place of the one he had lost. His aim was to replace the functions and movement of his original leg while maintaining comfort and with an objective of "passing": for the wearer to be able to blend back into society after an amputation. Victorian attitudes toward the absence of a limb perceived the changed anatomy as "feminizing" and questioned the physical and metaphysical effects on the mind of the amputee. A fully functioning mind was equated to a fully functioning and "whole" body. Palmer became accomplished in marketing his products internationally, emphasizing their practical and aesthetic benefits with a sensitivity to their ability to contribute to the wearer's confidence, sense of self, success, and "wholeness."

The "Palmer Leg" used springs and metal tendons to articulate the joint of the knees, ankles, and toes in an effective simulation of the movement of a real leg. The moveable elements were completely enclosed, giving the limb a more lifelike appearance, and its natural-seeming movement was a brilliant new addition to available prosthetics. The Palmer Leg was considered a triumph of American ingenuity and Palmer was granted U.S. Patent No. 4,834 for his artificial leg in November 1846.

B. F. Palmer's Patent Leg was immediately successful, lauded for its lifelike and elegant appearance and its smoothly articulated joints. The device won honors at American industrial competitions and was awarded a silver medal in 1851 at the event considered to be the first World's Fair in London, held at the Crystal Palace in Hyde Park. The "conspicuously inconspicuous" Palmer Patent Leg was acclaimed in the London *Times* and caricatured in *Punch*, the British humor and satire weekly magazine. By the start of the American Civil War, more than 3,000 of the appliances had been sold, with more than 500 of them purchased for women.

The Civil War, resulting in many thousands of amputees, forced a change in the public acceptance of prosthetic devices as well as the retail prospects for prostheses. The number of patents that were issued for artificial legs between 1861 and 1873 quadrupled from previous years. The problem of mobility was addressed by the Patent Leg for many amputees, but those who had lost arms experienced a difficult choice—without sophisticated prosthetic arms, their best options were prosthetics with hooks, and many veterans chose to deal with an empty sleeve rather than the cumbersome and frightening-looking hooks. The Palmer Company went back to work to create an acceptable prosthetic arm.

In 1862, with mounting numbers of amputees, the U.S. government committed to supplying artificial limbs to thousands of injured soldiers. Prosthetics companies vied for the lucrative government contracts, including Palmer's campaign featuring correspondence with the surgeon general of the U.S.A. and the chief of the bureau of medicine and surgery as well as endorsement letters from eminent surgeons. The Board of Surgeons decided that the best patent artificial limbs were those produced by Palmer, and that they would be adopted for use by the U.S. Army and Navy. In order to maximize the results of wearing a prosthetic limb, Palmer recommended that certain surgical procedures be followed by doctors when amputating a limb in order to leave the patient with a stump that would comfortably accommodate a prosthetic replacement.

The Palmer Leg was approved and performed well enough for some soldier amputees to return to active duty with the new limb. His advertising brochure now read: "The Palmer Arm and Leg, Adopted for the U.S. Army and Navy by the Surgeon-General, U.S.A." As the Palmer Company's offerings expanded to include workable arms and hands, the artificial arm produced by the company proved so superior that veterans petitioned the government to provide only the Palmer Patent Arm.

Companies like the B.F. Palmer Company and Jewett's Patent Leg Company grew rapidly as the federal Medical Department authorized the purchase of thousands of prosthetic legs and arms. Twenty percent of the 1866 budget of the state of Mississippi was spent on artificial limbs.

Another successful prosthesis company was launched in the South during the Civil War by a man who is popularly called the "first amputee of the war." Confederate soldier James Edward Hanger, born on his father's plantation, Mount Hope, near Churchville, Virginia, was eighteen years old in 1861 when he left his engineering classes at Washington College in Virginia to join the Churchville Cavalry. He enlisted on June 2, 1861, in Philippi, Virginia (now West Virginia), and on the very next day, while in the stable, a Union cannonball crashed into the building, shattering his left leg beneath the knee. Hanger's leg was amputated about seven inches below the hip bone, and after several weeks of recovery, he was sent to a Union prison at Camp Chase in Ohio. Later that summer after a prisoner of war exchange, he was returned to his family in Virginia.

Hanger's engineering education gave him the knowledge and impetus to design a new prosthetic leg for himself. He worked with barrel staves whittled into shape, metal, and rubber bumpers, and used hinges at the knee and ankle. Hanger patented his artificial limb in 1871, following it up with additional improvements and unique devices, earning an international reputation as to the excellence of his product. His company continued to receive commendations for their prosthetics, opening branches in Atlanta, Philadelphia, Paris, and London. Hanger Prosthetics & Orthotics remains a leader in the field today, where prosthetics have been advanced by technology to a degree allowing Olympic-level competition and performance.

The majority of Civil War doctors, no matter how well intentioned, were new to trauma surgery and to the practice of surgery in general, although the hordes of wounded requiring operations surely provided them with plenty of practice. Trained and reliable support staff was essential, and as skilled nursing had yet to come into existence on a large scale, members of the U.S. Army Medical Cadet Corps were extremely welcomed by the wartime hospitals.

On August 3, 1861, Congress approved the formation of the U.S. Army Medical Cadet Corps, a group of medical students detailed to be attached to the army as wound dressers and ambulance attendants. The act was titled "An act for the better organization of the military establishment" and the students were accorded the same rank and pay as the military cadets at West Point. Congress specified that the corps would be "composed of young men of liberal education, students of medicine, between the ages of eighteen and twenty-three years, who have been reading medicine for two years and have attended at least one course of lectures in a medical college. They shall enlist for one year, and be subject to the Rules and Articles of War." Applicants to the Cadet Corps had to submit testimonials to their character and physical fitness. At one point during the war years, there were no medical students at Harvard Medical College, as they were all engaged in the war, many as cadets.

The intention behind the formation of the Cadet Corps was to provide army doctors with a pool of trustworthy ambulance attendants and wound dressers. The roles of the cadets included assisting the physicians with any requested task, administering medications and anesthetics, keeping records, and performing postmortem examinations. The cadets assisted in surgery, and as the number of wounded grew, it's likely that many of these students made treatment decisions and performed surgery themselves, embodying an observation of Hippocrates's that "war is the only proper school of the surgeon."

Most of the cadets served in Army hospitals where they were usually paired with specific medical officers serving particular wards. The cadets were frequently housed at the hospitals with the surgeons, and their compensation included meals and quarters with wages of $30 per month (about $1,000 today). Their uniforms included frockcoats with green shoulder straps trimmed in gold lace and noncommissioned officers' belts and swords. Dr. Charles Leale, the first physician to reach President Lincoln after the shooting at Ford's Theatre, began his wartime service as a medical cadet, charged with taking care of two wards at the general hospital in Elmira, New York.

The medical cadets were in a military gray zone, as their rank fell between officers and enlisted men, and they sometimes had to pressure the authorities for some of the perks that were accorded to the officers, including a food allowance. Their service in the hospitals was remarkably valuable for both, as they provided trained medical assistants for the government at a low cost and their participation gave the cadets a dramatic wealth of knowledge and firsthand experience in military medicine. More than 200 medical cadets served the Union in the Civil War, and many veteran cadets continued to work in the Army medical department afterward.

One young medical cadet, Edward Curtis, composed a surprisingly upbeat song about the corps in 1863:

We're the Med. Cads gay and happy
Summoned from our homes to save
By the Surgeon's holy mission
Wounded warriors from the grave.

Military discipline and standards created a measure of order within the chaos. To organize, staff, stock, and administer the vast hospitals, the Army created elaborate and highly accurate record-keeping systems. For the purpose of future medical education, case histories were well-documented, follow-up was extensive, and many excellent postsurgical photographs were taken.

Record-keeping appears to be a mundane part of the medical experience, but its incorporation to the war effort made a huge contribution to medicine and to medical education. A need for quantification was an outgrowth of the huge numbers of soldiers, their wounds, illnesses, and treatments, making data analysis for the advancement of knowledge possible on a grand scale. Statistics became increasingly important in the work of managing hospitals, the administration of public health, and authenticating scientific results.

Dr. Jonathan Letterman, medical director of the Army of the Potomac and an experienced and creative trailblazer, brought meticulous and valuable record-keeping into the Union Army, creating a legacy for all future medical administration. He instituted compulsory reforms stating that the captains of the new ambulance corps had to provide an account after every action of transporting the wounded. The assistant surgeon of every regiment was required to submit a report for each case brought to the hospital, complete with patients' names, rank, company, regiment, type of injury, treatment given, and outcome.

In 1863, Letterman issued an additional decree that Army medical directors were to appoint inspectors to make monthly reports about issues being faced and deficiencies needing to be addressed. Weekly lists of men who were relieved of duty due to illness were required, as these calculations gave more accurate estimates for numbers of men who were still available to fight. The statistics obtained were directly relevant to the ordering of supplies and the preparation of facilities for treating troops. He believed that the importance of medical record-keeping was an integral component of the science involved and that the information obtained would help to avoid many of the organizational disasters that had plagued the Union Army at the beginning of the war.

Surgeon General William Hammond was a strong supporter of the philosophy that "the careful recording of vital medical events was as crucial to the management of medical affairs and institutions as bookkeeping was to the nation's commercial establishments." Hammond also began to order the medical officers to gather unusual anatomical specimens and foreign objects that had been removed during surgery including bullets and other projectiles. He required physicians to write and submit case histories, all of which would begin to form the collection of the Army Medical Museum (now the National Museum of Health and Medicine) and the invaluable six-volume *Medical and Surgical History of the War of the Rebellion.*

The statistics, descriptions, photographs, postmortem reports, and specimens were supplemented with surveys and studies. Dr. Joseph J. Woodward and Dr. John H. Brinton would eventually organize the vast quantities of material for the medical museum and library, creating a new foundation for the preservation of information contributing to the future of medical education and treatment in the West.

CHAPTER SIX

HOSPITALS:
A REVOLUTION IN CARE

One of the most dramatic progressions in American Civil War medicine was the evolution of hospitals. Monasteries had provided medical care for centuries in England and Wales until the 1530s, when King Henry VIII ordered their dissolution, at which point many town and city councils took over the running of hospitals to provide care for their communities. By the 1700s, hospitals began to enlarge their scope of treatments from the very basic care of the sick, adding simple surgeries and the setting of broken bones to their services. Some hospitals would also become training centers for doctors and surgeons.

F. Michael Angelo, archivist of Thomas Jefferson University, Archives and Special Collections, shined an unflinching light on the hospitals of the Middle Ages. "Most were more like hospices, where the monks and nuns would keep patients comfortable and clean until they died. No real treatment attempt. And they served as an important social net for the 'unclean'—lepers, plague victims, mentally ill—who became vagrants and homeless burdens on the citizenry for a few generations until the government finally took some responsibility."

Military hospitals appear early in American history. A hospital for sick soldiers and the West India Company's slaves was opened in 1658 in the territory then known as Manhattan Island. By 1679 this hospital would expand to five houses. During the American Revolution a century later, there is little recorded about the establishment of dedicated hospitals since private homes and other existing structures were commonly utilized for the sick and wounded. Medical understanding dating from the previous century is evident in these settings and in the few newer general hospitals. Wards were kept separate for cases of known communicable diseases; surgical cases were set apart and venereal and "itch" patients had designated wards.

In the 1800s, American hospitals became a haven for those patients who could not afford to call a private doctor to their homes. In U.S. cities and settlements, municipal almshouses were established to provide benefits for the poor, and, as many of the almshouse patients were elderly or extremely ill, they were frequently afforded basic housing and living services. Some of the early almshouses later expanded and became hospitals with more general treatment offerings. The 19th-century hospitals were far cleaner and better ventilated than the 18th-century institutions, and physicians emphasized the value of isolating potentially contagious patients from the general population to curb the spread of disease. The work of British social reformer and founder of modern nursing Florence Nightingale brought public attention to the deplorable conditions of most military hospitals during the Crimean War, and improvements were slow but visible.

Archivist Angelo characterized the hospitals of 1860 as having a great deal in common with the hospitals of 1760. "On the flip side, after the changes and advances during the Civil War, American hospitals of 1870 had more in common with those of 1970." It is a dramatic contrast and a testament to the growth and development of the field of medicine.

More than one million soldiers were treated in Union military hospitals during the course of the war, and despite less than perfect conditions, only a small percentage died. The South had a similar hospital recovery rate.

At the opening of the Civil War, existing military hospitals and medical care were dependent on the regimental field dressing stations, usually tents, which were responsible for the first line of care, and the field hospitals, which provided the second level. The injured who could not reasonably be sent back into battle were dispatched to the general hospitals. Pamphlets, books, and documents detailed the setting up of a field hospital:

> In locating a hospital the requisites are—1. Pure water; 2, wood; 3, good ground, dry and even surface; also, if possible near a wood where boughs may be obtained for beds. In making beds for the sick and wounded, a layer of pine boughs is first spread on the ground, upon that the gum blankets of the soldier, and then, the woolen blankets, using for the pillow anything that can be obtained.

Wounded Civil War soldiers usually received the first emergency attention at a field dressing station, which was generally set up behind the lines, but sheltered from enemy fire if possible. The stations were set up prior to any action on the battlefield, and some were identifiable by a red hospital flag or other visual marker to help guide the wounded and their rescuers. A sorting system that would become known as "triage" by World War I was employed—most head, chest, and abdominal wounds were considered to be untreatable, and those patients were made comfortable, frequently left to die, or they became the last to be evacuated. The slightly wounded and those needing surgery were separated and transported or treated onsite. Limb fractures were splinted, tourniquets applied to bleeding wounds until they could reach the surgeons at the field hospital, and gaping open wounds were packed with lint that had been scraped from linen or cotton fabrics, then bandaged until they could reach the field hospital or a general hospital. If the soldier's wounds were such that he was thought to have a strong chance of survival, he was transported to the field hospital farther back in the rear to be given further assessment and treatment.

The field hospital was the second stage of medical attention, a treatment center staffed by each regiment's surgeon and assistant surgeon. The surgeon's first goal was to stop bleeding; he then might administer morphine to address the pain and provide the victim with clean drinking water. Sometimes whiskey was given as well, then the patient was taken to an ambulance to be delivered to a general hospital for further treatment. The most common surgery at a field hospital was amputation, which was the most rapid way to save the life of a soldier wounded in a limb. During and after a large battle, the scene around a field hospital was a macabre vista of horribly wounded men, frantic bloody activity, and severed limbs. Most fighting took place in daylight, so there was an influx of injured brought in as night fell, when surgeons worked feverishly for hours on end, operating by candle or torchlight. Many field stations were set up in converted houses, barns, or other available structures; some were tents or simply open-air operating setups where the emergency amputations were performed in front of soldiers awaiting their own surgeries.

When the farsighted physician Major Jonathan Letterman became the medical director of the Army of the Potomac, he established the famed Ambulance Corps, and also reorganized and enlarged Union field hospitals, dramatically increasing the medical staffing of surgeons and assistants and sometimes adding men designated as nurses. An officer was assigned to arrange for food and shelter, and tents and medical supplies were issued to the medical teams. Letterman's new field hospital design and system organization, based on a brigade and divisional basis, became a standard of care for the wounded in American and European armies through World War II.

During the course of the war there was a discernible shift in the way medical care was delivered both on the battlefield and in the treatment facilities. In the earliest battles, stretchers had no appointed or trained bearers and were carried by any available, able men including musicians from the regimental bands. The reorganization of the medical department included the addition of designated, trained stretcher-bearers to the corps.

In the cities, large public buildings were refitted to serve as hospitals. Many Washington-area churches, halls, and hotels were appropriated for hospital purposes, including the Capitol building and the U.S. Patent Office. President Lincoln made visits to the wounded troops in some of the hospitals, a gesture repeated by every wartime president since.

When general hospitals with established buildings were filled with patients, tents were set up outside the structures, sometimes over an area of acres. In early 1861, the single military hospital in Washington, D.C., had been a two-story, six-room brick building that was set aside for smallpox patients.

As in the American Revolution, the Civil War still utilized many private homes and public buildings as hospitals. Dr. William Williams Keen of Philadelphia remembered being given orders to turn two Washington, D.C., churches into hospitals within five days. He was twenty-three years old, with less than two years of medical education.

> My assignment to this duty gave me another opportunity of learning how utterly deficient I was in training for my position . . . I was not lacking in ordinary intelligence and was willing to work, but I was utterly without training. To get those two churches ready as hospitals I had to have beds, mattresses, sheets, pillow-cases, chairs, tables, kitchen utensils, knives, forks, spoons, peppers and salts . . . all the drugs, appliances, and instruments needed . . . I needed orderlies, cooks, and the endless odds and ends of things which go to make up a well-organized hospital. I did not know how to get a single one. However, I inquired, and I set myself to work. For two nights I slept only about three hours each, and I had the satisfaction of reporting to Dr. Letterman at the end of

three days, instead of five, that I was ready. On the fourth day
I had one hundred wounded men in each hospital.

The paucity of hospital facilities was one of the first major issues of
innovation and construction during the war as it had become clear due to
the huge number of casualties that large, permanent hospital structures were
required. By 1864, America boasted almost 400 hospitals with approximately 400,000 beds, and federal military hospitals treated more than one
million soldiers during the course of the war. Civil War hospitals did have
a commonality with modern hospitals—the hospital hierarchies were based
on military structure, with regimented wards and a chain of order.

With the advent of major battles, the military and private citizens both
sought to provide and improve medical care for the growing numbers of
sick and wounded and to save as many lives as possible.

Both Union and Confederacy had established general hospitals by the
autumn of 1862. The designation "general" indicated that their services were
not restricted to specific regiments or corps, and were usually located in
large cities including Atlanta, Georgia, Lynchburg, Virginia, and Frederick,
Maryland, in the South; Philadelphia, Pennsylvania, and Washington, D.C.,
were major hospital hubs in the North, where large numbers of wounded
troops could be efficiently transported by train.

If a soldier's condition was mild enough for him to be released from a
field hospital in a short time, or if his condition was too critical for him to
be moved, he remained at the field hospital. Other victims would be sent
to the general hospitals for further treatment, convalescence, or rehabilitation. The general hospitals were intended to be permanent facilities in their
locations, although in several instances, Southern hospitals were relocated
in response to the movement of Union troops. It is estimated that two million patients were treated in the general hospitals during the war. Some of
the volunteers of the United States Sanitary Commission kept track of the
available hospital facilities.

Most of our volunteer medical officers knew nothing of military hospitals.

At first, when the sick accumulated in a regimental hospital beyond the capacity of the regulation canvas shelter, a neighboring house was converted into a hospital, and in like manner, a church, factory or other large building was extemporized into a brigade or general hospital.

In Alexandria, Virginia, hospitals were organized in abandoned dwellings, warehouses, churches, seminaries, etc.

Baltimore extemporized the National Hotel. The buildings of the Naval Academy at Annapolis were early converted to hospital uses.

The general hospitals had one surgeon in charge, a number of staff and assistant surgeons, and nurses who were assigned in proportion to the size of the hospital. These larger medical facilities usually employed cooks, stewards, laundresses, and other support workers. At first the hospitals were established in existing buildings including churches, schools, hotels, and courthouses, but the problems of poor ventilation, the lack of installations for toilets, bathing, large-scale food preparation, mortuaries, and the vast number of incoming patients called for far larger and specifically designed institutions.

One important evolution in the establishment of large general hospitals was the appearance of vast new "pavilion" hospitals in North and South, many of which were efficiently built like spokes on a wheel.

The "pavilion plan" for hospital design seems to have first appeared in 18th-century France, and was promoted in England in the mid-1800s. The British nurse and social reformer Florence Nightingale endorsed and supported the design in which she strongly believed—especially because it offered good ventilation, an aspect that had a strong correlation with a lower mortality rate. Nightingale had studied existing hospitals during her work in the Crimean War and collected data from her personal experience there. Pavilion hospitals offered many of the benefits of a tent, but had the stability and protection of a solid structure. They retained heat, offered cover from the elements, and the wards were easily accessible to hospital staff.

The design of the pavilion hospital featured long, narrow units or wards with multiple windows to provide the desired ventilation. The units were frequently connected by common passages that allowed personnel, patients, and supplies to move more efficiently through them. Frequently made of wood, the hospitals were familiar in Europe, especially in England and France.

At the onset of the Civil War, both Union and Confederate surgeons general began researching hospital designs that would provide the most efficient and effective structures and each decided independently upon the pavilion hospital, which had proven so successful in Europe. The design features were attractive in terms of maximum ventilation and sunlight, space requirements per patient, and nonporous building materials, and they allowed for the separation of patients with similar types of injuries or communicable diseases, thereby lessening the spread of diseases or infection. The choice of location was paramount, being based on available drinking water, access to supplies, and transportation, indicating that major cities offered the best availability of resources.

The Union called upon the United States Sanitary Commission to form a commission for reviewing hospital plans, and to suggest approved designs. U.S. Surgeon General William Hammond had always been a proponent of improved ventilation in health care facilities, and championed the choice of the pavilion design. In the Confederacy, Surgeon General Samuel Moore came to similar conclusions and created one of the South's largest and most well-organized hospitals, Chimborazo General Hospital in Richmond, Virginia. Chimborazo, with 150 pavilions, could accept up to 8,000 patients and boasted quite a low death rate. The hospital also claimed a unique position in the country by employing a woman, Phoebe Pember of North Carolina, as the first female hospital administrator.

The arrangements of the long wards of the pavilion hospitals were sometimes positioned in a rectangular configuration facing a central courtyard, but were varied in layout, including an elongated ellipse and a circular design with radiating spokes. The design functioned less effectively in colder climates as the increased ventilation made them impractical for heating. In Vermont, the pavilions were elevated and insulated with double floors to combat the low temperatures and the wind. Hospital grounds frequently contained detached outbuildings that served as laundries, administration buildings, officers' quarters, chapel, and "dead house." In the event of huge barrages of patients, outdoor tents still supplemented the main buildings. One Southern hospital was lauded for its excellence, as Confederate surgeon Dr. Herbert M. Nash remembered:

> In Chimborazo Hospital between 40,000 and 50,000 cases of wounds were treated. In it there was never a case of gangrene and not a case of smallpox. It had hot sulphur baths for skin diseases, in which the camp itch was successfully treated. Vaccination was constantly practiced in all hospitals. Out of the number of wounded treated at Chimborazo eight thousand died, during its existence—a moderate mortality.

Chimborazo in Virginia was the first of the pavilion hospitals to be constructed in the South, followed in the Union by Pennsylvania's West Philadelphia United States General Hospital (called "Satterlee"), which opened in 1862 with 3,519 patient beds. Philadelphia became a major Union hospital center with the addition of the Mower Hospital in Chestnut Hill the following year, a huge facility that had 3,100 beds in fifty pavilions. The Northern city also hosted the McClellan U.S. Army hospital with eighteen pavilions and 1,080 beds. Washington, D.C., was the other large hospital hub in the Union, with pavilion facilities including Campbell Hospital, Lincoln Hospital, and Armory Square. Nurse Amanda Stearns recorded in her diary that President Lincoln suggested that flower beds be planted between the eleven pavilions of Armory Square and, with his assistance, the landscaping was arranged.

The general hospitals were able to treat a variety of injuries and diseases, but as the war raged on and the casualty count rose, it became necessary to create specialty hospitals to handle large groups of patients with similar conditions.

The field of neurology was nonexistent in the American medical community until the Civil War years brought it under intensive study. In 1861 a neurological hospital was opened in Philadelphia by three young surgeons: Silas Weir Mitchell, William Williams Keen, and George Read Morehouse. The physicians had the backing and encouragement of Surgeon General William Hammond and their work would make the world aware of several formerly mysterious conditions that were caused by nerve injuries.

The brilliant, driven, and fastidious Dr. Silas Weir Mitchell noticed a similarity among many of the thousands of amputee patients. He petitioned for and received permission to establish a hospital in Philadelphia for the study of "nervous injuries," giving rise to the field of neurology. Known then as the nation's center of medicine and medical education, Philadelphia was also located conveniently to several railroads, and almost 157,000 wounded were brought to its hospitals during the war. The huge number of wartime sick and injured necessitated the establishment of specialty hospitals, including Turner's Lane for "nervous (neurological) injuries." Dr. Mitchell was fascinated by this work and pleased by the unique situation afforded by the specialty hospital.

The establishment of a single hospital for the reception of a single class of cases, in connection with the military service, was certainly a novel idea.

I began here to take interest in cases of nervous diseases, which at that time, nobody desired to keep for the reason that they were so little understood and so unsatisfactory in their results. I was therefore allowed to accept these cases from other wards. When this became known to the surgeon-general he was at once interested and set aside a larger ward for neural maladies. No sooner did this class of patients begin to fill our wards, than we perceived that a new and interesting field of observation was here opened to view.

The opportunity was indeed unique, and we knew it. The cases were of amazing interest. Thousands of pages of notes were taken. There were many operations and frequent consultations.

Turner's Lane, located on a country estate between Eastern State Penitentiary and Girard College, was the first hospital in the nation to be devoted specifically to nerve injuries. The many thousands of amputees who were sent to the institution gave the three founding contract surgeons a vast number of cases of the effects of modern warfare to study and compare, including spinal cord and brain injuries. They conducted research on narcotics, nerve injuries, and defined the phenomena that Mitchell labeled "phantom limb"—the sensation that an amputated limb was still present.

After the departure of Surgeon General Hammond, who had advocated for their work, Acting Surgeon General Barnes also became a supporter. He published their paper "Reflex Paralysis, the Result of Gunshot Wounds" in early 1864, and had it distributed to Union medical officers. The three doctors also published *Gunshot Wounds, and Other Injuries of Nerves* in the same year, a book that was still in use by the French Army during World War I.

Doctors Keen, Mitchell, and Morehouse "created a body of work that effectively founded American neurology," remarked Dr. Robert D. Hicks of the College of Physicians of Philadelphia.

Dr. Silas Weir Mitchell continued his research for decades after the war, contacting former patients to learn the effects of their wartime injuries throughout their lives, his son, Dr. John Mitchell, joining him in the work. In 1874, the American Neurological Association was founded by Dr. Mitchell and other physicians including former surgeon general Dr. William Hammond. The discipline of neurology remains a vitally important area of medicine.

With one million casualties to be addressed, both Union and Confederacy began to establish specialty hospitals to deal with specific injuries and illnesses. Eye and ear injuries were treated in the North by the Desmarres Hospital in Washington, D.C., Wills Eye Hospital in Philadelphia, Pennsylvania, and a dedicated eye infirmary in St. Louis, Missouri. Eye specialists in the South operated the Ophthalmic Hospital in Athens, Georgia, headed by Surgeon Dr. Bolling A. Pope. Eye ailments were usually attributable to injury, disease, or dietary lack including "night blindness" caused by a vitamin A deficiency. The Civil War eye specialists were using a very early version of the ophthalmoscope, but their methods and treatments were actually on a par with international standards of their time.

The widespread problem of venereal disease in both armies, primarily classified as "syphilis" or "gonorrhea" ("the clap"), was probably traceable to the large numbers of urban prostitutes. After the Union captured Southern cities Nashville and Memphis, the problem had become so pervasive that authorities legalized and regulated prostitution, including licensing. The sex workers had to agree to frequent medical examinations, and those found to be carrying or suffering from one of the diseases were sent to a specialty hospital in Nashville, Number 11, which was the former home of a bishop. Doctors were aware that the diseases were sexually transmitted and noted the correlation between a decrease in the number of cases when infected women were isolated. Nashville's Hospital Number 15, also known as the "Soldier's Syphilitic Hospital," was a huge 400-bed facility near Smokey Row, the infamous neighborhood that housed many of the city's brothels. It is estimated that as many as one third of the Civil War veterans living in veterans' homes died years later from the effects of venereal disease.

The huge number of amputee veterans created a need for a focused environment, and Union and Confederacy both established "stump" hospitals for soldiers who now needed artificial legs. In 1862 the Roman Catholic Sisters of Charity opened a specialty facility for amputees in New York City's Central Park. Housed in a converted building that had previously been St. Joseph's Convent School, it was referred to during the war as St. Joseph's Hospital, or Central Park Hospital.

The Civil War surgical situation was overwhelmed with orthopedic problems. One pervasive condition was the failure of a fracture to heal after treatment—"non-union." Some unhealed fracture sites developed motion similar to a joint, known as a "false joint" and some dislocations remained chronic. It has been noted that the majority of American military combat injuries dating back to the Revolutionary War and continuing to World War I have been orthopedic in type. Special hospital facilities were created to handle the difficult bone issues in both Union and Confederacy. The doctors' wartime experience in American combat orthopedics began to gain shape and emerge as a distinct area of specialization at this time, although it would be some years before it was formally recognized.

In a country that had previously had very few general hospitals, specialty hospitals began to emerge in North and South, necessitated by the extreme carnage of the war. Jaw and facial injuries could be treated in hospitals staffed with surgeons and dentists who worked with maxillofacial injuries. Memphis, Tennessee, had a facility for treating gangrene; Wilmington, Delaware, focused on feet and toes lost to frostbite; Philadelphia's Hahnemann Medical College and Hospital, founded in 1848, offered homeopathy, a popular form of alternative medicine.

African Americans, enslaved or free, suffered from many diseases and conditions related to living conditions and environmental factors; genetics deemed blacks to be victims of certain diseases more than they affected whites. The beliefs of the Southern medical community were frequently based on justifying slavery through describing blacks as inferior in health and physicality. The major causes of death for slaves were infectious diseases including tuberculosis and other respiratory illnesses like pneumonias. African Americans suffered greatly from gastrointestinal problems like typhoid fever and the many diseases that caused diarrhea and severe dehydration. Their death rate from disease was two and one half times the death rate of white soldiers suffering from the same illnesses.

Senator Henry Wilson of Massachusetts sponsored the District of Columbia Compensated Emancipation Act in April 1862, the passage of which freed slaves in the District of Columbia and compensated former slave owners up to $300 (approximately $8,200 today) for each freeperson. Following the enactment of the law, freedom was granted to 2,989 former slaves under more than 930 petitions. An influx of more than 40,000 escaped slaves flooded into Washington, D.C., seeking freedom and sanctuary. Regarded by their former owners as "stolen property," they became known as "contraband."

The sudden surge in the African American population created a new set of issues for the federal government and the Union Army, which were then also responsible for the defense of the capital and a victory over the Confederate Army. Suddenly, tens of thousands were in need of food, shelter, and medical care, and the Union Army, in a definitive move claiming responsibility for government-sponsored contraband relief efforts, established what was intended as a safe haven for them in the form of a camp and hospital.

The hospital was built in 1862 on the grounds of the former Camp Barker, a swampy site in northwest Washington, D.C., bordered by Twelfth, Thirteenth, R, and S Streets. The Union Army built one-story frame buildings and tented structures to serve as temporary housing and hospital wards for African American soldiers and civilians. Wards for men and women were separate, as were facilities for smallpox patients. The site contained a kitchen, laundry, dead house, ice room, stable, and living quarters for staff. Despite the Army's best efforts, the living conditions were poor, as the swampy ground created a damp, unhealthy atmosphere and there was a lack of fresh water. Overcrowding accelerated the rate of diseases that moved through the camp and hospital, and the temporarily built quarters did not stand up well to the weather. It seemed that everything was in short supply: food, clean water, stoves, blankets, tents.

Cornelia Hancock, born to Quakers of colonial descent in Salem County, New Jersey, received a quality education in academies there. After her brother and cousins enlisted in the Union Army, she volunteered as a nurse near Gettysburg in 1863, but was denied an assignment owing to her young age of twenty-three. Determined to participate in the relief effort, she made her own way to the battlefield, quickly winning acceptance and admiration for her dedication and work ethic. In the winter of 1863–64 she traveled to Washington, D.C., and volunteered at the Contraband Hospital, shocked by the terrible conditions and scarcity of supplies.

Contraband Hospital, Washington.
November 15, 1863.

To an unnamed friend:

I shall depict our wants in true but ardent words, hoping to affect you to some action . . .

Sickness is inevitable, and to meet it these rude hospitals, only rough wooden barracks, are in use—a place where there is so much to be done you need not remain idle. We average here one birth per day, and have no baby clothes except as we wrap them up in an old piece of muslin, that even being scarce. Now the Army is advancing it is not uncommon to see from 40 to 50 arrivals in one day. They go at first to the Camp but many of them being sick from exhaustion soon come to us. They have nothing that any one in the North would call clothing.

I always see them as soon as they arrive, as they come here to be vaccinated; about 25 a day are vaccinated. This hospital is the reservoir for all cripples, diseased, aged, wounded, infirm, from whatsoever cause; all accidents happening to colored people in all employs around Washington are brought here. It is not uncommon for a colored driver to be pounded [beaten] nearly to death by some of the white soldiers. We had a dreadful case of Hernia brought in today.

A woman was brought here with three children by her side; said she had been on the road for some time, a more forlorn, worn out looking creature I never beheld. Her four eldest children are still in Slavery; her husband is dead. When I first saw her she laid on the floor, leaning against a bed, her children crying around her. One child died almost immediately; the other two are still sick. She seemed to need most, food and rest, and those two comforts we gave her, but clothes she still wants. I think the women are more trouble than the men [when asked to donate]. One of the white guards called to me to day and asked me if I got any pay. I told him no. He said he was going to get paid soon, and he would give me 5 dollars. I do not know what was running through his mind as he made no other remark.

I ask for clothing for women and children, both boys and girls.

Cornelia Hancock, Volunteer Nurse

After the war. Hancock continued in her charitable efforts and moved to South Carolina to assist in caring for newly freed slaves. With funds requisitioned from the Freedmen's Bureau and donations from the Quaker organization, Philadelphia Yearly Meeting of the Society of Friends, she founded the Laing School for Negroes in Pleasantville.

The Contraband Camp was one of the very few hospitals in Washington, D.C., that treated black patients during the war. Initially, those in posts of authority including surgeons and head nurses were white, while positions like cooks and laundresses were black, but it later became one of the only facilities whose staff was largely African American, including surgeons and nurses, clerks, stewards, and matrons. In the spring of 1863, in a revolutionary action, the first African American surgeon in charge of any U.S. hospital was appointed. Dr. Alexander Thomas Augusta was designated to break through the long-held color barrier and be acknowledged in a position of command. During the Civil War, black troops were frequently stationed in unhealthy or swampy areas, and many regiments had trouble getting competent doctors who were willing to treat them. Although most of the twelve other degreed black doctors in the country were appointed to hospitals treating blacks, none was assigned to whites-only facilities.

Residents of the Contraband hospital made up most of the nursing staff. Washington, D.C., had more hospitals and beds than any other Union city, requiring the greatest number of nurses and other hospital workers. The newly arriving fugitive slaves provided an excellent source of additional labor, and the hospital hired nurses primarily from within their population. The men and women who served as nurses at the Contraband Hospital became paid workers and, including the largest number of black surgeons working in U.S. hospitals, made up the modernized staff of hospital workers.

The black-only facility received thousands of contrabands who found sanctuary and medical care, and within a year more than 15,000 people—black soldiers, freedmen, and escaped slaves—had been treated and the camp had 685 residents on its grounds. The camp was disbanded at the end of 1863, but the hospital remained in operation, providing medical care to African American soldiers and civilians. The facility moved several times over the next year, no longer an institution under the control of the U.S. Army and now called Freedmen's Hospital. It was the first hospital in America dedicated to the treatment of former slaves. In 1865, moving to the former Campbell General Hospital, Freedmen's Hospital became an official part of the Freedmen's Bureau, or Bureau of Refugees, Freedmen, and Abandoned Lands, and was the major general hospital for the African American community in Washington, D.C. Its facilities were much improved by the move, including its water supply and waste disposal.

Following the Civil War, in 1868 Freedmen's Hospital moved to the site of Howard University, which was chartered by the United States Congress in 1867. It became the teaching hospital for the university's new medical department, and was known as Howard University Hospital. Brevet Lieutenant Colonel Alexander Thomas Augusta, M.D., formerly surgeon in charge of the Contraband Hospital and the first black hospital administrator in U.S. history, joined the faculty of the Howard University medical school, where he remained until 1877. With many honors and successes to his name, Dr. Augusta died in Washington on December 21, 1890, and was interred at Arlington National Cemetery in Arlington, Virginia.

By the end of the Civil War, 179,000 African Americans had served in the Union Army and 19,000 in the U.S. Navy. Estimates are that almost 40,000 of them died during the war, most from infection or disease. Despite their service, black troops were often consigned the more difficult camp jobs like digging trenches, were paid less than white soldiers, were frequently issued old or faulty equipment, and their medical treatment in understaffed segregated hospitals was usually inferior to that in white hospitals. Black regiments, composed of many who had been enslaved, were also known as the "Corps d'Afrique." They began active service in the Union Army in June 1863 and demonstrated a higher mortality rate and suffered from more disease throughout the war than the white troops.

The Tenth General Hospital in Beaufort, South Carolina, housed in a large home that the Union Army had appropriated, treated most of the

146 wounded African American soldiers from the Fifty-Fourth Massachusetts Volunteer Infantry Regiment who were wounded in a disastrous attempt as part of a major campaign to secure a foothold at Charleston Harbor. Their story was memorialized in the feature film *Glory*.

The Union designated specific hospitals to care for black troops, the largest of which was located at City Point, Virginia, during the siege of Petersburg. More than 3,000 patients were treated at this hospital, an institution that was short of almost every supply and material furnishing including beds. In the white hospitals, convalescing men were commonly used as nurses, although the patients recovering in the black hospitals were at a severe disadvantage for distributing medicines, as most could not read.

The site of Summit House Hospital in Philadelphia was located on Darby Road and Woodland Avenue. In 1864, all of the white patients were moved to the Satterlee General Hospital to make room for 1,200 injured and sick black troops then arriving in the city at Grays Ferry. The 522-bed Summit Hospital reopened and was designated for the treatment of African American soldiers. A fundraising fair for the "Benefit of the Sick and Wounded Black Soldiers" at Summit Hospital was held by the Ladies of St. Thomas African Episcopal Church.

Early in the Civil War, the city of Alexandria, Virginia, was seized by Union forces, becoming a safe haven for those enslaved—making it to Alexandria meant making it to freedom.

L'Ouverture Hospital in Alexandria, Virginia, named for revolutionary Haitian leader Toussaint L'Ouverture, was opened in 1864 for black troops and contraband civilians. The grounds included long canvas tents for patients, barracks, cookhouse, office, deadhouse, sutler's store, and dispensary. The hospital was outside of the divisional structure of most of the other military hospitals in the city. The facility was built to house up to 600 patients at one time, and records indicate that in 1864 and 1865, about 1,400 patients were admitted, frequently staying for weeks or months, usually due to disease.

Chaplain Chauncey Leonard at the hospital opened a school for the soldiers, which was reported to have been well attended to the point of crowding, and he pursued funding to raise a real school building for the new students. L'Ouverture Hospital stood on the same Alexandria street as a structure known as the "Slave Pen," once the site of one of the South's largest slave trading market and a place where the basement served as a holding area for enslaved people being bought and sold. The building now houses the Freedom House Museum.

Relief worker, former slave, abolitionist, teacher, and writer Harriet Jacobs was the author of the largely autobiographical book *Incidents in the Life of a Slave Girl, Written by Herself*, published in 1861 and still regarded as one of the most celebrated narratives of life in slavery. At an August 1, 1864, hospital celebration of Freedom Day, marking the emancipation of slaves in the West Indies, Harriet Jacobs made the opening remarks and presented a flag to the hospital's surgeon in charge, Dr. Thomas Crombie Barker:

Physicians, Soldiers and Friends;

For the first time in Alexandria, we have met to celebrate a day made historical in our race—the day of British West Indies Emancipation . . .

Dr. Barker in presenting this flag to you for L'Ouverture Hospital—you, the soldier's physician and friend—you, who have by your many acts so endeared yourself to all within this place; upon you and this institution I invoke the blessings of Almighty God.

Soldiers, when you return from the field of blood and strife, sick, wounded and weary, you will find a welcome here. We will bind up your wounds and administer faithfully unto you. Then take the dear old flag and resolve that it shall be the beacon of liberty for the oppressed of all lands, and of every soldier on American soil.

Harriet Jacobs was instrumental in a successful petition drive to ensure that soldiers who died at L'Ouverture were buried as military men. A cemetery for the military dead had been opened in 1863, and in the following year, the African American soldiers who were or had been patients at L'Ouverture lobbied for those who had died there, arguing that they deserved burial at the military cemetery rather than in the Contrabands and Freedmen Cemetery. They wrote a petition that was presented to the surgeon in charge and eventually to Montgomery C. Meigs, quartermaster general of the U.S. Army. As a result of those actions, African American soldiers were accorded burial in Alexandria National Cemetery, and those who had already been buried at Contrabands and Freedmen's were disinterred and reburied in the military cemetery.

> We the undersigned Convalescents of Louverture [sic] Hospital
> & its Branches and soldiers of the U.S. Army:
> As American citizens, we have a right to fight for the protection of her flag, that right is granted, and we are now sharing equally the dangers and hardships in this mighty contest, and should shair [sic] the same privileges and rights of burial in every way with our fellow soldiers who only differ from us in color . . . We ask that our bodies may find a resting place in the ground designated for the burial of the brave defenders of our countries flag.

During the Revolutionary War in America, there were very few specific institutions serving as hospitals: private homes, barns, and businesses were more commonly utilized. The Civil War encompassed the use of existing structures as hospitals and also featured a wide array of treatment facilities, originally including small privately operated hospitals. In many cases after the first year of the war, the private hospitals were ordered to shut down, as they were not under military or government regulations and considered to attract corruption and "malingerers"—soldiers wishing to avoid battle by feigning illness. A few of the private hospitals did flourish and were given permission to operate and access military medical supplies.

The Robertson Hospital of Richmond, Virginia, held the distinction of being created and maintained by a woman. With permission, Sally Tompkins turned Judge John Robertson's city home into a hospital that accepted patients throughout the war, maintained a high standard of care, and had a remarkably low death rate. It was said that wounded soldiers frequently pleaded with their officers and doctors to be sent there. Captain Sally Tompkins at age twenty-eight was the first woman officially commissioned by the Confederate States Army, although she refused payment for her services.

The only other Southern woman to be commissioned and named a captain in the Confederate Army was the proprietor of another private hospital, Lucy Mina Otey, the wife of city leader Captain John M. Otey. Mrs. Otey had a long background in charitable work: before the war, among other volunteer activities, she served as president of the Ann Norvell Orphan Asylum of Lynchburg, which had been founded by her mother. Mina Otey was sixty years of age in 1861, a passionate volunteer and organizer who eventually lost her husband, three of her seven sons, and her son-in-law in the Civil War. She created the Ladies' Relief Society in Lynchburg, Virginia, directing its 500 members in a wide array of support activities, including making bandages, writing letters for patients, and preparing and delivering food to the hospitals. Upon arriving at a hospital one morning, Mrs. Otey was confronted by Dr. William Otway Owen Sr., head of the Lynchburg military hospitals, who ordered her immediate removal from the hospitals along with all other women, reportedly stating, "no more women or flies are to be admitted."

Undeterred, she traveled to Richmond and gained an audience with President Jefferson Davis, who provided his personal permission for her to found a hospital that would be operated by female nurses. She established the independent Ladies' Relief Hospital in the old Union Hotel on Main

Street in Lynchburg, stocked with beds for 100 patients. Over the course of the war the hospital maintained one of the lowest mortality rates of the regional military hospitals and a reputation throughout the South for excellence in care and organization.

The Confederate government eventually ordered all medical institutions to be under government control. In a similar solution to that found for Sally Tompkins, and to allow Mina Otey to keep her hospital open, she was commissioned and named a captain in the Confederate Army. Mrs. Captain Otey staffed the Ladies' Relief Hospital with the 500 members of the Women's Corps, of which she was the president. Her efforts certainly elevated the women of Lynchburg, and encouraged their contributions to the war effort, although her influence had limitations with the military—when she requested that the ladies who staffed her hospital be granted officers' permission to purchase supplies from the commissary, she was denied.

Lucy Mina Otey not only provided comfort, healing, and care for many Confederate soldiers, she also created an arena where several hundred women were able to gain skills and experience in expanded roles as hospital nurses and matrons, an invaluable education and preparation for their and the country's futures.

History has not always regarded children with a kindly or benevolent eye, or accorded them the human rights of adults. In antiquity, many babies born with deformities, or unwanted females, were frequently abandoned or left to die, as infanticide by exposure was condoned by many societies. Early history reveals few documents that acknowledge specifics for treating very young patients: one of the earliest rarities, from 1552 B.C.E., is the Ebers Papyrus, which discussed topics including breastfeeding and a cure for worms. By 400 B.C.E., Hippocrates had written about some pediatric ailments and suggested treatments for children's issues including asthma, diarrhea, clubfoot, and mumps. When Western attitudes toward the value, individuality, and health care of children began to change and diversify, it became apparent that the particular needs and diseases of children required specialized actions, facilities, and treatments. One of the first known volumes on pediatric medicine to be written in English, *The Boke of Chyldren*, was published in 1544 by the Oxford-educated lawyer, author, and early pediatrician Thomas Phaire.

The genesis of hospitals specifically for the care of children can be traced to Paris, France, in the very early 18th century. A Roman Catholic vicar at the late Baroque Church of Saint Sulpice transformed an old boarding school into a small parish hospital called the Hospital of the Jesus Child. This institution in the Rue Sevres was named a Royal Foundation in 1751, and during the French Revolution was converted to the National Orphan House.

Late-18th-century Paris saw statesman and banker Jacques Necker of Geneva become the finance minister to King Louis XVI's troubled France. The accomplished, romantic, and visionary Necker and his wife, the former Swiss governess Suzanne Curchod Necker, braved shockingly filthy and impoverished venues to visit French hospitals and prisons, working to improve the health and lives of the patients and prisoners. Necker was highly influential in a movement to reform the crowded hospitals and to create smaller neighborhood treatment centers to bring health care to the larger population.

In 1778, Madame Necker founded a hospital next door to the National Orphan House. In a radical departure from common practice, she designated a separate bed for each patient.

The compassionate actions of the Neckers helped to create a permanent acceptance of the need for specialized medicine for children. The first Western hospital devoted exclusively to the care of children was established in Paris in 1801 and named in honor of the devoted Madame Suzanne Necker. Hôpital Necker-Enfants Malades boasted 250 beds and had its own gardens. The hospital admitted children of both sexes under the age of fifteen years. This, the first true pediatric hospital, would come to provide the world with important medical discoveries and inventions, including the creation of the stethoscope by physician René Laënnec in 1816. The hospital inspired the establishment of similar facilities in countries including Germany, Austria, Poland, England, and the United States.

The early children's hospitals paired social welfare with health care. They commonly admitted not only children who were ill, but also those who were abandoned, orphaned, or indigent, offering food, clothing, shelter, and spiritual guidance. It was acknowledged at this time that poverty and poor health were closely related.

Prior to the mid–19th century, America's concern for its children offered negligible attention or scientific interest. Dr. Abraham Jacobi, a German pediatrician who immigrated to New York in 1853, brought progressive and wide-ranging ideas that would result in his becoming considered the father of pediatric medicine in the United States. Dr. Jacobi founded several organizations devoted to children's health and helped to confirm the need for that specialized field of health care. Jacobi emphasized the importance of children's hygiene and of disease prevention, and he pointed out that pediatricians could also facilitate the Americanization of international immigrants by educating children and parents about how to remain healthy.

The first pediatric hospital in the United States opened in Philadelphia in 1855. The new idea of an area of medicine devoted to the youngest citizens would forever change the perspective on health care for sick and injured children. Childcare had previously been viewed as a part of obstetrics; children were treated as "little adults" and their mortality rate had always been extremely high.

Dr. Francis West Lewis, a physician from Philadelphia's Pennsylvania Hospital, had visited the newly established Great Ormond Street Hospital for Sick Children in London, and was inspired to open a small hospital of twelve beds in his own city. In its first year of operation the hospital admitted sixty-seven children and charted 821 visits to its dispensary or clinic. Children's Hospital of Philadelphia would become and remain an inspiration and a model for children's hospitals across the country.

In the 21st century, the specialty of pediatrics is regulated and certified by organizations around the world and in the United States by the American Pediatric Society and the American Academy of Pediatrics. This field of medicine has continued to evolve and expand into highly specific subspecialties and facilities that are constantly created and updated.

America's first chartered hospital, Pennsylvania Hospital in Philadelphia, a beautiful enclave of classical brick buildings and landscaped gardens, began to provide its services to the community in the mid-1700s. The hospital was the culmination of an effort begun in 1709 by the Religious Society of Friends and a part of the hospital was intentionally set apart for the treatment of the mentally ill, the first patients being admitted in 1752. One unusual feature extant since the institution first opened its doors is largely concealed today by formal plantings but still intact—a "dry moat" more than seven feet deep and four feet wide. The moat was designed as part of the treatment for mentally ill persons who were cared for at the hospital, which accepted patients both rich and poor.

The dry moat was created to offer safe exercise for the mentally ill, and the local residents were fascinated, gathering on Sundays to watch the procession of patients. The hospital administration attempted to discourage the curious voyeurism, but after failing, they began to charge the uninvited gawkers 4 pence to view the patients. The money was put into a fund for caring for those afflicted physically or for the insane.

In the United States, the establishment of state asylums for the mentally ill began in New York with a law passed in 1842. The concept of creating a state institution dedicated exclusively to the treatment of African Americans with mental illness was examined in 1844 when it was suggested by Dr. Francis T. Stribling, superintendent of the Western State Lunatic Asylum in Staunton, Virginia, that an asylum for the "negro insane" should be established. In the same year, an article was published in the *American Journal of the Medical Sciences*, stating that the sixth census of the United States appeared to indicate that insanity was more prevalent in free African

Americans than in those enslaved, although the numbers and assertions cited were later proven to be false. Physician Samuel Adolphus Cartwright, practicing in antebellum Louisiana and Mississippi, created the term "drapetomania," which he claimed was a mental illness specific to slaves that manifested itself in the form of a desire for freedom. Cartwright asserted that his mythical "drapetomania" was caused by masters who "made themselves too familiar with slaves, treating them as equals."

In 1846, the Eastern Lunatic Asylum in Williamsburg admitted mentally ill African Americans in Virginia, housing them mostly in the basement of the building, and only after white patients had been accommodated. The superintendent of the asylum, Dr. John Galt, also supported the idea that an institution committed solely to the care of African Americans should be created. By 1848 enslaved people with mental illnesses in the state of Virginia could be admitted to private asylums if their owners could pay for it, although whites were given priority of admission.

Dorothea Lynde Dix was an American heiress who, in defiance of social mores and limitations, became an extremely strong and compelling advocate on behalf of the mentally ill. During the Civil War she served as superintendent of Union Army nurses, and prior to and after the war she lobbied state legislatures and the United States Congress to establish the first generation of hospitals dedicated to the treatment of the insane. In what was considered a rare and shocking pursuit for a woman, Dix traveled internationally and to several states in America, conducting serious investigations of the treatment of the mentally ill poor and the filthy, dark, and dangerous private hospitals and prisons where those destitute individuals were neglected, ill-fed and abused.

Dorothea Dix was a driving force and a leading figure for appropriate and humane housing and treatment of the mentally ill, working both internationally and in America with state legislatures and the U.S. government to pass bills for the establishment of adequate and dedicated state facilities. In 1854 she was granted an audience with Pope Pius IX, who, although Dix was a Protestant, took her findings seriously, visited asylums to witness them for himself, and thanked her for bringing his attention to these shocking institutions and cruelly treated people. She is credited with spearheading the reform movement in America that created compassionate care and housing for the mentally ill and was instrumental in the founding or expansion of more than thirty hospitals that treated mentally disturbed patients, including the Harrisburg State Hospital, the first public mental health facility in Pennsylvania, which included a library and reading room for the patients.

A 250-bed hospital was established in Washington, D.C., through the Civil and Diplomatic Appropriation Act of 1852. The Government Hospital for the Insane, later known as St. Elizabeth's Hospital, admitted its first patients in 1855. Its founder, Dorothea Dix, had written the law that outlined the hospital's mission "to provide the most humane care and enlightened curative treatment of the insane of the Army, Navy and the District of Columbia." She was a strong proponent of the moral treatment that had emerged in France and England. The therapy required the provision of comfortable circumstances and good food for the patients, with care that was based on kindness and respect. Some patients' restraints were removed and they were encouraged to exercise and spend time in the gardens that were part of many institutions' planning. The theories proposed that if mentally ill patients were removed from harsh conditions and treated with dignity and respect, they would stand a stronger chance of recovery.

The Washington hospital was the only federal mental health facility in the United States at the dawn of the Civil War. Soldiers were referred for a condition called "nostalgia," a despair so deep that some stopped eating, became listless, and sometimes died. There is a great deal of evidence that many Civil War soldiers exhibited symptoms of what would later be termed PTSD (post-traumatic stress disorder). St. Elizabeth's Hospital continued to care for Civil War veterans with mental illness for many years and is still in use as a psychiatric hospital in Washington, D.C. Dorothea Dix, in addition to her support for the institution, was also instrumental in the creation of more than thirty hospitals for the treatment of mentally ill patients.

Howard's Grove in Virginia, a Confederate war hospital that opened in June 1862, was typical of its time, composed of one-story wooden structures. The following autumn, another hospital was built adjacent to it, although the newer institution was set aside for the treatment of smallpox in African American patients. In 1865, when the Union Army captured Richmond, Howard's Grove was made part of the Freedmen's Bureau, an organization that assisted former slaves in their transition to freedom. The Freedmen's Bureau took particular interest in care of the mentally ill and supported separate institutions for their care.

The Civil Rights Act of 1866 required that African American mental patients must be accepted by state-operated mental health institutions, but many white hospital superintendents still refused to admit them. The control of Howard's Grove was transferred from the Freedmen's Bureau to the state, and the new hospital was renamed the Central Lunatic Asylum for the Colored Insane and believed to be the world's first hospital for the treatment of mentally ill African Americans. The facility was initially described as unacceptably crude, and improvements were undertaken to provide the patients with dedicated dining rooms and new bathrooms.

In the years after the Civil War, the country saw a sharp upswing in the number of veterans suffering from mental illness. In 1866, Congress passed an act permitting the Government Hospital for the Insane to admit all former Union soldiers who had served in the Civil War, and in 1869, a dedicated institution for the care of African American patients was established by the State of Virginia.

Care of the mentally ill remains a major problem in the United States today. It is estimated that state psychiatric facilities house approximately 45,000 patients, but many sufferers still populate America's prisons and streets. The dearth of adequate long-term care options remains an acute issue in the country and the world, although passionate reformers like Dorothea Dix have made it clear that the sad circumstance is one that should remain a serious public concern.

Few men who enlisted in the Union and Confederate armies had given much thought to the concept of being captured and held as a prisoner of war. In past conflicts in the country, many prisoners received paroles, but the Civil War broke new ground in every aspect of the practice. It is estimated that more than 410,000 soldiers were captured and held by enemy armies.

Northern and Southern prisons teemed with sick and wounded men, claiming 10 percent of all deaths during the Civil War. Most of these deaths were caused by disease or starvation. Captured enemy soldiers were often held in squalid prison conditions, with barely enough food to survive. Medical care was limited or nonexistent as disease and malnutrition ravaged the prisoners, and prison conditions in both Union and Confederacy were equally deplorable. Food supplies may have been abundant in the North, but that abundance did not always reach the prisoners.

Neither Union nor Confederacy really knew how to handle the growing number of prisoners, and after an initial exchange policy attempt was unsuccessful, both sides held on to the captured soldiers. More than 150 prisons were in operation during the war, and most featured crowded, filthy conditions, minimal food or clean water, and almost nonexistent health care. There was equal neglect, mismanagement, and cruelty on the part of both governments, and an incredible amount of needless suffering and death. The prisoners became sick and depressed, frequently to the point of suicide.

Henry Clay Trumbull was an author, editor, and a state Sunday school missionary employed by the American Sunday School Union. He was ordained in 1862 in order to qualify for an Army chaplaincy. Captured by Confederates while he was ministering to the wounded in Fort

Wagner, South Carolina, he was held prisoner in the state's Richland Jail in Columbia, accused of spying.

> An order came from General Beauregard's headquarters directing me to report for service among the wounded Union soldiers in the "Yankee Hospital." At the provost-marshal's I signed a parole, by which I agreed not to attempt to escape while on this duty.
>
> Wounded Union soldiers were in a large four-story brick building. This building was said to have been originally a private dwelling, then a warehouse, and for a time a slave mart, before its use as a prison hospital.
>
> What a sight met my eye as I entered that building! Our wounded men, shot on Saturday night, had, many of them, laid where they fell until the next day, exposed to the trampling of our retreating soldiers, and to flying sand half burying them by bursting shell, some indeed being again wounded by the enemy's rifles as they lay on the field. They were brought to this "Yankee" hospital. One hundred and sixty-three of them were here. As they were brought in, they were laid in rows on straw on the floor of the long lower room. Their blood-matted hair and beards, and their blood-saturated clothing, marked their need of care that could not yet be given them. In the yard of the building back of this room were six operating-tables, at which a force of busy surgeons was constantly at work. The severely wounded were taken, one by one, from their resting place on the straw to those surgeons' tables, where they were examined and operated on. After this treatment they were removed to hospital cots on the upper floors.
>
> The Confederate surgeons did everything in their power, with the means at their command, for the safety and comfort of the wounded Union soldiers, both white and black. Sisters of Mercy

were unceasing in loving ministry to the poor men. As I went from man to man, "to pour water on him that was thirsty," and to speak words of hope and cheer to the despondent, announcing that I too was a Union prisoner, while also an army chaplain. As I took dying messages from those prisoners to their home loved ones, or knelt by them in prayer and in counsel, I knew that I was a means of comfort to the needy, and I thanked God for the privilege.

Camp Sumter, the prison at Andersonville, Georgia, became almost mythic in tales of the horrors it contained. Originally a stockade to hold captured Union Army soldiers in a 26.5-acre plot, it was designed for maintaining a maximum of 10,000 prisoners. The prison opened late in the war—February 1864—and closed eighteen months later. During the time it was open, more than 45,000 Union prisoners were held in Andersonville and almost 13,000 of them died there.

Dr. John McKinney Howell from Houston County, Georgia, was an enlisted surgeon in the Confederate Army in 1862, and served until the end of the war. In July of 1864 he was appointed acting assistant surgeon and assigned to the Union Hospital in Camp Sumter Military Prison, also simply known as "Andersonville," infamous for the hideous effects of its brief existence. In the few short months the facility had been open, 4,576 Union soldiers had already died within its walls.

When Dr. Howell first arrived in the sweltering Georgia summer heat, he could hear cries and smell sickening odors that were coming from the prison pen. The space that had been allocated for 10,000 prisoners was regularly holding a population of 28,000 to 32,000. Many of the men were wounded, all were starving, and little shelter was available to shade them from the brilliant Southern sun or the winter rains. The available water was usually contaminated, and disease was rampant among the prisoners.

Dr. Howell's letters to his wife Emma reveal his frustration and helplessness:

> Today my dearest there is no sick call—reason, no medicine . . .
> Yesterday our orders were to send to the hospital all who could not
> walk and absolutely needed medical attention . . . nine hundred
> and fifty-seven . . . Such deaths as they are—men dying in the hot
> broiling sun. To those that are prepared, what relief death must be.

The surgeon in charge of the military prison at Andersonville was Dr. Isaiah Henry White, a prominent physician and citizen of Richmond, Virginia. He and Dr. Howell were members of a medical staff of fifteen people who were responsible for caring for an average prison population of 30,000. Each surgeon was expected to examine approximately 500 prisoners per day, and was only permitted to admit 200 prisoners to the overcrowded and disorganized hospital each day. The staff had to turn away a huge number of men who clearly and desperately needed medical attention, while those who were admitted were usually the sickest or the dying. The cemetery at Andersonville was also quite crowded.

Union physician Augustus Choate Hamlin of Columbia, Maine, served as a medical inspector in the U.S. Army. He described the scene at Andersonville:

> We must consider at length the details of this enclosure, with
> its hungry, emaciate, filthy mass of humanity, whence arose a
> stench of death so powerful as to be perceived at the distance of
> a league—the burning sky, the array of instruments of torture,
> the manifest design of cruelty.

The camp hospital stood on an uphill part of the prison grounds, a makeshift shantytown of sheds and tents that contributed to the waste runoff polluting the camp's primary water source, a small stream. The hospital had minimal medical supplies and never enough to treat the huge numbers of sick and dying prisoners. Many of the dying chose to remain within the prison stockade rather than being taken to the camp hospital, preferring to die among friends and companions rather than strangers.

Dr. Austin Flint Jr., of Massachusetts, reported on the state of disease in the Andersonville Camp for the United States Sanitary Commission. He found that the overcrowding in the camp meant that each prisoner had less food and clean water, and less space in which to lie down. The exposure to disease and insects dramatically increased the number of sick, and scurvy was a serious issue, affecting large numbers of the incarcerated. He witnessed sick soldiers washing clothes in a stream that was "a semi-fluid mass of human excrement, offal, and filth of all kinds." He noted that prisoners worked as hospital staff and that the sick were observed to be "literally incrusted with dirt and covered with vermin."

After the war had ended and the prison was shut down, Dr. Isaiah White, formerly of the Confederate States Army, participated in interview investigations about the conditions and the treatment of prisoners.

> These men on their arrival were broken down physically by previous hardships, hurried marches, want of sleep, deficient rations, and exposures in all kinds of weather, by night and by day that precede and attend the hostile meeting of armies. The prisoners seldom carried from the fields a sufficiency of clothing and blankets to protect them from weather changes. The depression of spirit consequent on defeat and capture, the home-sickness of the prisoners, and the despondency caused by the thought that they had been left by their own Government in the hands of the enemy with no prospect of exchange, conspired to render every cause of disease more potent in its action, and were the main factors in the production of disease and death.

Dr. White was questioned by a reporter about the availability of medical supplies for the prison.

> We were sadly deficient in medicines, the Unites States Government having declared medicines contraband of war, and by the blockade prohibiting us from getting them abroad, we were thrown largely on the use of indigenous remedies.

In further examination, it was confirmed that Dr. White had made repeated efforts to detail the condition of the prisoners to his superiors, had continually and without success appealed for medical supplies, additional medical personnel, tents, and adequate stores for cooking. The situation of the Union facilities appears to have been similar. U.S. secretary of war Edwin Stanton reported that Federal prisoners who died in Confederate prisons numbered 22,576, and that 26,436 Confederate prisoners perished in Northern prisons.

Andersonville was the largest of the Civil War prisons and has been the subject of the greatest number of observations and memoirs; its closest Union institution was the prison camp at Elmira, New York, which had similar reported atrocities and a comparable death rate.

Andersonville National Historic site was established in 1970, remaining in the 21st century a tribute and memorial to all American prisoners of war.

CHAPTER SEVEN

THE VOLUNTEERS: GENESIS OF A GREAT HUMANITARIAN MOVEMENT

As the Civil War blasted its way into existence, creating a trail of dead and broken bodies, there was a corresponding flood of responses. All over the country, small groups of women began to organize their energies in order to do everything within their power for the relief of the sick and wounded soldiers of the war. Women wrote letters to the men at the front, sent food to the hospitals, and in every town and city, women met to "sew for the soldiers." The efforts of the ladies would ultimately help to define the landscape of aid to the victims of the enormous conflict.

The huge war permeated every aspect of life for many civilians. It was literally in the front yards and parlors of homes across America. Another unique quality of the Civil War that had not been present in previous American conflicts was that communication had become far more sophisticated. The telegraph had been invented in the 1840s and was an important tactical and operational medium for the military, which handled 6.5 million messages during the war.

The war news was far more widely available to civilians than it had ever been before. Printing had advanced significantly and two weekly publications, *Frank Leslie's Illustrated Newspaper* and *Harper's Weekly*, brought the news of the war into many homes. These newspapers hired artists and sent them to the battlefields, resulting in shocking depictions of the violence and sentimental images of homesick soldiers and grieving families. In addition to carrying the war news, the papers included games, puzzles, and serialized stories and books, many with wartime themes. Sarah Weatherwax, senior curator of Graphic Arts at The Library Company of Philadelphia, pointed out that "the war infiltrated daily life."

The war occurred at a time when color printing had come into its own and photography was becoming cheaper and more accessible. It was possible to print multiple copies of the same image and to create colorful, inexpensive ephemera: cards, pictures, paper dolls, fans, and souvenirs, many of which had patriotic themes. Ms. Weatherwax observed that these were items that "brought the Civil War home to people at home." She indicated that the memorabilia and ephemera gave a strong sense of the period—the "everydayness" of it all, even in wartime. Everyone who read the newspapers was aware of the terrible conditions of the armies, and civilians on both sides of the conflict were inspired to offer their assistance.

The Confederate government, in its infancy when the conflict erupted, struggled to keep up with the needs of its armies, as it had no government-sanctioned commissions or agencies that had been created to support the soldiers' necessities. That lack was immediately obvious to the population of the Confederate states. On the home front, many wealthy Southern women had always relied on slaves to handle the duties of home and agriculture, but as the desperation of the troops became obvious, the women were forced to reevaluate the parameters of feminine behavior and accept more of the tasks they had formerly delegated. As men, white and black, were called to serve in the Confederate army, female slaves found themselves embroiled in a huge effort to preserve daily life and were now called upon to take on heavier tasks usually handled by men while also expected to support the cause of the fighting soldiers. The more moneyed women of the South made efforts through local auxiliaries and relief societies, cooking and sewing for the soldiers. Those who could afford it provided necessities like blankets, uniforms, and supplies for the troops and opened their homes to care for the wounded. It was an effort that would reverberate through both South and North.

Frequently titled "Ladies' Aid Societies" or "Soldiers' Aid Societies," volunteer groups in support of the wounded and sick soldiers began to appear all over the country. In the face of hundreds of thousands of casualties, it was clear that neither government was able to provide adequate medical supplies, food, or clothing for the men. Many families still at home when their men left for the army were struggling to feed their children, themselves, and their livestock. The desperation of the war years dissolved many of the old social mores and political limitations that had previously dictated the paths of lives. Women began to exercise an aggressive and assertive display of solutions and contributions outside of their familiar domestic worlds. Most of the women who worked in the relief effort had never, outside of their own households, spearheaded an effort, a movement, or an organization. In a bold display of compassion and patriotism they dared to step into leadership positions and to steer their new groups in unfamiliar and dangerous but essential seas.

Those who could afford financial aid contributed their own funds and solicited additional donations; they arranged events like concerts, dances, and dinners as fundraisers. Beautiful old inherited table linens and bedsheets were offered up for making bandages and wound packing. Nourishing food was prepared and taken to the hospitals. Records in the North indicate that women created about 20,000 aid organizations; Southern history includes at least one such society in virtually every city, town, and village. In another arena where they had never before ventured, Confederate women also worked in groups to make cartridges for their troops' weapons.

One of the earliest recorded Union women's aid organizations to be formally and officially established was a group of white women in Bridgeport, Connecticut, in April 1861. Black women sometimes joined white women's volunteer relief groups if they were welcomed, but it was not always offered as a comfortable option. Another reconfiguration of the social design emerged when President Abraham Lincoln's Emancipation Proclamation went into effect on January 1, 1863. Black men from the Southern states that were still in rebellion against the United States were officially permitted and encouraged to enlist as soldiers in the U.S. Army and African American women across the country began to form their own aid societies and relief organizations to support the men.

Black women faced a double serving of oppression for both their gender and their race, but they also exhibited remarkable strength and resilience in taking on essential roles in the newly changing landscape that was reflecting the advancement of women and of African Americans. Despite obstacles like limited mobility, illiteracy, and the captivity of enslavement, they worked to create networks to serve the needs of the black community and to elevate people out of oppression. Their roles were redefined and empowered during the Civil War as they created numerous support societies including the Ladies' Union Bazaar Association, Colored Ladies Soldiers' Aid Society of St. Louis, Missouri, and The Colored Women's Sanitary Commission. They collected supplies, raised funds, volunteered as teachers, and formed sewing groups, asserting themselves as powerful sources of assistance and relief. Their activism played a major role in providing for the care of black soldiers and for the transformation to freedom of untold thousands of Southern African Americans.

The Ladies' Refugee Aid Society of Kansas was formally founded in 1864 in Lawrence, Kansas, by black freedwomen, becoming the first known official soldiers' aid society in the West to be organized by African American women. It was followed by the Kansas Federation of Colored Women's Clubs, which was actually an umbrella organization for a number of state women's groups. The Kansas societies' goals were to provide food and shelter and physical and spiritual care for former slaves fleeing the dangerous tyranny in slave-owning states like Arkansas and Missouri. The resourcefulness, dedication, and passion of these women in wartime was a force that lit fires that could not be extinguished.

Sattira "Sattie" Douglas, born in 1840 to Alfred and Maria Steele, a free black middle-class Illinois couple, was provided with a good education and showed an early passion for abolitionism. She strongly supported the Union in the Civil War, and her husband, H. Ford Douglas, an outspoken abolitionist and one of the editors of Canadian newspaper *The Provincial Freeman*, served the Union in the Ninety-Fifth Illinois Regiment. Sattie Douglas frequently authored letters to newspapers, arguing for equal rights and encouraging enlistment and fundraising for black Canadians. She was a primary organizer of the Colored Soldier's Aid Society of Chicago, a teacher working with freed slaves, and she was also an organizer who assisted in the establishment of many confederations dedicated to helping and providing support to African Americans in Chicago and the American West.

Elizabeth Hobbs Keckley purchased her own freedom and that of her son George Kirkland for $1,200 in 1855 (comparable to $33,330 in 2020 USD) and moved to Washington, D.C. She had spent more than thirty years in slavery in Dinwiddie County, Virginia, and survived multiple beatings, whippings, and rapes. Her mother, Agnes, was a slave on the plantation of Colonel Armistead Burwell, and Elizabeth's father was the plantation owner, but despite her parentage, Elizabeth remained enslaved. She learned to sew at the age of three, later developing into an expert seamstress and brilliant designer, and it was her dressmaking talent that finally allowed her to earn the money to buy her freedom. In 1860 she moved to Washington, D.C., and established a dressmaking business with clients who included Jefferson Davis's wife, Vanna Davis, and Mary Anna Custis Lee, the wife of Robert E. Lee. Her designs and technique were beautiful and meticulous, her business flourished and at one time she employed twenty seamstresses. At the start of the Civil War she was working in Washington, D.C., where her principal client was Mary Todd Lincoln, the wife of the president. Elizabeth designed many dramatic and exquisitely made gowns for the First Lady.

Theirs began as a business relationship, but Elizabeth Keckley and Mary Todd Lincoln provided strong support for each other and bonded in mourning over the recent deaths of both of their sons—William "Willie" Wallace Lincoln died of typhoid fever in 1862 at age eleven, and Elizabeth's only child, George Kirkland, having joined the Union forces, was killed at Wilson's Creek in Missouri in 1861, his first battle.

Keckley was concerned about the former slaves, or "contrabands," who were fleeing in droves to the relative safety of Washington, D.C. during the war. Her memoir, *Behind the Scenes, or, Thirty Years a Slave, and Four Years in the White House*, published in 1868, revealed her original concept for a support organization:

> If the white people can give festivals to raise funds for the relief
> of suffering soldiers, why should not the well-to-do colored
> people go to work to do something for the benefit of the suffering
> blacks? I could not rest. The thought was ever present with me,
> and the next Sunday I made a suggestion in the colored church,
> that a society of colored people be formed to labor for the benefit
> of the unfortunate freedmen. The idea proved popular, and in
> two weeks "the Contraband Relief Association" was organized,
> with forty working members.

The Contraband Relief Association, headed by Keckley and beginning in 1862, collected funds, food, and clothing for impoverished former slaves and worked to find them shelter. Upon learning of the plan, the First Lady donated $200 (about $7,000 in today's dollars) and included Elizabeth on a trip to New York and Boston, where the dressmaker and designer met more people, white and black, who were interested in supporting her organization.

She raised an impressive amount of funding for the association on the trip, including a $200 gift from famed social reformer and abolitionist Mr. Frederick Douglass. In 1864, after African Americans began serving in the United States Colored Troops, the name of the group was changed to the Ladies' Freedmen and Soldier's Relief Association. In addition to supporting the soldiers, the women continued their efforts to assist recently released or escaped slaves, people considered "contraband" because they had been deemed by the Confederacy not to be legally free and were considered to be "seized property of war."

The association used the local independent African American churches for their events and meetings, hosting fundraisers, concerts, and speeches. Elizabeth Keckley convinced prominent blacks including Frederick Douglass; John Sella Martin, a pastor in Boston who had escaped slavery; and minister, educator, and orator Henry Highland Garnet, as well as noted white abolitionist Wendell Phillips to support them. The group hosted Christmas dinners for the sick and injured soldiers in local hospitals, shared food with other organizations, and were instrumental in placing African American teachers in the new schools for blacks.

Three years after the Civil War, Elizabeth Keckley wrote and published her autobiography, in which she included descriptions of her enslaved past, but the book met with mixed responses owing to the information she revealed about the Lincolns' private lives. She continued to support herself by dressmaking and in 1892 accepted the offer of a faculty position as head of the Department of Sewing and Domestic Science Arts at Wilberforce University in Ohio. Upon her retirement, suffering from the effects of a mild stroke, she returned to Washington, D.C., and lived at an institute she had helped to found, the National Home for Destitute Colored Women and Children, until her death in 1907.

Those who knew Elizabeth Keckley remembered her cultured, polished intelligence and her artistic gifts. She was an invaluable catalyst in helping the black community to achieve autonomy and in encouraging intra-ethnic networking. Her spirit and passion for freedom and equality affected untold thousands of freed blacks and invited white supporters to the movement. Her association was one of the first organizations in the United States created by and for African Americans.

Black women and white women devoted their efforts to every level of work, from rolling bandages to organizing fundraising events. Ladies began to appear in venues where they had never before been seen: hospitals, administrative offices, and on the battlefield.

All throughout the North and South women were organizing compassionate efforts to support their fighting men and those at home who were devastated by the violence and losses. In Tennessee, Mrs. Felicia Grundy Porter set up a Women's Relief Society that grew to serve the entire Confederacy. The Contraband Relief Society in Washington, D.C., addressed the provision of food and clothing to former slaves fleeing to Union camps. Women of all ages on both sides of the war worked to feed and care for the soldiers, and to encourage their spirits. Mrs. D. Giraud Wright, a Confederate senator's daughter, was the former Louise Wigfall, and remembered her teenage volunteer participation in relief measures.

> Charlottesville is in a whirl of excitement and the ladies go in crowds to the depot to assist the wounded, who come in train after train. We are all going this afternoon laden with icewater, buttermilk, etc., to see what we can do, as upwards of four or five thousand are expected.

The Ladies' Union Aid Society of St. Louis, Missouri (L.U.A.S.), was formally established on August 2, 1861. Initially getting together in the homes of the founding members, the group became quite large and began to meet weekly in the military hospital in downtown St. Louis in order to go over reports from the hospitals and to plan their support activities.

When the hospitals of the city were inundated with shockingly huge numbers of wounded, the members of L.U.A.S. worked to help care for them, and provided burial expenses for those who would not be going home. The women raised large amounts of money to support the group's expenses and some of them went into the field personally to provide nursing services. Two of the L.U.A.S. members who worked directly on the battlefields, Mrs. Margaret Breckinridge and Mary Palmer, died of conditions termed exhaustion, and other members suffered wounds and frostbite.

At home, the ladies strove to bring comfort to the men who were convalescing in fourteen of St. Louis's hospitals. They made gift baskets for the soldiers, some of which might contain fresh bread and fruit, clothing, eyeglasses, and books to read.

L.U.A.S. members petitioned the Western Sanitary Commission, a separate but similar association to the United States Sanitary Commission, to support the manufacture of clothing for the men. Receiving $5,000 from the Commission, they arranged to sew 75,000 garments and hired soldiers' wives who needed the income to do the sewing. Their work did not go unheralded, and they subsequently received a $6,000 contract from the medical purveyor to produce an additional 128,000 pieces of clothing as well as an order for 261,000 yards of bandages.

In 1864, the Ladies' Union Aid Society collaborated with the Western Sanitary Commission to hold a fundraising Sanitary Fair for the benefit of the hospitals and the wounded soldiers then being shuttled through St. Louis. Although the Western Sanitary Commission's committee chairs were mostly men, it was acknowledged that the women of L.U.A.S. did most of the actual preparation and personally worked in the booths during the event. The Mississippi Valley Sanitary Fair and its popular range of exhibits was open from May 17 to June 18, 1864, and raised $550,000 (worth almost $9.7 million in 2021 U.S. dollars). The newspapers noted that the most popular kiosk had been a fortune-telling booth called "The Delphic Oracle."

The Southern citizens' volunteer efforts resounded across the Confederacy—small soldiers' aid societies sprang up in every city and town. One organization in Charleston, South Carolina, was focused on blockade running to procure the medications that their wounded and sick needed so desperately. The Union's naval blockade was also a target for daring sailors in Wilmington, North Carolina, who managed to bring some desperately needed supplies in and out of Southern ports while navigating under the guns of Union vessels. It was said that wounded Confederate soldiers passing through any Southern town would be welcomed, fed, and cared for by the custom of families in private homes who would take in convalescent soldiers. Volunteer organizations distributed Bibles and religious tracts with the intention of providing hope in a very discouraging situation.

The scarcity of money and men that was beginning to devastate the South did not allow it to create such a well-organized and powerful organization as the North was able to do. Despite the dedication and patriotism of the Southern civilians, the Confederacy, owing to its far smaller population, had nothing that could equal the gigantic civilian volunteer response from the North, the United States Sanitary Commission.

Virtually every American family was touched by the war, and in the North, private citizens rallied to a volunteer effort in huge numbers. Women organized thousands of small groups dedicated to supporting the Army, and in 1861 a preliminary meeting was held at the New York Infirmary for Women where Unitarian minister Henry Whitney Bellows addressed more than fifty female attendees. That initial gathering led to a far larger meeting in New York in April 1861 at the Cooper Union for the Advancement of Science and Art, a distinguished institution of higher education. The meeting attracted between 3,000 and 4,000 women and became the foundation of the Women's Central Association of Relief. Katharine Prescott Wormeley was a passionate supporter of the women's participation.

As the men mustered for the battlefield, so the women mustered in churches, school-houses, and parlors. Time and the Sanitary Commission were to show that by a great united effort their work was to broaden out into a fundamental good to the whole army, that lives were to be saved, the vital force protected; and that women were to bear no small part.

The earliest of these associations of women was formed within fifteen days after the President's call for seventy-five thousand men.

The women had a passionate desire to help the condition of the soldiers, but there was a lack of hard information or a direct connection to the government. Finally, the dire situation of the U.S. troops became fully apparent with the devastation from the First Battle of Bull Run on July 21, 1861, a loss that illuminated the Union Army's disastrous lack of medical supplies and organized rescue and evacuation plans and sanitation concerns. New York City's leaders and activists from sectors of the civic to the medical joined the wave of action to provide civilian support for the government and the military.

A variety of plans for initiatives were discussed, and the association leadership began to shift from the women to the men, and acquired a new name while promoting similar goals of support, although much expanded. The work of the new United States Sanitary Commission would create improved opportunities for women throughout the war and afterward, both paid and volunteer, giving them previously unavailable and valuable experience in business, administration, and the medical field. Through the Sanitary Commission and other volunteer organizations, women were able to work openly for the relief movement.

With no precise consensus for the goals and structure of a new organization reached among the participants, a delegation traveled to Washington in May 1861. "A Commission of Inquiry and Advice in respect of the Sanitary Interests of the United States Forces" was appointed to work with the U.S.

War Department and Medical Bureau. With the approval of Secretary of War Edwin Stanton and President Abraham Lincoln, the United States Sanitary Commission was officially established. The Reverend Henry Whitney Bellows was appointed president, Alexander Dallas Bache, a powerful voice in American science, was vice president, and prominent New York attorney George Templeton Strong was named treasurer.

The small ladies' aid groups had snowballed and morphed into larger organizations that now made up the United States Sanitary Commission, the private civilian relief association that operated across the North, focusing on supporting sick and wounded soldiers and targeting areas where the government could not effectively provide. It obtained supplies, provided food, raised funds, inspected army camps, and instructed troops on the importance of hygienic conditions. A strong focus of the Commission was the sanitary condition of the troops and educating the military and the government on the importance of health and cleanliness. The organization sought to bring supplemental relief in a variety of ways, including staffing field hospitals and organizing and sponsoring huge public events that raised millions of dollars. The main objective was for the Commission to work with the U.S. War Department to provide medical supplies and care for wounded and sick Union soldiers. The Commission also planned to train nurses who would work in the military hospitals. It was a revolutionary effort and it was the only civilian-led organization that was recognized by the federal government.

Much of the design of the Sanitary Commission was inspired by the successful work of Florence Nightingale in the Crimean War, although Nightingale's efforts were supported and funded by the British government. The U.S. Sanitary Commission did not receive its finances from the federal government, instead soliciting donations of cash and supplies from private citizens at home, insurance companies, and other businesses. Its work was also supported by the smaller soldiers' aid societies and the fundraising Sanitary Fairs that were held in many large cities.

The work of the Commission extended across the Union and eventually provided care, food, and lodging for those soldiers returning from service at the fronts. They worked to create and distribute pamphlets about sanitary practices for army camps and helped veterans to apply for benefits and pensions. Delegates of the U.S.S.C. were empowered to advise on matters concerning the health of their volunteer forces, the inspection of recruits, and the provision of cooks, nurses, and other workers for the military hospitals.

Upon the official establishment of the Commission in Washington, D.C., the U.S. government agreed to provide a room in the city for the use of the new organization. The distinguished landscape architect Frederick Law Olmsted, the designer of New York City's Central Park, was chosen first as resident secretary, later as general secretary.

Olmsted, born in Hartford, Connecticut, in 1822, became known to many as the father of American landscape architecture and was lauded for his high standard of excellence. Olmsted designed or codesigned city parks across America from Buffalo, New York, and Detroit, Michigan, to Berkeley, California. In Washington, D.C., he worked on the Capitol Building's surrounding landscape.

An ardent abolitionist who examined the effects of slavery on the social structure and economy of the South, Olmsted was also a prolific journalist. He was commissioned by the *New York Daily Times* (now *The New York Times*) to travel through the Southern states and from 1852 to 1857 he sent detailed dispatches of his observations of the antebellum South. His articles were eventually collected into three volumes: *A Journey in the Seaboard Slave States*, *A Journey Through Texas*, and *A Journey in the Back Country in the Winter of 1853–4*.

> My own observation of the real condition of the people of our
> Slave States, gave me . . . an impression that the cotton monopoly
> in some way did them more harm than good, and although

the written narration of what I saw was not intended to set this forth, upon reviewing it for the present publication, I find the impression has become a conviction.

New York City's Central Park was one of Olmsted's grand projects: a team effort with the more experienced English architect Calvert Vaux, and a concept that supported Olmsted's belief that all citizens should have access to a common green space that is not subject to private development. His vision was revolutionary at the time, and formed the basis for the future planning of public parks and urban park systems.

Olmsted was serving in the position of superintendent of works of Central Park when the Civil War broke out. Unable to enlist in the army as a result of an 1860 carriage accident that left him permanently disabled, he took leave of his New York responsibilities to accept the duties of coordinating the administration of the United States Sanitary Commission. He moved to Washington, D.C., where he structured a medical effort for the relief of the sick and wounded and became actively involved with major efforts of the Commission including supplying hospital ships for the Union Army and organizing a fair that raised more than $1 million for the relief effort. He coordinated the distribution of donations to the Commission and supplied U.S.S.C. support personnel throughout the Union Army.

Patterned on the British Sanitary Commission, which had been formed in the 1850s to clean up the dregs of the Crimean War, the U.S. Sanitary Commission organized volunteer branches in many cities. The Commission arranged for examinations of troops, camps, and medical facilities, and found unsanitary conditions and poor diet everywhere. They began a traveling outpost with the Army of the Potomac to speed the delivery of sanitary supplies to its field hospitals. Due to government shortages, the Sanitary Commission provided the majority of medical supplies to the battlefields of Antietam, Fredericksburg, Chancellorsville, and the Second Battle of Bull Run.

The volunteers of the U.S. Sanitary Commission dedicated themselves to filling the gaps and voids in the Union's wartime machine. The volunteer Western Sanitary Commission, a related organization in St. Louis, specialized in establishing and equipping hospitals. The Northwestern branch of the Sanitary Commission created a goal of preventing scurvy among the soldiers by collecting and transporting fresh vegetables to the camps and hospitals. Nationwide branches of the organization in larger cities coordinated the efforts of their smaller local aid societies. The United States Sanitary Commission volunteers supplemented the efforts of the Medical Bureau and provided invaluable support at no cost to the federal government, basing all of their efforts on donations and fundraising.

The Commission requested a draft of powers from President Lincoln and Secretary of War Edwin Stanton, successfully lobbying for changes to be instituted by the government for the improvement of conditions regarding the health of Union soldiers:

> The general object of the Commission is . . . to bring to bear
> upon the health, comfort, and morale of our troops, the fullest
> and ripest teachings of Sanitary Science in its application to
> military life.

In 1862 and 1864, the Commission provided and staffed hospital ships to evacuate the sick and wounded of the Army of the Potomac. In response to thousands of civilian letters inquiring about dead, wounded, and missing soldiers, members of the Commission began a hospital directory that included the names of the patients in every general hospital. Members also collected food, clothing, bedding, and financial contributions and commissioned and distributed pamphlets on sanitation and hygiene. During its existence, the United States Sanitary Commission raised an estimated $15 million in cash and collected supplies of immeasurable value. A volunteer summed up the impact of some of the fundraising events sponsored by the U.S.S.C.

The history of the great enterprise popularly called "Sanitary Fairs," forms one of the most curious and characteristic chapters of American life. The great instincts of patriotism and humanity have been successfully appealed to.

The outpouring of compassion gave rise to even larger relief efforts, notably the fundraising "Sanitary Fairs" in cities including New York, Chicago, Boston, St. Louis, Cincinnati, Cleveland, and Philadelphia. Individual fairs frequently raised over $1 million to improve the hygienic habits of the troops and the deplorable condition of the camps.

The Sanitary Fairs were some of the most successful philanthropic, humanitarian efforts in American history. Organized by civilians, they were a combination of grand-scale expositions, bazaars, and entertainment venues. The fairs ran for weeks and were hugely popular fundraisers for the benefit of soldiers' relief and support, making possible a patriotic way for those who could not serve in the military to contribute to the cause.

The Sanitary Fairs were a means for citizens to provide a communal event in support of the medical care of wounded and sick Union soldiers, and each city worked to outdo the others with lavish displays and exciting events. They featured art exhibits, musical performances, games, parades, and auctions, and usually lasted from ten days to two or three weeks. They were run by the U.S.S.C.'s regional auxiliaries and took place in large cities between 1863 and 1865. Many of the fairs published a daily newsletter for distribution to attendees announcing the schedules and times for theatrical acts, dances, cattle shows, and exhibitions. They stirred a patriotic fervor and positive excitement among the population, and donations of every kind poured in. Chicago was the first city to hold a fair, calling it the "Northwestern Soldier's Fair" and raising more than $80,000 (with a relative worth of more than $2.6 million today) in its two-week run.

The contributions to the Fair, to be sold for the benefit of our sick and wounded soldiers, were large. The farmers from miles around kept streaming in with their wagons by hundreds, loaded down with their farm produce; others came leading horses, or driving before them cows, or oxen, or mules which they contributed; others brought live poultry. Some wagons were loaded with butter and cheese by the ton. The mechanics brought their machines—mowing machines, reapers, threshing machines, pumps; and nails by the hundred kegs—and plate glass, hides, and cases of boots, native wine in casks—a steam-engine made by the working-men in Chicago.

Loaded wagons came in long processions, bearing marks of frontier service, and most of them told of war.

The success of Chicago's fair inspired New Yorkers to organize a similar event, and Sanitary Fairs followed in many Union cities, fostering a spirit of friendly competition. The largely female-run events publicly established the ability of women to function in business and to do battle from the home front. They gave women valuable experience as organizers and managers as well as the inspiration to prepare for taking a larger role in business and society after the war. The president of the United States Sanitary Commission announced in August 1865 that the funds raised at the fairs had been crucial to the Commission's work in supporting hospitals and troops throughout the war.

Women responded by the thousands to volunteer for work with the Sanitary Commission. Taking on brand-new roles for their gender, and frequently treading in unfamiliar territory, women provided service at field hospitals and Army camps. Receiving rudimentary training onsite, they worked as nurses and served as assistant caretakers with the ill and wounded, taking on tasks they had never before imagined doing. Some women worked as fundraisers and managers within the organization, and some actually became paid employees. The U.S. Sanitary Commission provided opportunities for women as professionals and wage earners, and many of the women volunteers found paying work after the war, utilizing the skills and confidence they had gained. Women were acquiring a new sense of their own value without compromising their femininity. They were learning that they could organize, administer, handle business, and save lives.

General Secretary Frederick Law Olmsted of the Sanitary Commission found himself working side by side with many privileged white women who became strong supporters of the organization and developed into leaders themselves in the process. British-born Katharine Prescott Wormeley, a resident of Newport, Rhode Island, and one of the best-known translators of French literature in her time, joined the Newport Women's Union Aid Society at the start of the war. The following year she volunteered with the Sanitary Commission and became a superintendent of nursing, working closely with Olmsted and serving on hospital ships. She spent a great deal of time in Virginia with the Peninsular Campaign and, as a fundraising effort, she wrote *The United States Sanitary Commission: A Sketch of its Purposes and its Work*, a history of the organization. She also published a collection of her letters after the war, titled *Letters from Headquarters during the Peninsular Campaign: The Other Side of War*, and remained involved in nursing as head nurse at the army hospital at Portsmouth Grove in Rhode Island.

The war created a huge void in the workforce of the nation and in the families at home. It also created a great need and opportunity for women to step into leadership roles.

Some of the few American women holding medical degrees joined in the relief effort. Dr. Elizabeth Blackwell, the first woman to graduate from an American medical school, was a strong believer in the power and energy of women's groups. Blackwell had worked with her sister, Dr. Emily Blackwell, in founding the New York Infirmary for Women and Children and in publicizing and stressing the importance of education for girls. She brought her gifts and strengths to the Civil War relief movement in 1861, recruiting female volunteers and endeavoring to create a huge nationwide network of trained nurses to work with the wounded.

Blackwell's early efforts to establish the Women's Central Association of Relief (W.C.A.R.) in New York were met with resistance from the male-led United States Sanitary Commission, which was not supportive of a relief organization headed by women and particularly not if it involved the notoriously volatile Blackwell sisters. Elizabeth's description as a strong and very critical personality kept her interpersonal and business relations on a rocky footing, and she even had a serious falling out with her British friend, nursing reformer Florence Nightingale. The W.C.A.R. was eventually absorbed by the Sanitary Commission, but Blackwell still managed to arrange for the New York Infirmary to work with the pioneer Dorothea Dix to train nurses for the North's relief movement. Their combined efforts educated large numbers of nurses in medical techniques, sanitation, and hygiene. These trained nurses were an invaluable addition to the Union's medical teams and improved the quality of battlefield and hospital care for thousands of soldiers.

Dr. Blackwell's difficult disposition was not a hindrance to her impressive body of work and legacy of positive change, which finally did earn her the respect of the medical community. A passionate activist for her entire life, after the war she continued to lead and participate in reform movements including medical education, sanitation and hygiene, preventative medicine, women's suffrage, and family planning. She was a beacon for countless other 19th-century women choosing to study medicine in America, England, and Wales.

The United States Christian Commission, an important support organization working for the relief effort, was founded in New York in 1861 in response to the devastation of the troops in the First Battle of Bull Run. The military and civilians had accorded little attention to the spiritual and emotional needs of the troops before the war, but it became apparent that an opportunity existed to devote an organization to their psychological and spiritual well-being. A joint effort of the Young Men's Christian Association (Y.M.C.A.) and Protestant ministers, the Christian Commission furnished supplies, medical services, and religious support and literature to Union troops.

The Commission provided Protestant chaplains and social workers to contribute to "the spiritual and temporal welfare of soldiers and sailors" and to serve without payment. They were supported by five thousand volunteers or "delegates" who included seminary students and concerned Christian civilians. Their original plan was to assist the military clergy in their daily work, as the existing clergy and chaplaincy program (with only thirty members) was overwhelmed by deaths and casualties on an incredible scale. The delegates of the Christian Commission dove into the void and were soon found on many battlefields, assisting at medical stations and providing food, supplies, and Bibles to the men.

> The Commission gives help that saves life and relieves anguish
> on the field and in the hospital.
> The work begins while the battle rages. The delegate assists
> in gathering the wounded from the field, even under the guns
> of the enemy if need be, and at the hospitals assists the surgeons at
> the amputating table, or strips off the bloody garments from the
> mangled men, washes them, and puts clean clothes upon them,
> or prepares and gives food or drink to them.

Members of the Commission found themselves in completely unfamiliar locations and situations, performing tasks amid extreme violence and bloodshed. These civilians were relying on their faith and continuing to offer any possible assistance to the wounded men. The delegates were onsite at major battles including Antietam, in Washington County, Maryland, in September 1862.

Several of our delegates with four ambulances loaded with stores and medicines, arrived at Antietam in advance of any other stores, at a time when the destitution was almost entire, and the calls for aid overwhelming. At the same time, delegates were sent from Philadelphia and Baltimore, until there were over seventy Christian men at work upon these battlefields, and among the hospitals.

Some of them worked all day during the battle of Antietam, the shells often passing over the place, doing whatever good sense, sympathy, and Christian love could suggest; dressing wounds; giving nourishment and stimulants to sustain the men; bathing them, taking their last messages and tokens of love, praying by the dying, and pointing to Jesus.

After the battles, they sought out the wounded, aided in bringing them in, and in many cases, buried the dead with their own hands. Some of them were the means of great comfort, by finding the bodies of the dead, and bringing home some mementoes from them.

The Commission's beliefs included a focus on fresh food and a varied diet as part of the process of enhancing spiritual and emotional benefits. Annie Turner Wittenmyer was a wealthy widow living in Keokuk, Iowa, when the war began. A lifelong philanthropist and reformer, Mrs. Wittenmyer organized the Keokuk Soldiers' Aid Society, later becoming its secretary, visited Army camps, and coordinated a statewide system for collecting hospital supplies from local aid associations. She garnered notice and respect, inspiring Union secretary of war Edwin Stanton to issue an unusual order in July 1862, stating:

Permission is hereby given to Mrs. Annie Wittenmyer, Special Agent of the Iowa Sanitary Association, to pass with such goods as she may have in charge, to add within the lines of any of the

Armies of the Departments of Kansas and of the Mississippi,
for the purpose of visiting the sick and wounded soldiers of the
Iowa Regiments in either of those Armies.

Encountering disagreements between the Keokuk organization and
the Iowa Army Sanitary Commission, Annie chose to devote her relief
work to the U.S. Christian Commission, where she focused on developing
special diet kitchens, the first such facilities in Union Army hospitals. The
Commission supported her concept and the first kitchen was created in
Nashville, Tennessee. Her intention was to provide improvement in the
health of soldiers who seemed to be dying from inadequate nutrition, and
also to train women interested in missionary work who might then be able
to gain access to working in hospitals. The new "lady managers" met with
a great deal of initial resistance to their presence and their plans, but by the
end of the war they had created almost 100 diet kitchens in large military
hospitals and the Union Army Medical Department had incorporated
Mrs. Wittenmyer's ideas as a necessary part of healing. The kitchens also
represented a new opportunity for women to work in an area outside of
nursing and home front fundraising. After the war Annie Wittenmyer wrote
about her experiences in her book, *Under the Guns: A Woman's Reminiscences of the Civil War,* and continued her reform work. Concerned with the
orphans of soldiers killed in the war, she founded orphanages, requesting
that the government donate the then unused army barracks in Davenport,
Iowa, for use as a home for children orphaned by the war. Secretary of War
Stanton again supported her by applying to Congress for bed linens, pillows,
and other items to provide comfort at the orphans' home, and Congress
approved the transfer of the camp and its equipment to the Iowa Soldiers'
Orphans Association in January 1866. She also lobbied Congress for a bill
granting pensions for nurses who had served in the Civil War.

The Christian Commission worked to improve the soldiers' morals as
well as their physical conditions, finding them to be related. The U.S.C.C.

delegates distributed tens of thousands of Bibles, religious books, tracts, and newspapers, and they purchased copies of popular magazines to be sent to the men. The volunteers established reading rooms stocked with recent newspapers in the permanent Army camps and furnished the soldiers with writing materials and postage stamps, encouraging them to send letters home to their families and to hopefully send part of their pay.

The Commission competed with the sutlers who sold liquor by setting up coffee wagons near the camps. They procured steam-powered machines that were said to be able to prepare 1,200 cups per hour. The wagons could travel at eight miles per hour through rows of tents and stretchers, a journey both novel and welcome. The president of the Christian Commission, George Stuart, was very proud of the work of the coffee wagons:

> How many lives of men wet, muddy, battle-worn, lying down
> on the ground, without shelter or fire, have been saved by the
> hot draught of coffee thus administered to them?

The Commission sought to "bring men to Christ," providing pastoral care and assisting in arranging worship services to further their mission of improving the state of men's souls. They became particularly adept at helping to construct chapels in the Army camps and offered prayer services in hospitals and battlefield regiments. Delegates were sent to the South for six weeks at a time to distribute millions of religious tracts and hymn books, organize Bible studies, preach sermons, and engage in religious conversation with the soldiers. They sought to comfort new recruits to the Army: young men who were frightened, confused, and homesick at finding themselves in a foreign and hostile environment.

Over the course of the war, the United States Christian Commission estimated that its expenses including the supplies it provided were in excess of $6.25 million (worth more than $110 million today).

Both of the civilian relief organizations, the United States Sanitary Commission and the United States Christian Commission, were essential to the Northern war effort. They analyzed the situations and conditions that the government could not address, created viable solutions to problems, and raised their own funding to support their work. Their philosophies and areas of interest and strength were different, but they proved that civilians could support their armies and their government and that, despite any adversity, humanitarian motivations are the actions that truly make a difference.

One of the most honored women in American history, Clarissa Harlowe Barton, who preferred to be called "Clara," was born on Christmas Day 1821 in Oxford, Massachusetts, the youngest of five children. Her father, Captain Stephen Barton, was a successful businessman and community leader who had served in the Indian wars and regaled his children with stories of his wartime service. When Clara was eleven, her brother David fell from the rafters during a barn raising, suffering serious injuries, and the young girl became his devoted nurse for the next two years, forgoing school in order to care for him. She was acutely shy and timid, but took full responsibility for her brother's care, administering his medicines, even applying and removing the leeches his doctor recommended for "bleeding" him as part of the treatment. David Barton eventually recovered with the help of a "steam doctor" who treated him with vapor baths, and he grew up to serve as an assistant quartermaster with the rank of captain for the Union Army during the Civil War.

Clara's devoted nursing experience seems to have stayed with her and stirred a desire to heal and comfort. It was likely the touchstone that sparked her dedication to humanitarian work, although her timid nature was a hindrance. It was suggested to Clara's mother that in order to cure her excessive shyness, her daughter should train as a teacher.

Clara Barton proved to be popular as a teacher, and after several years she enrolled at the Clinton Liberal Institute to enhance her own education. She then moved to Bordentown, New Jersey, where she opened a free public school, attracting about 200 pupils. The success of her school was such that the community became involved and, to her surprise, hired a man to run it at twice Clara's salary. Declaring that she would never work for a lesser amount than a man received, she resigned from teaching and moved to Washington, D.C., in 1854.

Clara Barton was hired as a recording clerk at the United States Patent Office in Washington, becoming their first female clerk, and was paid $1,400 annually, which was the same amount her male colleagues received. She was the first woman ever appointed to such a post, and met some serious opposition from her coworkers, especially for her outspoken stance on abolitionism. Her job was reduced and her salary lowered, then finally her position was eliminated and she went home to Massachusetts.

After the election of Abraham Lincoln in 1860, she returned to Washington and to the Patent Office as a copyist. When the Civil War began, her fierce desire to help with the effort led her to make an offer to her superiors at the Patent Office. She suggested that she would do the work of two clerks, but draw only her original salary for one, in order that more men could be released to fight for the war effort. Her offer was refused, so Clara resigned and dedicated herself to service for the relief endeavor.

The city was quickly flooded with units of the first, newly recruited federal troops and the residents of Washington were besieged with a chaotic display of thousands of men in uniform, hungry, without bedding or spare clothing, and many were already wounded.

Her initial efforts were to collect and distribute supplies for the troops—food, clothing, medicine—and to tend to the wounded. She wrote to friends in New Jersey, New York, and Massachusetts asking them to help in the relief effort and soon built up a network of volunteer suppliers and donors who remained involved throughout the war. As the newly recruited soldiers poured into Washington, she ran into many she knew personally, including some of "her boys" whom she had previously taught in her classrooms.

Clara Barton provided a wide range of supplies and services to the Union troops on behalf of volunteer organizations including the U.S. Sanitary Commission, but she never formally aligned herself with any specific agency or group. She took the suffering of the soldiers personally, and strove to provide comfort and support in hopes of keeping their spirits up. She wrote letters for the soldiers, read to them, listened to their thoughts and problems, and prayed with them.

Moved by the plight of the war wounded, she received permission to go to the battlefields as a nurse, and often followed the Army into action. Barton considered herself to be a "relief worker" and supply organizer rather than a nurse. She worked as a fundraiser and had a special interest in finding lost individuals. She was present at many battles, including Second Bull Run, Antietam, Fredericksburg, and the siege of Charleston, and the troops called her the "Angel of the Battlefield." Clara provided nursing care and supplies to the Union troops from 1861 to 1865. She received a military pass from U.S. surgeon general William Hammond that allowed her to go inside military lines in order to provide care to the soldiers.

After the terrible Union defeat at the First Battle of Bull Run in July 1861, she was among the first volunteers to tend to the wounded as they poured into Washington, D.C. She knew that the worst suffering was occurring on the battlefields, and she was intent on bringing supplies and relief to the sites. Military regulations and long-held societal mores were restricting the field hospital staffs to male-only personnel, but she was determined to deliver aid directly to those who needed it most.

Clara Barton appealed to the government for permission to execute another idea and finally she and wagonloads of supplies appeared blessedly on battlefields including Antietam, in Maryland. Records indicate that she usually brought supplies to the battlefields, then stayed for some days to assist in nursing the wounded from both sides. During the Battle of Fredericksburg, Virginia, in December 1862, she assisted at the Lacy House, a hospital more than a hundred miles away in Chatham, Virginia, where the wounded were being brought. The overwhelmed physicians were too busy to enter data in their records, so while Clara was there, she listed in her diary the names of the men who died and where they were buried.

Barton was focused on bringing wagonloads of supplies into a designated battlefield as early as possible, making every effort to pull ahead of the medical units, which were at the rear of a column. On the way to Antietam, she ordered her drivers to travel through the night, following the cannons. She and her team were ready with relief by the time there were casualties on the field.

She was at every battlefield in Virginia, South Carolina, and Maryland, bringing in supplies and staying to nurse the wounded. Although she had no formal medical training, General Benjamin Butler named her the head nurse for one of his units in 1864. Barton risked her life by her mere presence on the battlefields, and had more than a few narrow escapes. On one occasion during the Battle of Antietam, she was taking care of a wounded man when a bullet passed through her sleeve, leaving her uninjured but killing her patient.

President Abraham Lincoln was concerned with the lists of thousands of missing men: lists that kept growing. In March 1865, he appointed Clara Barton to "search for missing prisoners of war," in order to help families reunite with their loved ones or learn their fates. He wrote:

> To the Friends of Missing Persons: Miss Clara Barton has kindly offered to search for the missing prisoners of war. Please address her . . . giving her the name, regiment, and company of any missing prisoner.

Using her own funds, Clara set up an organization called "Friends of the Missing Men of the United States Army" and recruited several volunteers to help with the searches. Of necessity, the searches soon included grave identifications. Years later, the American Red Cross would establish an important tracing service that continues the essence of Barton's work into the 21st century.

A few months after beginning the huge task of searching for the missing, Clara Barton was contacted by Dorence Atwater, a former Union Army soldier who had been captured by Confederates as a teenager and was among the first group to be imprisoned at the infamous camp at Andersonville, Georgia. While he was incarcerated, he approached the head surgeon to request parole to work as a clerk in the prison hospital. He became one of several prisoners with the duties of maintaining the death register, which he began to secretly copy, concerned that the Confederates would not turn over the list at the end of the war.

Atwater, who later became a businessman and a State Department consul, had kept his secret copy of the list of the dead, which became known as the "Andersonville Death Register." The document allowed him to work with Barton in marking graves of many of the unknowns, and they both spent a great deal of time writing letters and notifying the families of missing and dead soldiers. Clara's Washington connections allowed the case to be presented to Secretary of War Edwin M. Stanton, who agreed that the almost 13,000 Andersonville graves should be appropriately marked and honored. Andersonville National Cemetery was dedicated on August 17, 1865, and Clara Barton was given the honor of raising the flag during the ceremony.

She testified before Congress in 1866 about the condition of the Andersonville prison grounds, an open stockade without shelter or running water, where so many had suffered and died. She also testified about the plight of freed slaves who had not been told about their freedom or guided in how to survive in the postwar country. Clara continued her work in locating missing soldiers until 1869, responding to more than 63,000 letters from families and friends and identifying about 22,000 missing men.

In need of rest after her work in the Civil War, Barton's doctor prescribed a trip to Europe for her to relax, but it turned out to be a journey that would galvanize her next humanitarian efforts with a fresh dose of inspiration as she was introduced to a group known as the Red Cross in Geneva, Switzerland. While visiting the country, she met Dr. Louis Paul Amédée Appia, a Swiss surgeon with a specialization in military medicine. In 1863, Dr. Appia had joined the Geneva "Committee of Five," a group that constituted a precursor to the International Committee of the Red Cross, and six years later his work would make a huge impression on the American relief worker, educator, and humanitarian.

Barton, in her lifelong effort to reduce the suffering of humanity, was electrified by events unfolding overseas, events that offered a larger field of service, notably the Red Cross and the Geneva Convention. She read a book that had been published in 1862, *A Memory of Solferino*, by the founder of the global Red Cross network, Swiss businessman and humanitarian Henri Dunant. Dunant espoused the need for international agreements to protect the injured and sick during wartime. He felt the agreements should be forged without regard to nationality, and for national societies to give aid voluntarily and on a neutral basis.

Dunant's concept led to an 1864 treaty that was first negotiated in Geneva, Switzerland, and ratified by twelve of the European nations. The agreement was known by several names including the "Geneva Treaty," the "Red Cross Treaty," and the "Geneva Convention." Clara Barton would later aggressively lobby the United States to ratify the treaty as well. When the Franco-Prussian War broke out in 1870, she went to the battlefields with European volunteers from the International Red Cross. The emblem of the organization and the movement was a red cross on a white background: the reverse imagery of the Swiss flag. Barton's work was sponsored by Grand Duchess Louise of Baden, the daughter of Kaiser Wilhelm I; Clara served as a nurse and was able to help distribute much-needed supplies to the defeated city of Strasbourg on the border of Germany and France, later organizing a similar relief effort in Paris. Clara Barton wholeheartedly endorsed the effort:

The International Committee assumed that there should be a relief association in every country which endorsed the treaty.

In most countries the co-operation of women has been eagerly sought. It is needless to say it has been as eagerly given.

On her return to the United States, Clara Barton corresponded with the Red Cross officials she had met and worked with in Switzerland. They acknowledged her remarkable leadership and organizational abilities and supported her wish to include her country in the global Red Cross Network, urging her government to sign and endorse the Geneva Treaty. She worked to build support for an American society of the Red Cross, lecturing, writing, and meeting with President Rutherford B. Hayes and influential friends and colleagues including Frederick Douglass. It took years, but the American Association of the Red Cross was finally formed in May 1881 and Barton, at age fifty-nine, was elected president the following month. A year later, the United States joined the International Committee of the Red Cross as Barton continued to lobby American presidents, and finally, in 1882, President Chester Arthur signed the Geneva Treaty, which was ratified by the Senate a few days later. The American Red Cross received its first congressional charter in 1900.

Clarissa Harlowe Barton led the U.S. delegation to St. Petersburg, Russia, for the Seventh International Conference of the Red Cross. She served as president of the American Red Cross until 1904, resigning at the age of eighty-three, and for the rest of her life resided at her home in Glen Echo, Maryland, passing on at the age of ninety. She was buried in her family cemetery in North Oxford, Massachusetts, and her Maryland home was restored and opened to the public as a memorial to her selfless service, revolutionary vision, and devotion to the needs of people in distress. In 1975, Clara Barton's Maryland home was designated a National Historic Site, the first in America to be dedicated to the achievements of a woman.

The 21st-century American Red Cross continues in its traditional commitment to relief, serving as a means of communication between members of the American military and their families and providing international disaster relief and mitigation.

The man who would define world-changing humanitarianism was the first son born to a wealthy home in Geneva, Switzerland, in 1828. Jean-Henri Dunant's parents were devout Calvinists, civic-minded, charitable, and influential in Geneva society. His mother did volunteer work with the poor and sick and his father was active in helping with the welfare of orphans and parolees. Dunant grew up with a value system based on religion and social work, and as a teenager, he joined the Geneva Society for Alms Giving. At nineteen he cofounded an informal organization called the "Thursday Association": young men who met for Bible studies and to work with the poor.

Dunant's youth paralleled a period of religious awakening known as the Réveil, and he took his societal concerns very seriously, spending time to make prison visits and performing social work. In 1852, inspired by the international youth group Young Men's Christian Association, or Y.M.C.A., which had been founded in London in 1844, he established a Geneva chapter of the organization. The concept of practicing Christian principles by developing a healthy "body, mind, and spirit" resounded well with the young man, and three years later he took part in the association's First World Y.M.C.A. Conference in Paris, an international event.

Dunant became a driving force for the international Y.M.C.A. movement, always encouraging its growth. He spent some time as a representative of the group, traveling in Holland, Belgium, and France and corresponding with Y.M.C.A. chapters in almost thirty different towns in Europe and North Africa. In 1854, Henri entered the business world, and in 1858 published his first book, which contained travel observations for the most part, although one chapter was issued separately in 1863, titled *L'Esclavage chez les musulmans et aux États-Unis d'Amérique* (*Slavery among the Mohammedans and in the United States of America*).

Dunant moved further into the business world by creating a company that could operate in foreign colonies, beginning with a land concession in French-occupied Algeria. The water and land rights for the tract were not clearly delineated, and Dunant decided to appeal directly for assistance to French emperor Napoleon III, creating a document of praise for the leader and planning to deliver it personally. The emperor and his army were fighting against the Austrians, who were occupying much of what is today's Italy.

Henri Dunant traveled to Napoleon's headquarters in Solferino, in northern Italy, arriving by chance on June 24, 1859, the same day as a great battle between the two forces had occurred, leaving 40,000 dead, wounded, and dying on the battlefield. It did not appear that the military was going to make any attempt at caring for the men, and Dunant began to organize the local civilians, especially women and girls, to give help to the injured soldiers. No materials or medical supplies had been provided and Dunant personally organized the purchase of needed goods, helped to erect makeshift hospitals on the field, and successfully gained the release of captured Austrian doctors to assist with the terrible aftermath.

Dunant returned to Geneva in July, the course of his life having been profoundly changed by the events in Solferino. The horrific scenes and circumstances had inspired him with a novel idea that would eradicate the chances of such human destruction and chaotic suffering ever occurring again. He decided to write a book about his experiences and thoughts and in 1862 published *Un Souvenir de Solferino* (*A Memory of Solferino*) at his own expense. He had 1,600 copies of the book printed and sent it to many of the leading military and political figures in Europe. The book, in addition to providing graphic details about the aftermath of the Solferino battle and estimates of its cost, presented the concept for the creation of a neutral organization that would provide care and protection to wounded soldiers in wartime.

The book contained Dunant's plan: a specific vision for the nations of the world to agree to form relief associations designed to provide and oversee the care for the wounded on the battlefield and through their convalescence. He caught the attention of many in Europe and, in February 1863, the Société genevoise d'utilité publique (Geneva Society for Public Welfare) appointed Dunant and four other men including, Swiss Army general Henri Dufour, physicians Louis Appia and Théodore Maunoir, and jurist Gustave Moynier, president of the Geneva Society for Public Welfare, to form a committee to review the possibility of promoting such a plan. It was, in effect, this committee of five that created the Red Cross, memorializing their first meeting on February 17, 1863, as the founding date of the International Committee of the Red Cross.

Dunant's belief in the proposal was strong enough that he funded his own campaign to promote it, traveling throughout Europe and working to obtain promises from the various governments to send representatives to a planned conference in Geneva, Switzerland, in October 1863. Sixteen nations sent thirty-nine delegates to the conference and worked on establishing groundwork and resolutions agreeing to guarantee neutrality to the wounded and to medical workers and to make supplies available for their use. They also agreed to adopt the emblem of a red cross on a white field, the reverse colors of the flag of the host country. Twelve nations signed an international treaty, familiarly known as the Geneva Convention, on August 22, 1864, at a conference organized by the Swiss government. It was noted that Henri Dunant was responsible for arranging accommodations for the delegates.

Dunant persevered with the treaty and the proposed scope of the Red Cross, extending it to include naval personnel in wartime and to address natural disasters in peacetime. In 1872 he arranged a conference to recognize the need for an international agreement on the handling of prisoners of war and for settling disputes between countries through courts of arbitration rather than by warfare.

In 1901, for his compassionate vision and humanitarian creations, Jean-Henri Dunant, and Frédéric Passy, French economist and "dean" of the international peace movement, were awarded the first Nobel Peace Prize ever given. Dunant was the recipient of many additional honors, but, unfortunately, his later life took a dark turn, leaving him lonely, ill, and no longer welcome in Geneva society. He lived extremely frugally, never spending the Nobel Prize money or other rewards he had received. When he died in October of 1910, his estate was made up of legacies to individuals who had cared for him at the end of his life, establishing medical attention for the local poor who were sick, and supporting charitable organizations in Norway and Switzerland. For more than 150 years, his compassion and humanitarian actions have remained in global evidence every day through the benevolence of the Geneva Convention and the work of the International and American Red Cross.

CHAPTER EIGHT

THE LEGACY

The unique phenomenon known as Civil War medicine actually extended its reach beyond science and medicine, impacting education, humanitarianism, and society, and marking distinct changes in Western medicine and culture.

The legacy of Civil War medicine is not an exclusively clinical story, nor is it just about the thousands of medics and volunteers who served. It is the far broader story about a need that transcended into a movement and would change lives, perspectives, and techniques in a revolutionary way. The echoes of Civil War medicine are in every ambulance, every vaccination, every woman who holds a paying job, and in every African American who pursues higher education. Those echoes are in every response of the International and American Red Cross and they are in the recommended international protocol for the treatment of prisoners of war and wounded soldiers.

In examining the various aspects of the legacy of Civil War medicine, it is impressive to review progress that was made in the field during and as a result of the conflict. As with most wars, medicine evolved to keep up with advances in weaponry. The Civil War occurred at a dramatic period in arms technology, and medicine struggled painfully to match the pace of the resulting damage. The challenges, changes, and learning curve resulting from the tragedy of those thousands upon thousands of surgeries and illnesses became the foundation and the launching pad of modern Western health care and medical education.

The necessity to provide for massive armies and gigantic battles led to a reimagining and reorganization of emergency medical rescue, field medicine and surgery, convalescent care, and medical record-keeping. The assembling of those huge armies and the creation of a gargantuan number of victims forced a massive change in social and professional status for women and African Americans. The legacy of this war marks the early beginning of acceptance for female and black physicians, and the ending of slavery opened access to literacy for millions of people. The story and its accompanying phenomena present a multifaceted view of the many angles of an American event that lit the fuse of an explosion that changed much of the Western world in profound and permanent ways.

The experience and educational level of thousands of doctors was advanced and upgraded as they became familiar with the use of anesthesia, innovative surgical procedures, new observations, practices, and treatments, and the importance of sanitation and hygiene. They created and implemented dramatic new standards of care that vastly improved the quality of medical education and practices in America.

One of the most important and far-reaching advances of the American Civil War was the evolution of hospitals. The medical community of the Civil War achieved an outstanding record for survival rates from disease and wounds as they designed, built, and operated state-of-the-art hospitals and marked the beginning of the modern elevation of medicine.

The new weapons technologies created a wholesale mechanical slaughter at a time when organized, systemized medical care and trained nursing staffs did not exist. There were no established methods of getting huge numbers of wounded men from the battlefield to places of care and there were few large-scale treatment facilities.

The great American journalist and poet Walt Whitman noted his observations as he visited numerous hospitals while serving as a nurse in the Civil War. After the Battle of Fredericksburg, Virginia, in 1862, a very large brick home was used as a hospital. After viewing the facility as he visited the wounded he wrote that it was

> quite crowded, upstairs and down, everything impromptu, no system, all bad enough, but I have no doubt the best that can be done, all the wounds pretty bad, some frightful, the men in their old clothes, unclean and bloody.

His visits to the makeshift division hospitals found them even more shocking in their bleak desolation:

> merely tents, and sometimes very poor ones, the wounded lying on the ground, lucky if their blankets are spread on layers of pine or hemlock twigs or small leaves.

The Civil War changed the long-held tradition that government did not have responsibility for the health of the individual soldier. Before the war, no one who was injured had expected to be nursed by a trained professional. No one had expected hospitals to be clean, or anesthesia to be given before surgery. No soldier who was wounded had anticipated the swift arrival of an ambulance. Expectations on the part of the patient, military, and civilian had transformed forever.

Owing to the unprecedented number of casualties, the perception and vision of hospitals expanded by orders of magnitude. The few forty-bed military hospitals of prewar America, long considered to be large institutions, gave way to massive facilities that could treat many thousands of patients, and the growth of general hospitals became rapid and permanent. Specialty hospitals appeared in profusion: "stump" hospitals for amputee patients, eye- and ear-focused hospitals, hospitals for the treatment of maxillofacial injuries with daring new techniques including dental surgery and "plastic operations."

The work of doctors Silas Weir Mitchell, George Read Morehouse, and William Williams Keen at Turner's Lane Military Hospital in Philadelphia laid the groundwork for the field of neurology during the war. The postwar emergence of neurology as an important and distinct specialty area of medicine is the direct result of that specific hospital and the doctors' daring explorations into previously unknown areas supported by their dedicated data collection and analysis.

Dr. Jonathan Letterman, the medical director of the Army of the Potomac, known for his ingenuous solutions, reorganized military hospitals—he created a standard staff and hierarchy to be implemented in all military hospitals. Each individual hospital would have one surgeon in charge with two assistant surgeons. Within the hospital, officers with the highest levels of medical skills, rather than the highest ranking in the military, would be chosen to perform surgical operations. Medical supplies now came under the aegis of the Medical Department rather than the quartermaster.

The American Revolutionary War had utilized private homes and existing buildings as hospitals. The Civil War, with its huge armies and equally large number of casualties, required a new kind of hospital dedicated to the care of thousands of patients who were suffering from various diseases and the vicious wounds that were being created by the improved weapons of the war. They needed permanent structures that were faster and easier for medical personnel to move through.

"Pavilion" hospitals were in use in Europe and were seen favorably as an improvement to existing health care, the design being strongly endorsed by British nurse and social reformer Florence Nightingale. The surgeons general of both North and South independently decided on the pavilion hospitals as the most efficient and effective design available, and the two governments built their new facilities from pavilion plans. The long, narrow wards with many windows improved the ventilation of the buildings and allowed supplies to move smoothly throughout. As the new hospitals came into use, a noticeable drop in the death rate began to occur, and the medical professionals were making valuable connections between cleanliness and better health.

Mobile army hospitals were pioneered in the South by Dr. Samuel Hollingsworth Stout, surgeon and medical director of hospitals for the Confederate Army of Tennessee. Dr. Stout, a native of Nashville, had acquired his medical education in part at the University of Pennsylvania and Pennsylvania Hospital, both in Philadelphia. In his position as medical director, he was responsible for coordinating the management of doctors, the procurement of medical supplies, and the safe relocation of wounded and ill soldiers as battles occurred closer to them. As the Union Army invasions penetrated deeper into the South, Stout had to marshal the almost constant relocation of sixty hospitals in Mississippi, Georgia, and Alabama. During the war he was continually on the move inspecting, organizing, and arranging the hospitals that fell under his responsibility. Stout's new hospital structure was specific as to special orders, hospital stewards, nurses, and other employees, as well as reports of supplies of food, medicine, hospital equipment, and the details of patients who were admitted.

He kept and preserved meticulous records of the medical and hospital matters, hoping to publish them with conclusions after the war, and his papers give a detailed picture of the daily life and conditions in Confederate military hospitals. Dr. Samuel Stout was a creative thinker and a gifted administrator who developed streamlined mobile hospital units that could be moved with the armies, a system that has been adapted in all American conflicts since.

The United States Sanitary Commission created a system of waterways for moving soldiers to Northern hospitals as quickly as possible. Hospital ships formed a highly effective manner of transporting the wounded to general or specialty hospitals in the larger cities. The Navy has always been a strong proponent of medical research and activity in both wartime and peacetime, and during the Civil War it provided a major source of support to the medical departments.

Women nurses were permitted to serve on hospital ships, ushering in a new era of the repeal of some gender prejudices. Systems were developed for the loading and transport of the patients, and hospital ships became a more scheduled and organized part of the relief effort, allowing at one point for the conveyance of 20,000 patients per month from Virginia to hospitals as far away as New York.

The Union's first hospital ship, the side-wheel steamer U.S.S. *Red Rover*, was a former Confederate ship that had been captured by federal forces and refitted to move the wounded. The ship's first voyage as a floating United States hospital was in June of 1862. Her final journey was in December 1864 and she was decommissioned on November 17, 1865. The *Red Rover*'s log showed that she had transported and provided treatment for 2,947 patients in her career as a Civil War hospital ship.

Hospital ships have remained an important component of the Navy's response to the medical needs of its personnel and of those with whom its missions have interfaced. The peacetime achievements and contributions of hospital ships continue to provide humanitarian aid and support in a global arena.

The American Civil War marked the country's first use of railroads to transport large numbers of casualties away from field hospitals and bring them to facilities that could offer them better care. In 1861, thousands of troops and huge quantities of supplies were moved by rail over the more than 20,000 miles of railroad tracks in the North and 9,000 in the South.

The U.S. Army utilized the railroads in a haphazard and disorganized manner at the beginning of the war, lacking coordinated schedules and failing to designate the specific uses of the cars. In January of 1862, President Lincoln granted the government the authority to centralize the management and administration of the railroads and the ability to commandeer train lines as necessity dictated. The reorganization of the railroads gave the North a powerful system that would help them win the war. It also generated the far more rapid mass evacuation of wounded troops.

In the first months of use of the railroads by the medical department, supplies from ammunition to animal forage were shipped in boxcars, which returned bearing wounded soldiers. On the first of the hospital trains, straw was used to pad the boxcar floors, along with pine branches and any available blankets. The closed cars had little or no ventilation and the jostling of the swaying and jolting ride caused even more pain for the battered men.

A member of the U.S. Sanitary Commission, Dr. Elisha Harris, rode on one of the early hospital trains and was horrified by the additional suffering caused by the paltry accommodations. During the trip he designed and sketched out a system for hanging the men's stretchers using India rubber rings as shock absorbers. Dr. Harris envisioned cars that would make it possible for medical attendants to move easily through them and to go from car to car.

In October of 1862, the Philadelphia, Wilmington and Baltimore Railroad outfitted and donated a hospital car designed by Dr. Harris. Other companies followed suit, and the U.S. Army soon had hospital trains composed of specially designed cars to connect battlefields and hospitals.

Trains became a primary means of transporting the Civil War wounded, and later they began to be upgraded and supported by mobile medical facilities during World War I. Trains continued to provide medical service throughout World War II, by then enhanced with onboard surgical wards. In many parts of the modern world where people live far from large cities in sparsely settled areas, hospital trains are relied upon to bring their mobile treatments and examinations.

The changing face of medicine during the Civil War was necessitated by wartime conditions and was paralleled by another huge change happening in the social, political, and professional status of American women. The mid-19th-century "sentimental domestic" image of females faded quickly into obscurity as the needs of the country and its men became more and more desperate. Women who had never worked outside of the home and the requirements of their households were suddenly in a brand-new environment. As they became aware of the wartime devastation, they were intent on being part of the effort for providing comfort in helping to nurse and care for the many thousands of sick and wounded soldiers. They took over running businesses, learning on the fly, while keeping life going at home. They were tenacious and persistent in overcoming the gender bias so prominent at the military hospitals and on the battlefields, insisting on being part of the relief actions.

Women began to found aid organizations and agencies and to emerge in some leadership roles despite the prejudicial state of society. White women and black women staffed the hospitals, some as paid workers and thousands as willing volunteers. The importance of skilled nursing care had become quite clear by the beginning of the Civil War with its endless injuries and illnesses among the troops. Clara Barton, Dorothea Dix, Elizabeth Blackwell, and untold numbers of inspired women transformed nursing from a menial service to a respected profession.

The Civil War marked the beginning of social acceptance of American women as doctors. In the 1860s, most medical schools wouldn't admit female students, and many men refused to be treated by female doctors. Slowly, but persistently, women continued to demand medical education and to be allowed to assist on the battlefield and in the hospitals. As the medical community slowly accepted female physicians, it also began to acknowledge the need for trained, skilled nurses in all medical settings, and, slowly, support for the establishment of civilian nursing schools for women was finally given.

The American Civil War's legacy includes one woman doctor who would break dramatically through numerous barriers and receive an astonishing and singular honor for her wartime service. Dr. Mary Edwards Walker of Oswego, New York, a graduate of Syracuse Medical College, was awarded the Congressional Medal of Honor by President Andrew Johnson in November 1865. Dr. Walker, surgeon, feminist, suffragist, prisoner of war, and suspected spy for the Union, is, and to this date remains, the only woman ever to have been honored with the renowned accolade and tribute.

The lives of American women were profoundly changed by the Civil War as they faced new challenges and expanded duties and responsibilities at home, on the battlefield, in medical facilities, and in business. Women entered a dramatically different arena, one with more freedoms and opportunities for participation, education, and the pursuit of professional careers.

At the beginning of the war, no formal training, standards, or requirements for nurses existed, a situation that was addressed by the vigorous efforts of women including Dorothea Dix, Elizabeth Blackwell, and many others who were influenced by the work of British nurse and reformer Florence Nightingale.

Nursing, in addition to being an extremely necessary part of medical care during the war, presented a way for women to participate in the relief effort in a manner that was outside of the home and opened new doors for work for them. Thousands of women simply traveled to the battlefields and hospitals to offer their services in caring for the overwhelming number of sick and wounded men. For many, their domestic experience gave them grounding in basic care—feeding, comforting, administering medicine, writing letters, and praying with the patients. As the conflict wore on, the new nurses became more adept at changing bandages and washing patients. Much of the work was physically demanding, dirty, and usually heartbreaking. Nurses who worked behind the scenes in the heavier jobs in the hospital kitchens and laundries were frequently assigned those duties based on race and class; the discrimination was familiar in both North and South.

Civil War nursing was a dangerous job at best. Nurses were exposed to patients suffering from numerous diseases, some of them communicable, they handled patients with ferocious infections, and some nurses died from the conditions and illnesses they contracted. Nurses frequently gave aid directly on the battlefield, rendering them vulnerable to the firing of weapons from both sides.

As the wartime hospitals became more organized and systems were instituted, the role of the nurses became increasingly defined and grudgingly accepted. There was more training available for them, either by working with authorities like Dorothea Dix and Dr. Blackwell, or from women who had gained some experience in the hospital tasks and shared their knowledge. It quickly became clear that trained, professional nurses were a vital asset to the patients, the hospitals, and medicine in general. Many Southern women nursed patients in their homes and had no formal ties with the military or hospitals. Their numbers are unknown, but their compassion was tangible and invaluable.

Although Florence Nightingale had established the world's first training school for nurses in London in 1860, it would be 1873 before the first nursing school in America opened at Bellevue Hospital in New York. More than 800 American schools offer degrees in nursing today. Nursing is a vital and necessary profession that has helped to advance medicine throughout history. One young Civil War Union nurse, Ella L. Wolcott, put its value in perspective:

> I have been a "female nurse" since a year ago last October and only regret that I did not go in the beginning when a mistaken humility is all that withheld me . . . I went in with many misgivings—but now I KNOW that women are worth in the hospitals. It is no light thing to hear a man say he owes you his life and then to know that mother, wife, sister, or child bless you in their prayers.

After the war, many of the women who had taken leadership positions in the volunteer and humanitarian agencies as well as in the local aid groups went on to become part of the movement for women's suffrage. Their vision for themselves had been greatly expanded by their work in wartime relief.

The women who served as Civil War nurses proved that nursing is an extremely important profession and one worthy of great regard. They faced inexperience, discrimination, rejection, and disrespect, but their tenacity and devotion demonstrated the indispensable nature of their worth and illuminated our world's wholehearted need for them.

One of the greatest legacies and most dramatic successes of the American Civil War is its ambulance system. In a stunning avalanche of violent attacks, the America military learned how to handle their casualties of war. The condition of the medical corps of the Army of the Potomac in 1861 could be described as disastrous. Any wagons or conveyances in use as ambulances came under the command of the quartermaster and were used not only for the transport of wounded soldiers, but also for supplies and equipment. Drivers and stretcher-bearers were untrained, usually those men not involved in the fighting due to ill health, irresponsibility, or "malingering." No precedents were established for the transport of the wounded and no vehicles were specifically dedicated to that purpose.

The injured men in the very early days of the war were often simply left to fend for themselves, and without the assistance of a comrade or anyone who could be summoned into service as stretcher-bearers, the victims could lie helpless on the field of battle for days, suffering the effects of exposure and thirst in addition to their injuries. Virginia's First Battle of Bull Run in July 1861 caught the Union Army, which was expecting a mere skirmish, by surprise. It was the first major battle of the war, a full-scale victory for the Confederate Army and a crushing defeat for the Union. More than 1,000 federal soldiers were wounded and the vehicles expected to serve as ambulances after the battle had disappeared on the retreat.

Nathaniel Bowditch, whose brigade had been dispatched to Kelly's Ford, Virginia, was the son of physician, abolitionist, and humanitarian Dr. Henry Ingersoll Bowditch. Nathaniel had been wounded during the battle, lay abandoned on the field for hours, and then died of his injuries. The sad scenario was echoed at other battles. Many of the Bull Run casualties lay where they had fallen on the field for more than a week. Dr. Bowditch had traveled to Virginia to visit his son, arriving only to find that he had died. The grieving father railed against the lack of reliable vehicles and drivers, stating that most of the civilian ambulance drivers were not trained and "of the lowest character," and adding that many were "cowards or drunks." His son's terrible death reignited Dr. Bowditch's activism and he worked to turn Nathaniel's loss into a cause for creating a reliable ambulance corps to transport wounded soldiers in future. He found support from the medical community, including the venerable Dr. Samuel D. Gross of Philadelphia.

> Every regiment, or body of military men, should be amply provided, in time of war, with the means of conveying the wounded and disabled from the field of battle. For this purpose suitable carriages and litters should constantly be in readiness.
>
> A proper number of men should be detailed for the purpose of rendering prompt assistance to the wounded, carrying them off the field of battle to the hospitals or tents. Unless this be done as a preliminary step, much suffering will inevitably be the consequence.

In 1862 Major Jonathan Letterman was assigned to the Army of the Potomac, later becoming its medical director. With approval from Surgeon General William Hammond, President Abraham Lincoln, and General George McClellan, Letterman was given permission to do whatever was needed to create a system that provided substantial support to the men in the combat zone. His actions would change the course of the war and of American medicine.

Dr. Letterman was appalled by the lack of resources for the wounded, and in just six weeks he implemented a system to evacuate the injured and to provide them with well-planned transportation and care. He replaced the quartermaster's command over ambulances with the supervision of the medical department. He established caravans of dedicated ambulance vehicles, each with a driver and stretcher-bearers, to convey the disabled men to field hospitals, ensuring that only the wounded soldiers and medical necessities would be transported by those designated vehicles. He arranged for and hired private wagons to carry medical supplies, introduced spring suspensions to the ambulance vehicles, and had lockboxes installed under their drivers' seats, making it harder for medicines and supplies to be stolen. He instituted training for stretcher-bearers in order to inflict the least amount of additional discomfort to the injured men. Letterman's innovations radicalized rescue and evacuation as part of medical treatment on battlefields and made it possible for soldiers to receive transportation to a hospital and care far more quickly than the Bull Run debacle had allowed.

Surgeon General Hammond supported Letterman's plan, ordering one ambulance per 150 soldiers and two medical supply wagons for each regimental corps. Stretchers were provided and men were trained to carry them with instructions to bring the victims to field dressing stations. The superb new ambulance system proved itself resoundingly well at the Battle of Antietam, near Sharpsburg, Maryland, in September 1862, the bloodiest day in American history. The staggering butchery of 23,000 casualties in the ten-hour battle resulted in more than 2,000 Union soldiers killed and almost 10,000 wounded. The new rescue system evacuated all of the wounded men from the field within twenty-four hours. It was an incredible demonstration of the power of an organized ambulance corps. Major Letterman was pleased that the ambulances were efficient and effective.

[It] affords me much gratification to state that so few instances of apparently unnecessary suffering were found to exist after that action and that the wounded were removed from that sanguinary field in so careful and expeditious a manner.

Letterman also instituted an early concept of "sorting" the wounded that would in the next century become known as "triage"; a tiered system of care. The procedure prioritized the prognosis and treatment of each injured soldier. It was a process that would begin to define emergency medicine. The doctors at the field stations quickly evaluated every wounded man, decided whether he should receive immediate attention (usually amputations), be taken to a general hospital for further care, or, if wounded in the chest, head, or abdomen and deemed too critical to survive, made comfortable and left to die.

In March 1864, the United States Congress implemented Jonathan Letterman's new systems across the entirety of the U.S. Army. Letterman's ambulance corps saved thousands of lives and created the basis of a legacy for future casualties, medics, and the military. Ethical concerns for the treatment of the sick and wounded gained new strength and respect. Ambulances, later including those that operate by air or sea, have become a staple of combat zones, were adopted by hospitals, and are now an integral standard of modern U.S. military battlefield medical management. Dr. Letterman is remembered today as the "Father of Battlefield Medicine" for his dedicated humanitarian concerns, his prescient concepts, and his unflagging work to improve conditions for the sick and wounded of his time and those in future conflicts. In responding to a need by creating a system, Letterman's concept also moved medical care from the actions of individual doctors to a practice that included multiple providers, teams, and interactive patient transport and care. Dr. Jonathan Letterman's efforts are still visible in the U.S. standard of military medical operations that affect the lives of soldiers and veterans today.

Probably the most important available drug during the Civil War was anesthesia, which is estimated to have been used in 95 percent of all wartime surgeries. Fortunately for the mid-19th-century soldiers, anesthesia had been explored in America since the 1840s, although its use was most common by dentists. Union dentist Dr. William Thomas Green Morton was one of the earliest pioneers in the use of anesthesia, even bringing its temporary relief to the wounded lying on the Civil War battlefields as they awaited rescue and evacuation. Morton is frequently credited with championing anesthesia into common medical usage and he served as one of the only dedicated anesthetists of the Civil War.

I have been the instrument of averting pain from thousands and thousands of maimed and lacerated heroes, who have calmly rested in a state of anesthesia while undergoing surgical operations, which would otherwise have given them intense torture.

Military surgeons were very quick to adopt its use, and anesthesia was actually utilized in almost all Civil War surgeries. President Abraham Lincoln was said to have brought his own chloroform to a dental appointment in Washington, D.C.

Although anesthesia quickly developed widespread use during the war, there was serious opposition to the practice from some clergy, and there were doctors who still maintained the belief that pain was a valuable stimulant to men in shock.

Anesthesia serves three purposes during painful surgical procedures: it relaxes the muscles, making it easier for the surgeon to work on the patient, it is an analgesic, which brings a state of painlessness, and it creates amnesia, or memory loss, during a traumatic episode like invasive surgery. Ether and chloroform, the available anesthesias during the Civil War, were a boon not only to the physician, but as a means of preventing shock and pain to the patient. Anesthesia remains a vital component of surgical procedures today and has allowed the incredible advancement of surgical techniques and solutions.

The crude application of a chloroform-soaked cloth placed over the nose and mouth of a patient made it impossible to administer the drug with any dosage accuracy until Southern physician Dr. John Julian Chisolm invented a device to deliver anesthesia with greater precision. The 2½-inch "Chisolm Inhaler" made it possible to use a fraction of the usual quantity of the drug for an effective result. Dr. Chisolm's device was the first step in a progression of applications that would lead to the accurate and precise administration of anesthesia to patients preparing for 21st–century surgery.

The single procedure credited with saving the lives of thousands of wounded men was the most common surgical operation performed during the Civil War—amputation. In the absence of the surgeons' available time, instruments, and techniques to repair damaged limbs, amputation was the fastest way to keep badly wounded victims from experiencing increasing pain, infection, and a likely miserable death to follow. The number of victims and the pace at which they arrived at field hospitals and general hospitals made the execution of delicate and complex surgeries an impossibility. Required to operate on countless casualties, with many of the surgeries carried out under severely adverse battlefield conditions, Civil War surgeons quickly discovered that an almost immediate response of amputation for a wounded limb created the most hopeful outcome for saving the patient's life. They also learned that the farther the site of the amputation from the torso, the better odds for recovery. Despite the prevalence of infection after the operations, it's remarkable that approximately 75 percent of the amputees survived their surgery and convalescence.

The wartime surgeons began to perfect their amputation techniques, with many of them able to perform the operation within six minutes, and as the war progressed, they developed more sophisticated closures for the wounds to prepare their patients for the use of prosthetic limbs upon recovery.

As the fields of plastic and reconstructive surgery exploded, Civil War doctors began to develop new techniques for addressing a huge surge in nerve injuries and the chronic pain accompanying them, opening a new area of focus and treatment. Dr. Silas Weir Mitchell reflected on the medical solutions still to be discovered.

> There are those who suffer and grow strong; there are those who suffer and grow weak. This mystery of pain is still for me the saddest of earth's disabilities.

Neurology was another discipline of medical specialization that became available for wide-ranging study as a result of doctors having access to thousands of patients with similar wounds or symptoms. The disorders and new classifications were localized and identified by Dr. Silas Weir Mitchell during his work in the Civil War. A brilliant young man, Mitchell was born in Philadelphia to a prominent doctor and his wife. He attended courses half-heartedly at the University of Pennsylvania but did not finish his program of studies, although he eventually completed and received his M.D. degree from Jefferson Medical College at age twenty-one. In the manner of those who could afford it at the time, he pursued additional studies in Paris, a city known for medical innovation.

Bright, curious, and multitalented, Mitchell had many friends and colleagues from the South and was a somewhat reluctant participant in the wartime effort. He was initially employed as a contract surgeon in the Union Army and while working in hospital service in Philadelphia, began to acquire a particular and intense interest in patients whose wounds left them with "nervous diseases" (nerve disorders), also noting that these were some of the least understood conditions and that they did not respond well to most treatments.

The huge number of wartime amputees brought a menu of similar pains and discomfort, including the phenomenon of "phantom limb"—the sensation that an amputated arm or leg was still extant and functional and frequently painful. Fortunately for Dr. Mitchell, the young surgeon general, William Hammond, was open to new ideas and granted his requests for increasingly larger hospital facilities to be set aside for these patients. Turner's Lane Hospital was the last and largest of his nervous disease hospitals and it was here that Mitchell began his serious studies of these injuries and a search for their remedies. His team gathered data from the victims of a wide variety of injuries—from guns, artillery shells, bladed weapons, and falls. He was the first to use electrical stimulation and massage on damaged muscles and began to explore and prescribe his "Rest Cure."

Turner's Lane Hospital welcomed soldiers with all kinds of nerve injuries. The hospital provided invaluable opportunity for study in the newly emerging field. A passionate researcher, Mitchell knew that he had an extraordinary situation for intensive examination:

> No sooner did this class of patients begin to fill our wards, than
> we perceived that a new and interesting field of observation was
> here opened to view.

Dr. Mitchell's extensive interests and abilities proved him to be quite a Renaissance man—he published numerous scientific papers of great value not only on nerve injuries but also on a wide range of topics including the effects of rattlesnake venom, uric acid generation, and his own experience ingesting mescal buttons. He certainly established himself as the "father of neurology," but furthermore as an "evidence-based" or "scientific" pioneer. Mitchell also produced a rich literary bequest that included his original novels, short stories, and poetry. His many accomplishments in both science and the arts are a stunning trove of creations, but he is most remembered and lauded for his Civil War service and its enduring value to science and medicine. Dr. Silas Weir Mitchell's studies and efforts propelled the field of neurology into existence and into the future.

Modern plastic surgery made its debut during the American Civil War, although its application in the period was far more survival-based than cosmetic.

Nearly 10,000 cases of gunshot and shrapnel wounds to the face were counted during the war, although only thirty-two "plastic operations"— plastic in the sense of shaping or sculpting—to repair them were recorded. The techniques of maxillofacial reconstruction were new, delicate, and unfamiliar; they needed to be performed with meticulous care and were limited to using skin flaps and bone from the patient's own body to reshape or repair massive damage from the highly effective new weapons. With the field of plastic operations in its infancy and a minimum number of experienced practitioners, it was unfortunately impossible to address most of the Civil War's victims of facial wounds.

Dr. Gurdon Buck, called the "father of modern plastic surgery," an 1830 graduate of Columbia University College of Physicians and Surgeons, was a pioneer in the new field of facial reconstructive surgery. Some of the techniques he incorporated had actually been described in 1000 B.C.E. India, then again another 1,000 years later in Rome, after which they were presented as theory in the English medical journal *The Lancet* in 1837. The projections seemed unrealistic to medical practice in mid-19th-century America, and Buck was one of the only Civil War surgeons who had investigated the information and had prior knowledge of transposing flaps of skin to cover large facial deformities. His innovations in technique, such as using very tiny stitches to minimize scarring, were novel contributions to a new Western area of medical specialization.

Gurdon Buck authored the first American textbook on plastic surgery, *Contributions to Reparative Surgery*, and is also known as the first physician to record clinical "before" and "after" pre- and postoperative photographs, including them as illustrations in his publications. His achievements created a revolutionary foundation for the highly advanced plastic surgery offered today and opened the floodgates for the now-expected publication of educational surgical photographs. Dr. Buck was a surgeon associated with New York Hospital for most of his life and a founding fellow of the New York Academy of Medicine.

Before the American Civil War, chest wounds were deemed among the most difficult to treat and were usually fatal, with victims having only an 8 percent survival rate. Sustaining a wound from a projectile that punctured the chest resulted in the deadly "sucking chest wounds" that allowed air to travel into the lungs, usually leading to a lung collapse and death. The young British-born Union assistant surgeon Benjamin Howard, M.D., had an idea for preventing the collapse, a concept that turned out to be surprisingly successful. Dr. Howard had volunteered his services to the Army and was mustered into service as an assistant surgeon in the Nineteenth Regiment of New York Volunteers, later known as the Third New York Light Artillery. After his appointment in the regular Army, he came up with the technique of closing a chest wound with metal sutures, then layering it with bandages saturated with an ointment called collodion, which dries into an airtight seal. Surgeon General William Hammond, who knew Dr. Howard, gave him permission to experiment with the method. Dr. Howard's method quadrupled the survival rate for chest wounds and soon became a standard treatment to prevent lung collapse, the principles of which are still applied in some circumstances today.

The culture of mid-19th-century America equated physical disability with defect of character. A whole and healthy body was a mark of manliness, while an amputated limb or a serious limp could be construed as evidence of moral degeneration. The Civil War's terrible harvest of limbs forced changes in the perception of those who had been harmed and spurred the prosthetics industry to create newly advanced solutions for restoring movement to thousands of devastated soldiers.

The field now known as "rehabilitative medicine" was originally developed and enhanced to meet the needs of the huge number of Civil War amputees. It is a branch of medicine that seeks to restore function and quality of life to people with physical impairments or disabilities. Prosthetic limbs had been available for centuries, but the sophistication of the new American and European innovations made them far superior to any that had been produced before.

In response to the shockingly large number of amputees, the proprietors of Northern and Southern companies strove to improve the technology and appearance of prosthetics. It was extremely important to the surviving amputees that they could once again fit inconspicuously into civilian life. Oliver Wendell Holmes Jr. served the Union Army as a soldier in the Civil War, later becoming an associate justice of the Supreme Court of the United States. His observations were pithy and sometimes poetic.

At an age when appearances are reality, it becomes important
to provide the cripple with a limb which shall be presentable in
polite society, where misfortunes of a certain obtrusiveness may
be pitied, but are never tolerated under the chandeliers.

The federal government subsidized the purchase of artificial limbs
for verified Union soldiers who had served in the war, although Confederate veterans were not eligible for federal aid. Some of the former
Confederate states created their own programs to provide prostheses for
their veterans.

Soldiers who had lost arms could be considered to be at a greater disadvantage than those whose legs had been sacrificed. Many of the artificial legs
provided mobility to the wearer, but prosthetic arms tended to be affixed
with metal hooks, and many veterans preferred the appearance of an empty
sleeve to the hook. Prosthetic limbs provided slight compensation for the lost
body part, but they could not ameliorate the emotional and psychological
damage that was another scar of amputation surgery.

The age of the simple wooden peg leg was ended as the Civil War heralded the era of modern prosthetics and the birth of an advanced industry
to design and manufacture artificial limbs. The U.S. government's commitment to support its veterans continues through programs to ensure
ongoing progress in prosthetics design, customization, and manufacture
with the goal of providing independence, mobility, and dignity to 21st-
century wounded warriors.

The field of dentistry made significant strides in the 19th century: it
detached from the general area of medicine and became a distinct and separate profession. In the early part of the century most dentists gained their
educations by apprenticing themselves to more experienced practitioners,
but by 1840, the Baltimore College of Dental Surgery in Maryland had
become the first independent educational institution for training dentists.
At the start of the Civil War, the North had a total of four dental schools,

where students from both North and South attended and studied from the same textbooks.

When the war began, the many thousands of casualties forced all medical practices to rapidly evolve and develop. Soldiers still sustained the normal scope of problems with their teeth, but now the medics faced incoming patients with grave facial wounds as well. Although its available resources and funding were superior, and despite the protests of the American Dental Association, the Union Army remained staunchly and stubbornly without a dental corps. During the Civil War it would be the Confederate Army's Dental Corps that shined in its dedication to emphasizing and maintaining dental care in its troops, an attitude that has since been fully adopted by the entire country.

Wartime dentists created a solution to a particularly difficult type of injury when Dr. James Baxter Bean in the South and Dr. Thomas Gunning in the North both independently created a hard rubber interdental splint that likely saved the lives of many soldiers. Some men who had been shot in the face or jaw were fitted with the device, which, in a pre-intravenous or tube-feeding world, allowed them to consume sustenance during their convalescence and hopefully prevented major facial deformities from occurring as a result of their injuries. For many dentists-turned-military-surgeons, the field of maxillofacial surgery rapidly opened its realm of possibilities throughout the war.

Although the Union Army never acknowledged the value of good dental care or required it during the length of the conflict, the Confederacy continued to emphasize the importance of dental health and hygiene throughout the war, educating its soldiers to proper care and encouraging them to brush their teeth.

Americans have long had a reputation for generosity of spirit and fighting for the "underdog." The philanthropy of the citizens of the United States is an impressive testament to a population of well-intentioned people open to supporting important causes, and that history is nowhere more evident than during the Civil War era.

The citizens' organization that was called the United States Sanitary Commission was created to take care of those aspects of the war that the government could not. It was a model of reform for the medical services, inspiring the War Department to drastically reorganize, update, and upgrade its medical policies. When the Civil War began, acquisition and distribution of supplies presented a major problem, and no quality controls existed. Military uniforms were poorly made and there was extensive profiteering in food and horses. Surgeons and the wounded sometimes waited for days after a battle before medical supplies arrived, if they arrived at all.

The Sanitary Commission began a program of inspecting the conditions at camps and hospitals and they published reports, pamphlets, and circulars written by Commission agents and physicians. They published a hospital directory with the names of over 600,000 hospitalized men, including the black soldiers, who were frequently treated in segregated hospitals. The Commission advocated the adoption of sanitary principles by the United States Army.

By late 1863, the work of the Sanitary Commission had made remarkable improvements in the evacuation and treatment of the wounded, demonstrated at the Battle of Chattanooga. Volunteer J. S. Newberry worked with the United States Sanitary Commission, frequently on the battlefields:

> I was at Chattanooga through all the exciting scenes of the recent battles, and was able to contribute something to the efforts of the Agents of the Commission to relieve the wants and sufferings of the wounded.
>
> I am quite sure that I do not exaggerate when I say that the wounded in no considerable battle since the war began have been so well and promptly cared for; and I can say also with equal confidence, that the aid rendered by the Sanitary Commission has never been more prompt and efficient, more heartily welcomed, or more highly appreciated.

The United States Sanitary Commission laid a foundation for some of the discoveries that were proven and revealed after the war. They knew that cleanliness mattered, although they weren't sure why. They knew that sanitary conditions led to fewer infections, slowed the spread of disease, and lowered the mortality rate. The Commission's work paved the way for the acceptance of the revolutionary discoveries from Europe: Dr. Louis Pasteur's germ theory of disease and Dr. Joseph Lister's treatments for infection.

After its official termination in 1865, the Sanitary Commission's remaining funds continued to be distributed to veterans, although assistance to widows and orphans was left to the local aid societies, but the legacy of the United States Sanitary Commission as a leader in humanitarian aid continued long after the Civil War ended.

The founding president of the Sanitary Commission, Reverend Dr. Henry Whitney Bellows, led a new organization, the American Association for the Relief of Misery on the Battlefield. The Association was a branch of the Geneva-based International Society for the Relief of Wounded Soldiers, the organization that would contribute to the formation of the International Committee of the Red Cross.

Some great and enduring acts of humanitarianism were directly related to the American Civil War. The United States Sanitary Commission served in many respects as a model for the Geneva Convention in October of 1863, a treaty among nations agreeing to provide for the humane care of wartime wounded and those who tended to them.

The remarkable efforts by both sides to rescue the wounded in the American Civil War had been dramatically mirrored by events in Europe. In 1859, two years before the Civil War began, Jean-Henri Dunant, a wealthy businessman, traveled to northern Italy in hopes of meeting with Emperor Napoleon III. The emperor was in the area to pursue military action against the Austrians.

Dunant unintentionally became a witness to the horrifyingly bloody battlefield of Solferino, Italy. More than 40,000 were killed or wounded in a single day. Just as was true in the Civil War, newly improved weapons had drastically raised the number of casualties. Dunant thereafter dedicated himself to lessening the carnage of war, calling for a meeting in Geneva to start the Association for the Prevention of Misery on the Battlefield. He was a recipient of the first Nobel Peace Prize in 1901.

Henri Dunant was one of the five founders of the International Red Cross in 1864 and he was the primary force behind the international meeting of diplomats who drew up the Geneva Convention—the agreement among nations on rules covering the care of those wounded in battle and the protection of those who provide that care. The Geneva Conventions are regarded as one of humanity's greatest accomplishments of the post–Civil War period. This body of international law seeks to regulate the protection of people who are not participants in the hostilities, as well as those sick or wounded who can no longer fight. The rules have been expanded to include the humane treatment of prisoners of war and to prohibit murder, mutilation, torture, the taking of hostages, and unfair trial.

The creation of the Geneva Convention was a revolutionary humanitarian event and movement and it influenced the missions of the International Committee of the Red Cross and the American Red Cross, all directly tied to alleviating the type of terrible suffering caused by the Civil War. Clara Barton, having experienced war firsthand, was deeply impressed with the stipulations of the treaty.

> The Sanitary Commission of the United States served as an excellent example to the relief societies of Europe.
>
> A permanent international committee with headquarters at Geneva was formed.
>
> One of the first objects desired by the International committee was a treaty which should recognize the neutrality of the hospitals established, of the sick and wounded, and of all persons and effects connected with the relief service.

The treaty provides for the neutrality of all sanitary supplies, ambulances, surgeons, nurses, attendants, and sick or wounded men, and their safe conduct when they bear the sign of the organization, viz: the Red Cross.

The Red Cross was chosen out of compliment to the Swiss republic, where the first convention was held, and in which the central committee has its headquarters. The Swiss colors being a white cross on a red ground, the badge chosen was these colors reversed.

One of the most esteemed women in American history, educator and humanitarian Clarissa (Clara) Harlowe Barton of Massachusetts, embodied the heart of a healer. From childhood she exhibited extraordinary compassion and nursing abilities, and she created a lifetime of devotion to and advocacy for those in distress. Throughout her life she helped guide people through the darkest of times, and she opened new paths for others to offer volunteer service. She created a remarkable and resilient movement for the betterment of humanity, and her legacy is especially evident in the American Red Cross.

Barton overcame crippling shyness to become a gifted educator and a popular teacher early in her career. She went on to organize a huge relief effort during the American Civil War, collected and delivered supplies, cooked for the troops, and nursed the wounded on many battlefields. She was shocked by the disorganization and lack of medical supplies at the Union field hospitals, on one occasion noticing that the hospital had no more bandages and was covering open wounds with corn leaves. She arranged for wagonloads of supplies and equipment and personally delivered them to the sites of many major battles, risking her life in the process each time.

She engaged in a massive effort to locate and identify missing soldiers. Her efforts to find the graves of prisoners culminated in an investigation of the prison and cemetery at Andersonville, Georgia, and its subsequent designation as a National Historic Site and memorial to all American prisoners of war.

Clara continued her work with the missing soldiers and their families until well after the war ended, and then traveled to Europe at her doctor's suggestion. She visited Geneva, Switzerland, where she was introduced to the International Committee of the Red Cross and its humanitarian work. Upon her return to the United States she was determined to create an American Red Cross with the same philanthropic goals. It took almost twelve years, but she was finally successful in 1881, and accepted the position of president, which she held for twenty-three years. Early in the existence of the organization, she amended the charter of the Red Cross to include the provision of relief for all disasters, whether natural or man-made.

Barton was a strong supporter of the Geneva Convention, the international treaty protecting the war injured and their caretakers, and she was one of the most vigorous voices urging the United States to ratify the treaty. She wrote a twelve-page letter to the U.S. Senate's Committee on Foreign Relations about supporting and protecting the Red Cross and its goals, especially emphasizing the importance of the country's joining the Geneva Convention.

> Perhaps no more advanced step than this, in the march of civilization and humanity had ever been taken, nor a more unique or touching sight of its kind had been looked upon, than this body of twenty six men representing the Heads of the war-making powers of the world . . . performing journeys of thousands of miles to sit down in calm counsel to try to "think out" if some more humane and reasonable methods might not be found, and *agreed upon* by the governments of the world for the treatment of the unfortunate and helpless victims of the wars.

The United States Congress finally ratified the Treaty of the Geneva Convention in 1882. The document had a huge international impact overseas and in the United States. Nations around the globe still strive to abide by the agreements endorsed by the Convention. The International Committee of the Red Cross and the American Red Cross have both grown exponentially and provide relief and aid in the face of wars and disasters, and the image of the lifesaving Red Cross remains strong as a powerful bequest of the Geneva Convention.

Clara Barton, a passionate public supporter of suffrage for women, had a strong impact on the acceptance of women in medical care and their ability to provide it during times of war, which accelerated women's access to paying jobs in health care. She was also a frequent speaker on public health and health interventions and wrote at length about her nursing experience and the importance of health as a global issue. In 1898, she wrote *The Red Cross: A History of This Remarkable International Movement in the Interest of Humanity*. Clara remained with the Red Cross until 1904, guiding the organization in helping with disasters, aiding the poor and homeless and educating the public about emergency preparedness.

Clara Barton's huge legacy of service to humanity is evident every day in the work of the American Red Cross, one of the world's most important humanitarian and disaster aid organizations. Her personal example of a devotion to serving others has proven to be a life source for millions over the years and has opened new opportunities for philanthropists and concerned citizens around the globe.

Military precision proved a blessing to medical record-keeping, providing structure within the chaos. To organize, staff, stock, and manage the huge hospitals, the military and the Sanitary Commission created new record-keeping systems; case histories were well-documented and autopsy reports were made for the future of medical education. Follow-up was extensive, and many postsurgical photographs were taken.

Institutions like the Army Medical Museum, the Army Institute of Pathology, and their many descendants including the National Library of Medicine and National Institutes of Health owe their lineage to the Civil War. In 1870 through 1888, the records created during the Civil War were published in the six-volume *Medical and Surgical History of the War of the Rebellion (1861–65)*, which documented virtually all cases of gunshot wounds, broken bones, communicable diseases including chicken pox, measles, and yellow fever, amputations, therapies, and pharmaceuticals. Illustrations of every type of stretcher, every ambulance vehicle, every surgical instrument, every bandaging technique were recorded. Nothing like it had ever been published, and Europe regarded it as America's greatest contribution to medicine. The noted German pathologist Rudolf Virchow was a leading figure in late-19th-century medicine. He reviewed the first volume in 1879:

> Whoever takes up and reads the extensive publications of the American medical staff will be constantly astonished at the wealth of experience found therein. The greatest exactness in detail, careful statistics, and a scholarly treatment are here united, in order to preserve and transmit the knowledge purchased at so vast an expense.

Surgeon General William Hammond established the Army Medical Museum in May of 1862. It was the first federal medical research facility and its mission was to study and improve medical conditions during the Civil War. The material collected by the museum in the course of the conflict would be the basis for the revolutionary six-volume reference work, detailing every medical condition encountered during the war. Hammond's vision and legacy would be continued by some very able men.

Joseph Janvier Woodward received his M.D. from the University of Pennsylvania in 1853. He had an intense interest in photographic research on microscopic images and many of his photomicrographs were later published in *The Medical and Surgical History of the War of the Rebellion*. At the outbreak of the Civil War he offered his services to the government.

Woodward was put in charge of the Army Medical Museum in Washington. He supervised the collecting of the material that would be presented for publication and the education of new generations of physicians. He became famous around the world for his publications in the fields of microscopy and photomicrography, and in 1881 was elected president of the American Medical Association. His devotion to the museum was legendary, as noted by Dr. James Ewing, also of the Army Medical Museum.

> In a history of the Army Medical Museum, the author states that during the Civil War, Woodward, failing to get material from the army camps, gathered up a company, hired some mule teams, drove to the battlefields near-by, exhumed buried limbs and bodies, and brought the pathological specimens to Washington himself.

The men who amassed the formidable collections making up the Medical Museum and Library were passionate about the work. Four of the massive volumes of *The Medical and Surgical History* were completed under U.S. Army Surgeon General Joseph K. Barnes's administration. Barnes planned to reimagine the surgeon general's library as a national medical library that could be accessible to the public, envisioning a medical version of the Library of Congress. He was equally devoted to the Army Medical Museum, intending it to become the greatest medical museum in the world.

> The materials in the office relating to the surgery of the late war consist of the reports of the medical officers, and of illustrations of pathological specimens, drawings, and models.

The extent of these materials is simply enormous. The result has been the accumulation of a mass of facts and observations of unprecedented magnitude.

In January, 1863, several artists were engaged; a colorist; a draughtsman; and two engravers. A valuable collection of drawings had been accumulated; draughtsman having been sent to battle-fields and hospitals to portray the effects of recent wounds, or the results of surgery. Numerous patients in hospitals were photographed, and the Museum now possesses over a thousand photographic representations of wounded or mutilated men.

All of these have either been bound, or indexed and filed in a convenient and accessible form. Lastly, the great treasures of the Army Medical Museum, comprising over five thousand illustrations of military surgery, having been so far classified and arranged as to be available for scientific inquiry.

After the war and into the 20th century, the museum staff engaged in medical research, including important work on infectious diseases like yellow fever, and made contributions to research on vaccines for typhoid fever. They led campaigns for health education including information on combating sexually transmitted diseases.

The museum research focused increasingly on pathology, and in the 1940s it evolved into the Armed Forces Institute of Pathology and the National Museum of Health and Medicine. The library became the National Library of Medicine. Today's National Museum of Health and Medicine has a collection of over one million items; its concentration reflects the history and practice of American medicine, military medicine, and current medical research issues.

The Civil War marked the beginning of modern advancements in medicine that were generated in response to the new weapons technologies that created an unprecedented mechanical massacre.

The medical community of the Civil War achieved an outstanding record for survival rates from disease and wounds. They designed, built, and operated revolutionary new hospitals. They served as the medical directors of huge armies and completely reorganized the medical corps. They initiated programs and research and left a legacy of skill and honor.

Organized, systemized medical care did not exist in the America of 1860. Skilled nursing as a profession or a staff position did not exist. Methods of getting wounded men from the battlefield to a place of care were haphazard at best and nonexistent at worst. There were no large-scale treatment facilities and surgery was rarely performed in the country. By the end of the war, there were great hospitals like Chimborazo and Satterlee, hospital trains and ships, skilled nurses, and a working ambulance corps.

The Civil War doctors embraced a practical approach to medicine, setting up new systems and methods, sometimes learning surgical techniques in camps and hospitals from the diagrams in books. Many of the physicians and surgeons were recent medical school graduates with no practical experience, but they were able to share ideas and information with their more experienced colleagues. They quickly implemented the discoveries of other men, and what they hadn't learned in the medical schools, they learned on battlefields and in field hospitals. The more immediate the care, the greater the likelihood of survival.

Many more lives were saved than was possible in earlier wars, and many lives were saved later because of knowledge gained during the Civil War. Both the Confederate and Union medical departments exercised good, solid, logical organization and changed the vista of health care. The war trained thousands of surgeons at a time when there were very few doctors in America who knew how to treat gunshot wounds. The technology of the time also gave them options that had not been available in earlier wars: surgical tools, anesthesia, and improved conveyances for the wounded.

The Civil War changed the long-held tradition that government did not have responsibility for the health of the individual soldiers. Before the war, no one who was injured had expected to be nursed by a trained professional, had envisioned that hospitals would be clean, or counted on the administration of anesthesia before surgery. The arrival of an ambulance was not anticipated by anyone who was wounded either in war or in peacetime, but by the end of the Civil War, expectations on the part of the patient, the military, and civilians had changed forever. Confederate General Alexander E. Porter of Georgia looked back at the medical outcome of the terrible conflict.

> Was all our blood shed in vain? Was all the agony endured for the Lost Cause but as water spilled upon the sand? No! A thousand times, no!
>
> We have set the world record for devotion to a cause. We have taught the armies of the world the casualties to be endured in battle; and the qualities of heart and soul developed both in our women and men, and in the furnace of our afflictions, have made a worthier race, and have already borne rich reward in the building up of our country.

These medical departments gained great insights and understanding from the horrific bloodbath. They grouped patients with similar injuries and made revolutionary observations. They worked with astonishing efficiency, saving lives by getting the wounded off the battlefields more quickly and transported to hospitals faster. They created centers of medicine that did not exist before the Civil War. They changed the substance of health care in America.

Dr. Robert D. Hicks of the College of Physicians of Philadelphia noted that "Before the war, an M.D. was someone who attended a year of medical lectures and then repeated them for a second year. The war created a new process with measureable standards. A military doctor not only had to graduate with an M.D. and show apprenticeship to an established physician but had to pass an oral and written examination. Before the war, doctors were all M.D.s; after the war, specialisms began in neurology, trauma management, and ophthalmology, for example. Doctors became specialists. Hospitals were no longer just for indigent and dying people. Today, when we see an injured person transported to hospital emergency care via ambulance, we are witnessing Civil War medicine."

In retrospect, it seems remarkable that despite primitive surgical conditions and desperate supply shortages, so many of the casualties survived—a victory of both science and spirit. Although the bodies had lain "thick as leaves," revolutionary changes in health care had emerged from the ashes of the war.

Like the killing power of weapons, medical science has soared in many ways. No subsequent war has taken the lives of as many Americans; a result of improved medical education, advanced surgical techniques, the understanding of neurology, and faster evacuation of the wounded. Women and African Americans have achieved prominent roles in medical science and society, the terms of the Geneva Convention still seek to protect medics and the wounded in times of war. The American Red Cross and the International Committee of the Red Cross have grown to provide emergency relief for a myriad of natural and man-made disasters. These profound human achievements, as well as the record of the hideous carnage, are the legacies of the American Civil War.

GUNSHOT WOUNDS

AND OTHER

INJURIES OF NERVES.

BY

S. WEIR MITCHELL, M.D.
GEORGE R. MOREHOUSE, M.D.
AND
WILLIAM W. KEEN, M.D.

ACTING ASSISTANT SURGEONS U.S.A.,
IN CHARGE OF U.S.A. WARDS FOR DISEASES OF THE NERVOUS SYSTEM, TURNER'S LANE
HOSPITAL, PHILADELPHIA.

PHILADELPHIA:
J. B. LIPPINCOTT & CO.
1864.
373

LEFT: *Gunshot Wounds and other Injuries of the Nerves,* by S. W. Mitchell, G. R. Morehouse, W. W. Keen, M.D.s. Published in 1864, this landmark work by surgeons at Turner's Lane Hospital was the first to observe and report on such nerve damage–related indications as RSD (Reflex Sympathetic Dystrophy Syndrome), neuralgia, and "phantom limb." BELOW: Surgical Instrument Set, maker: V. W. Brinckerhoff, N.Y., ca. 1860. This case of amputation instruments was found on the field after the first battle of Fair Oaks, Va., as inscribed on the lid. *Both images courtesy of Thomas Jefferson University Archives, Philadelphia.*

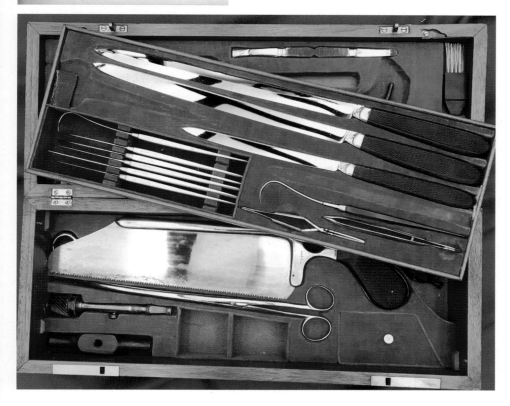

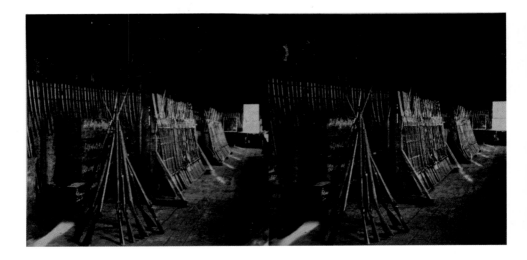

ABOVE: Bayoneted rifles on racks at the arsenal of the 134th Illinois Volunteer Infantry, Columbus, Ky. From Carbutt's Garden City Photographic Gallery, 131 Lake Street, Chicago, 1864. Photographic print on stereo card; albumen, stereograph. BELOW: Photograph of view of the defenses of Washington between 1860 and 1865. Arlington, Va., 1st Connecticut Artillery drilling at Fort Richardson. Stereographs, wet collodion negatives. *Both images courtesy of The Library of Congress.*

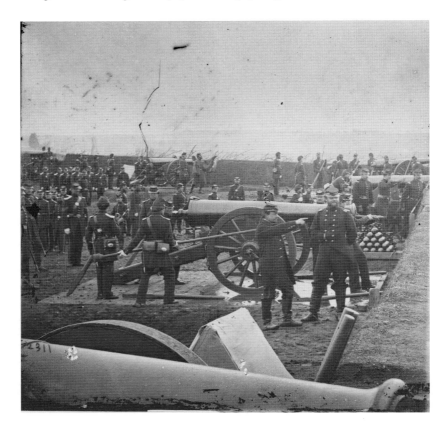

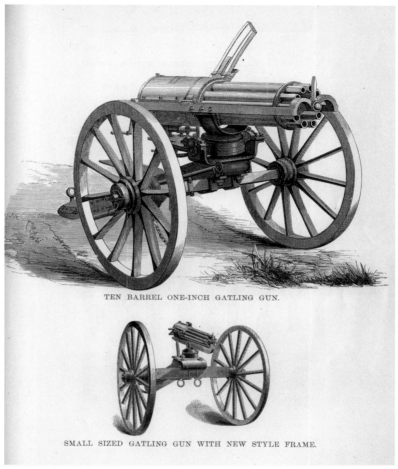

TEN BARREL ONE-INCH GATLING GUN.

SMALL SIZED GATLING GUN WITH NEW STYLE FRAME.

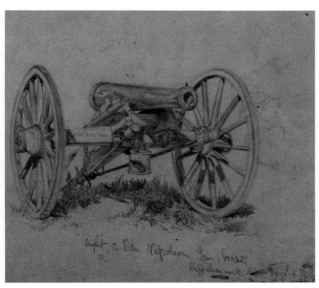

ABOVE: Gatling Gun. Printed paper image of an early machine gun invented in 1861 by Dr. Richard Jordan Gatling. It was a rapid-fire multiple-barrel firearm, a forerunner of the machine gun. *Courtesy of The Library Company of Philadelphia.* LEFT: Light "12-pounder Napoleon Gun, brass, in position covering the ford" on mount. A versatile cannon developed in France in 1853 and widely copied in America by North and South. Pencil drawing, 1863, Edwin Forbes, artist. *Courtesy of The Library of Congress.*

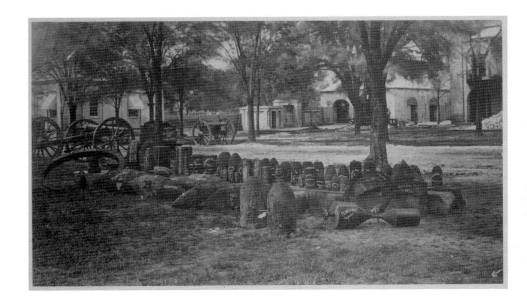

ABOVE: Confederate torpedoes, shot, and shells in front of the arsenal, Charleston, S.C. Photographic print by Mathew Brady, ca. 1865. *Courtesy of the National Archives.* BELOW: *The Battle of Gettysburg, Pennsylvania, July 3, 1863.* Currier & Ives, American printmaking firm, hand-colored lithograph. New York, 1863. *Courtesy of The Library Company of Philadelphia.*

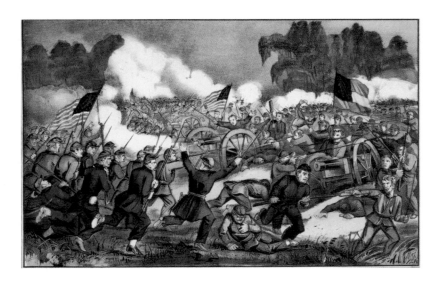

PROPOSALS

FOR THE REMOVAL OF THE DEAD ON THE
GETTYSBURG BATTLE-FIELD.

SEALED proposals will be received at my Office in the Borough of Gettysburg, until the 22d inst., at 12 o'clock, noon, for the following two contracts, viz:

1st.   For disinterring the bodies on the Gettysburg Battle Field and at the Hospitals in the vicinity, and removing them to the Soldiers' Cemetery on the south side of the Borough of Gettysburg.

2d.   For digging the graves, and burying the dead in the Cemetery.

☞The specifications of work for each contract, to be strictly complied with by the Contractor, can be seen and examined at my office.

DAVID WILLS,
Agent for A. G. CURTIN, Governor of Pennsylvania.

Gettysburg, Oct. 15, 1863.

PRINTED AT THE "SENTINEL OFFICE," GETTYSBURG.

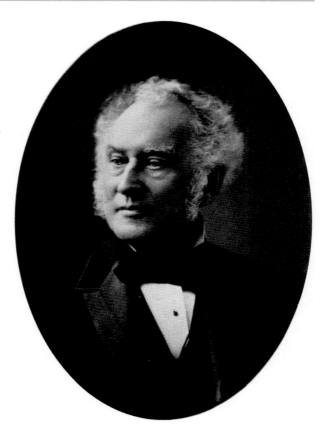

ABOVE: "Proposals for the Removal of the Dead on the Gettysburg Battle-field." Created by David Wills, who was President Abraham Lincoln's host while Lincoln was in Gettysburg. The Gettysburg Address was completed by the president in an upstairs bedroom of Wills's home. David Wills was key in establishing the National Cemetery at Gettysburg, Penn. Printed on paper, 33 x 48 cm. Originally part of a McAllister scrapbook. *Courtesy of The Library Company of Philadelphia.* RIGHT: Dr. Samuel David Gross, an academic trauma surgeon, professor, and author, taught generations of medical students and is immortalized in Thomas Eakins's painting *The Gross Clinic. From Wikimedia Commons.*

RIGHT: Surgeon General Samuel Preston Moore of the Confederate States of America was a brilliant visionary and administrator who reorganized and transformed the medical corps of the Confederate army into one of the most efficient and effective divisions of the Southern military. *From Wikimedia Commons.*

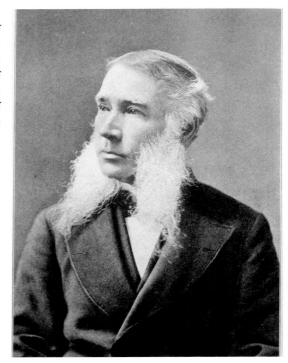

BELOW: Surgeon General William Alexander Hammond served a relatively brief tenure with the Union Army, but his huge impact on the medical corps would leave an indelible stamp. Hammond encouraged the creation of an ambulance corps, the keeping of meticulous medical records, the Army Medical Museum, and later, the American Neurological Association. *From Wikimedia Commons.*

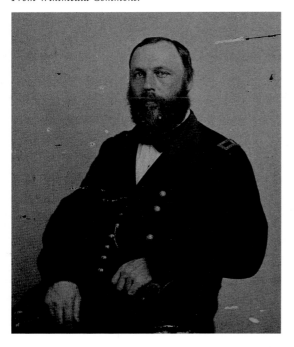

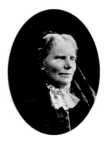

ABOVE: Dr. Elizabeth Blackwell was a brilliant and determined woman who became America's first degreed female medical doctor. A passionate and effective advocate for many causes in England and America, her dedication and her temper were equally respected. *From Wikimedia Commons.*

A BOOK FOR ALL TIME!

Will be ready in June, 1882.

EYERY LADY SHOULD OWN ONE

——OF——

DOCTRESS R. CRUMPLER'S

Book of Discourses

ON THE

Cause, Prevention and Cure of Infantile Stomach and Bowel Complaints, from birth to the close of the teething period.

EMBRACING AN EXPERIENCE OF NEARLY 30 YEARS.

REFERENCES.

" Dr. Rebecca Crumpler's manuscript contains very valuable information for women, and if published in book form I hope it will have a wide circulation."

Mrs. F. W. HARPER, Philadelphia, Pa.

" The subject matter of Dr. Rebecca Crumpler's manuscript is of very great importance to young mother's, and if published in book form should become a household companion of every family."

ISAAC J. WETHERBEE, M.D.

Boston, Nov. 3d, 1881.

" The manuscript of Dr. Rebecca Crumpler's book exhibits an excellent treatise to young mothers."

H. STACY, M.D.

Boston, Nov. 3d, 1881.

MAY BE OBTAINED OF

Doctress R. Crumpler, Readville, Mass.

Or any of her Agents.

ABOVE: At the time of the Civil War, Dr. Rebecca Lee Crumpler was the only African American woman in the country to hold a formal medical degree. In another singular effort, she published a textbook geared to the care of women and children, an area infrequently addressed in the mid–19th century. *Courtesy of The Library Company of Philadelphia.*

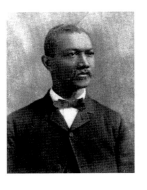

RIGHT: Dr. Alexander Thomas Augusta was the first African American physician commissioned as an officer in the U.S. Army. Denied a medical education in the United States owing to his race, Dr. Augusta moved to Canada where he earned his medical degree. His return to America would create his personal legacy of breaking barriers in medicine, the military, and medical education. *Courtesy of the National Park Service.*

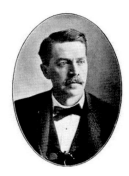

LEFT: Dr. Hunter Holmes McGuire demonstrated a lifetime of excellence as a surgeon, teacher, orator, and soldier. He served as a brigade surgeon to General Thomas "Stonewall" Jackson, becoming Jackson's close friend and personal physician. McGuire treated his commander after Jackson was shot by friendly fire, but was unable to save his good friend. For the rest of his life, Dr. McGuire wrote and spoke about Jackson's life and achievements. *From Wikimedia Commons.*

BELOW: Assassination of President Abraham Lincoln at Ford's Theatre, Washington, D.C., April 14, 1865. A depiction of the murder from the Rare Book And Special Collections Division, Broadside Collection, 33.8 x 42.8 cm. Date unknown. *Courtesy of The Library of Congress.*

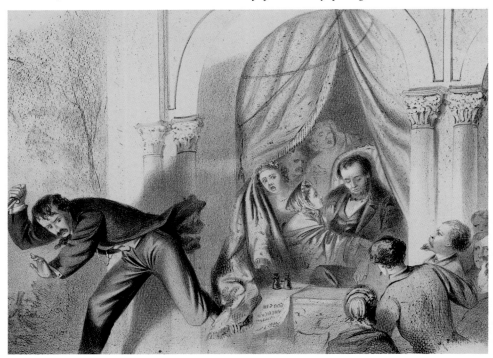

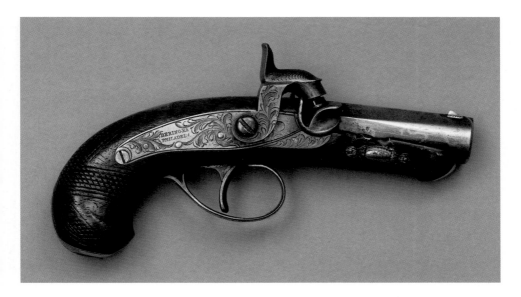

ABOVE: Derringer gun used by John Wilkes Booth to assassinate Abraham Lincoln. It is a .44 caliber pistol that fired a single round lead ball weighing almost an ounce. Photograph 2007. BELOW: *The "Bullet," With Which Our Martyr President A. Lincoln Was Assassinated By J.W. Booth, As Seen Under A Microscope.* Lithograph, Chicago Lithographing Co., Chicago, ca. 1867. Text on banner at top of print: "Death is not death, tis but the ennoblement of mortal man." *Both images courtesy of The Library of Congress.*

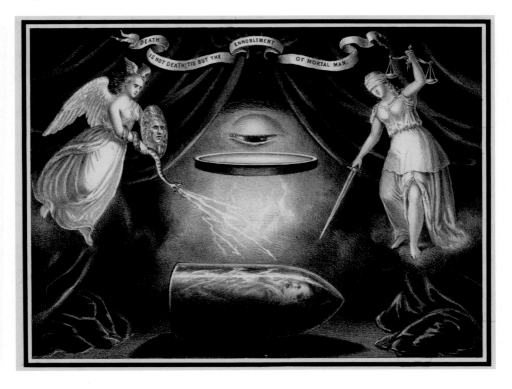

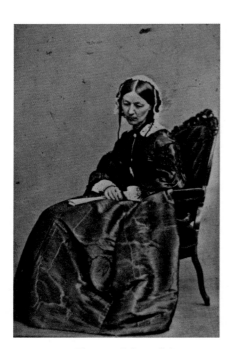 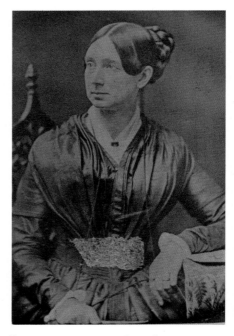

ABOVE LEFT: *Florence Nightingale/By appointment, Mr. Kilburn, 222 Regent Street.* Carte de visite portrait of the founder of modern nursing who served as an inspirational model for the American Civil War nurses. William Edward Kilburn, photographer. Albumen print, London, 1854. ABOVE RIGHT: *Dorothea L. Dix, Superintendent for Nurses for the Union Army During the Civil War.* Over the course of the war Dix appointed more than 3,000 nurses, approximately 15% of all Union Army nurses who served. G. K. (George Kendall) Warren, photographer. Boston, Mass., between 1861 and 1865. Cartes de visite, albumen print. *Both images courtesy of The Library of Congress.*

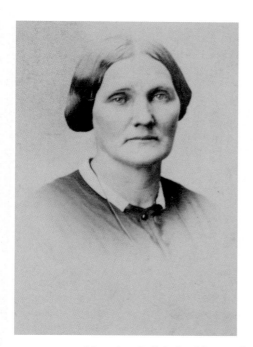 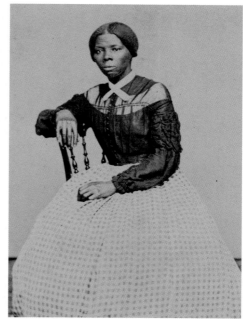

ABOVE LEFT: *Mary Ann Ball Bickerdyke, Civil War nurse and agent for the United States Sanitary Commission*/Fassett's Gallery, 122 & 124 Clark St., Chicago. Albumen print, carte de visite. S. M. (Samuel Montague) Fassett, photographer, Chicago, ca. 1860–1870. Beloved by the soldiers, she cared for wounded men on nineteen battlefields and improved or established almost 300 hospitals. ABOVE RIGHT: Portrait of Harriet Tubman, nurse, Union spy, scout, and conductor on the Underground Railroad, guiding people on the perilous journey to escape enslavement. Benjamin Powelson, photographer, Auburn, N.Y. 1868 or 1869. Albumen print, carte de visite. *Both images courtesy of The Library of Congress.*

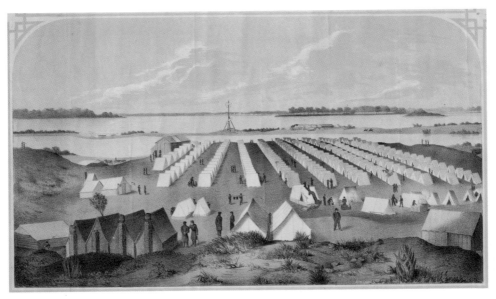

REMINISCENCES OF
MY LIFE IN CAMP

WITH THE 33D UNITED STATES
COLORED TROOPS LATE 1ST
S. C. VOLUNTEERS

BY

SUSIE KING TAYLOR

WITH ILLUSTRATIONS

BOSTON
PUBLISHED BY THE AUTHOR
21 HOLYOKE STREET
1904

ABOVE: *Camp of 104th Penna. Vol.'s Morris Island, S.C.* Susie King Taylor and her uncle escaped slavery and found their way to the Union-occupied Morris Island. The young teen began to hold classes, teaching children and adults how to read. Lithograph, tinted. Creator: Hoffman, Abram J., lithographer, Albany, N.Y., 1863. LEFT: As a young child, Susie King Taylor risked her life to learn to read. Escaping slavery at age fourteen, she served as a nurse, cook, and laundress in the Civil War, but perhaps her most important legacy was teaching literacy. She was the only African American woman to publish a book about her wartime experiences. *Both images above courtesy of The Library Company of Philadelphia.*

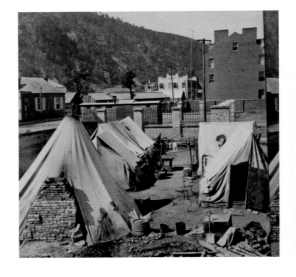

RIGHT: Contraband Camp, Harper's Ferry, Va. Stereograph shows a tent camp occupied by escaped slaves. John P. Soule, photographer. Albumen print. Boston, Mass., 1862. *Courtesy of The Library of Congress.*

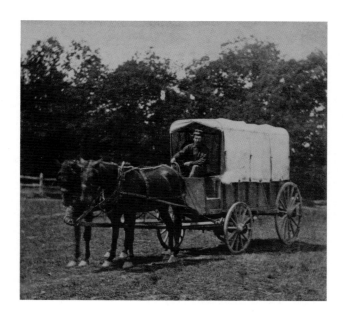

ABOVE: Ambulance wagon on the battlefield of Bull Run, where the Union troops suffered terrible losses. Stereograph showing soldier driving horse-drawn ambulance. Albumen print, stereograph format. Brady's National Photographic Portrait Galleries, photographer. E. & H. T. Anthony (Firm), publisher, 1861, New York. BELOW: Battle of Antietam—Army of the Potomac: Gen. Geo. B. McClellan, comm., Sept. 17, 1862. The single bloodiest day of the Civil War with 23,000 killed or wounded. Color lithograph, Kurz & Allison, Art Publishers, Chicago. ca. 1888. *Both images courtesy of The Library of Congress.*

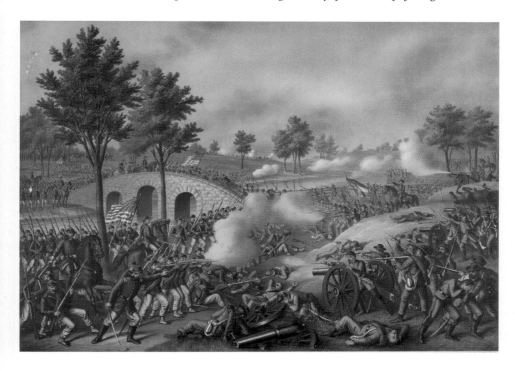

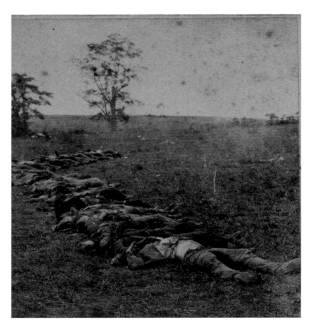

LEFT: *Gathered together for Burial after the Battle of Antietam*, showing dead bodies on the ground. Albumen print, stereograph. Alexander Gardner, photographer. Published E & H. T. Anthony, New York, 1862. *Courtesy of The Library of Congress.*

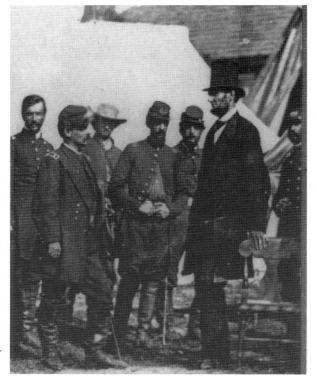

RIGHT: *Abraham Lincoln on battlefield at Antietam, Maryland*, cropped version that highlights McClellan and Lincoln. From left, Col. Alexander S. Webb, chief of staff, 5th Corps, Gen. George B. McClellan, and Lincoln. Photographic print, gelatin silver. Alexander Gardner, photographer, Washington, D.C., October 1862, printed later. *Courtesy of The Library of Congress.*

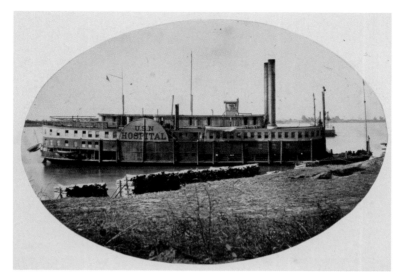

ABOVE: The U.S. Navy's first Union hospital ship, U.S.S. *Red Rover*, was a captured former Confederate vessel. The staff of the ship included female nurses—African American women and nuns from the Catholic order Sisters of the Holy Cross. Albumen print, stamped on verso: "Frank F. Raciti, 273 King George Road, Warren, New Jersey." Published between 1862 and 1865. *Courtesy of The Library of Congress.* BELOW: Camp Scene, Trestle Bridge at Whiteside, Va. Both armies shipped supplies in boxcars, and returned them filled with wounded soldiers. Creator, War Department, Office of the Chief Signal Officer, 1866. Photographer, Mathew Brady. *Courtesy of the National Archives.*

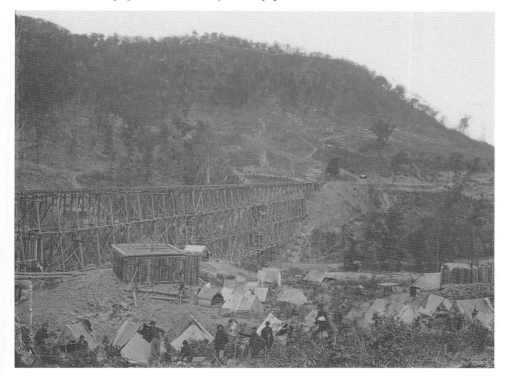

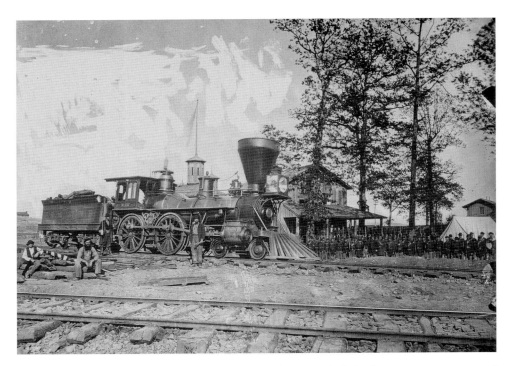

ABOVE: Engine No. 137, U.S. Military R.R. The Civil War marked the first time trains were used as ambulances in America. Creator: War Department, Office of the Chief Signal Officer, Mathew Brady, photographer. ca. 1860–1865. *Courtesy of the National Archives.* BELOW: Lincoln Hospital, Washington, D.C., was a temporary hospital established during the Civil War in an area of the city known today as Lincoln Park. Hand-colored lithograph, published by Charles Magnus, New York and Washington, ca. 1864. *Courtesy of The Library of Congress.*

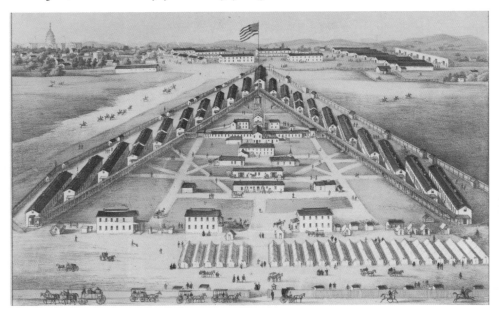

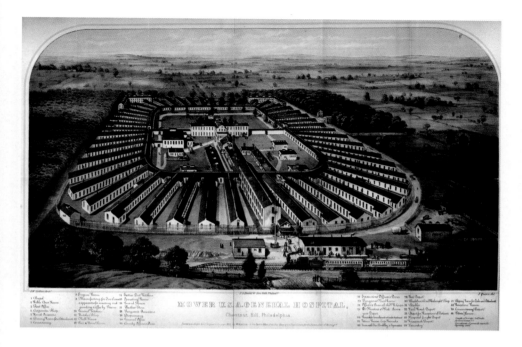

ABOVE: Mower U.S.A. General Hospital, Chestnut Hill, Philadelphia. James Fuller Queen, artist. Lithograph, color. P.S. Duval & Son, publisher, Philadelphia ca. 1865. One of the largest military hospitals in the North, Mower had 3,600 beds. *Courtesy of The Library Company of Philadelphia.*
BELOW: Hicks U.S. General Hospital, Baltimore, Md. Jun Caldwell, architect. Print by E. Sachse & Co., Baltimore. Color lithograph, Bar Kane, ca. 1864. *Courtesy of The Library of Congress.*

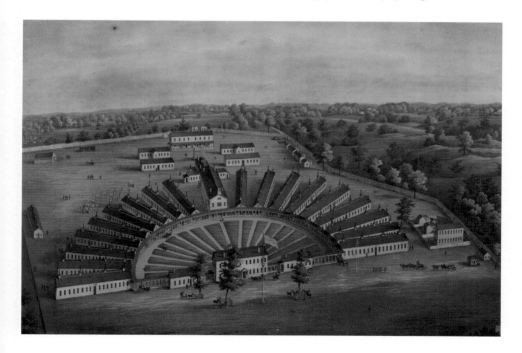

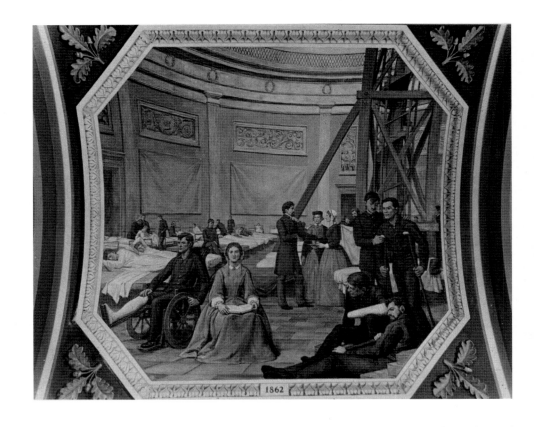

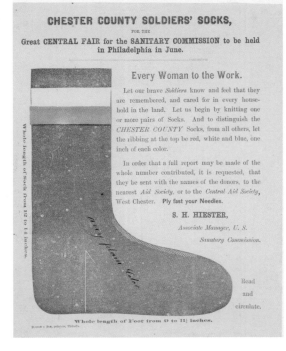

ABOVE: The Capitol used as a hospital during the Civil War. Photographic print, artist unknown. Many public and private buildings in Washington, D.C., were utilized as hospitals during the war. *Courtesy of National Library of Medicine.*

LEFT: *Chester County Soldiers' Socks, for the Great Central Fair for the Sanitary Commission to be held in Philadelphia in June.* The shortage of supplies for the soldiers was serious, especially for items that were created by hand. Women from North and South volunteered to knit socks and mittens for the troops from patterns that were distributed or printed in the newspapers. Lithograph, published by P.S. Duval & Son, Philadelphia, 1864. *Courtesy of The Library Company of Philadelphia.*

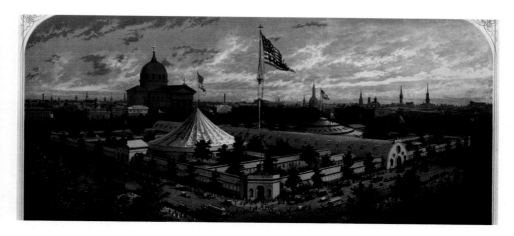

ABOVE: *Buildings of the Great Central Fair, in aid of the U.S. Sanitary Commission, Logan Square.* Lithograph, James Queen, creator. Published by P.S. Duval & Son, Philadelphia, 1864. BELOW: The "Sanitary Fairs," organized to aid the work of the United States Sanitary Commission, were large events that frequently lasted one to three weeks in Union cities. A special daily newspaper like *Our Daily Fare* was issued at many of them, listing the times and places of events including musical performances, auctions, and restaurant hours. *Both images courtesy of The Library Company of Philadelphia.*

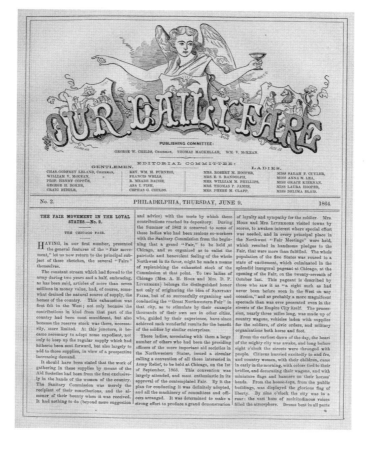

OUR DAILY FARE

PUBLISHING COMMITTEE:

GEORGE W. CHILDS, Chairman, THOMAS MACKELLAR, WM. V. McKEAN.

EDITORIAL COMMITTEE:

GENTLEMEN.

CHAS. GODFREY LELAND, Chairman,
WILLIAM V. McKEAN,
PROF. HENRY COPPÉE,
GEORGE H. BOKER,
CRAIG BIDDLE.

REV. WM. H. FURNESS,
FRANCIS WELLS,
R. MEADE BACHE,
ASA I. FISH,
CEPHAS G. CHILDS.

LADIES.

MRS. ROBERT M. HOOPER,
MRS. R. S. RANDOLPH,
MRS. WILLIAM M. PHILLIPS,
MRS. THOMAS P. JAMES,
MRS. PHEBE M. CLAPP,

MISS SARAH P. CUYLER,
MISS ANNA M. LEA,
MISS GRACE KIERNAN,
MISS LAURA HOOPER,
MISS DELIMA BLAIR.

No. 2.   PHILADELPHIA, THURSDAY, JUNE 9.   1864.

THE FAIR MOVEMENT IN THE LOYAL STATES.—No. 2.

THE CHICAGO FAIR.

HAVING, in our first number, presented the general features of the "Fair movement," let us now return to the principal subject of these sketches, the several "Fairs" themselves.

The constant stream which had flowed to the army during two years and a half, embracing, as has been said, articles of more than seven millions in money value, had, of course, somewhat drained the natural source of supply, the homes of the country. This exhaustion was first felt in the West; not only because the contributions in kind from that part of the country had been most munificent, but also because the reserve stock was there, necessarily, more limited. At this juncture, it became necessary to adopt some expedient, not only to keep up the regular supply which had hitherto been sent forward, but also largely to add to those supplies, in view of a prospective increasing demand.

It should have been stated that the work of gathering in these supplies by means of the Aid Societies had been from the first exclusively in the hands of the women of the country. The Sanitary Commission was merely the recipient of their contributions, and the almoner of their bounty when it was received. It had nothing to do (beyond mere suggestion

and advice) with the mode by which these contributions reached its depository. During the Summer of 1863 it occurred to some of those ladies who had been zealous co-workers with the Sanitary Commission from the beginning that a grand "Fair," to be held at Chicago, and so organized as to enlist the patriotic and benevolent feeling of the whole Northwest in its favor, might be made a means of replenishing the exhausted stock of the Commission at that point. To two ladies of Chicago (Mrs. A. H. HOGE and Mrs. D. P. LIVERMORE) belongs the distinguished honor not only of originating the idea of SANITARY FAIRS, but of so successfully organizing and conducting the "Great Northwestern Fair" in that city, as to stimulate by their example thousands of their own sex in other cities, who, guided by their experience, have since achieved such wonderful results for the benefit of the soldier by similar enterprises.

These ladies, associating with them a large number of others who had been the presiding officers of the more important aid societies in the Northwestern States, issued a circular calling a convention of all those interested in Army Relief, to be held at Chicago, on the 1st of September, 1863. This convention was largely attended, and most enthusiastic in its approval of the contemplated Fair. By it the plan for conducting it was definitely adopted, and all the machinery of committees and officers arranged. It was determined to make a strong effort to produce a grand demonstration

of loyalty and sympathy for the soldier. Mrs. HOGE and Mrs. LIVERMORE visited towns by scores, to awaken interest where special effort was needed, and in every principal place in the Northwest "Fair Meetings" were held. The whole population of the five States was roused to a state of excitement, which culminated in the splendid inaugural pageant at Chicago, at the opening of the Fair, on the twenty-seventh of October last. This pageant is described by those who saw it as "a sight such as had never been seen in the West on any occasion," and as probably a more magnificent spectacle than was ever presented even in the streets of the Empire City itself. The procession, nearly three miles long, was made up of country wagons, vehicles laden with supplies for the soldiers, of civic orders, and military organisations both horse and foot.

From the earliest dawn of the day, the heart of the mighty city was awake, and long before eight o'clock the streets were thronged with people. Citizens hurried excitedly to and fro, in early in the morning, with colors tied to their bridles, and decorating their wagons, and with miniature flags and banners on their horses' heads. From the house-tops, from the public buildings, was displayed the glorious flag of liberty. By nine o'clock the city was in a roar; the vast hum of multitudinous voices filled the atmosphere. Drums beat in all parts

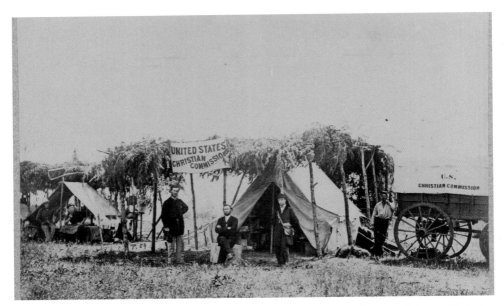

ABOVE: *Headquarters of the U.S. Christian Commission in Virginia.* The United States Christian Commission was created by a convention of the Young Men's Christian Association (Y.M.C.A.) in response to the terrible losses at the First Battle of Bull Run. The U.S.C.C.'s agents provided religious support to the troops, and also brought chaplains, social workers, and recreation to the soldiers suffering under wartime conditions. Unknown author. *From Wikimedia Commons.* BELOW: The Executive Committee of the U.S. Sanitary Commission. From left: Dr. William Holme Van Buren, George T. Strong, Rev. Henry Whitney Bellows, Dr. Cornelius R. Agnew, and Prof. Wolcott Gibbs. Glass negative, wet collodion, photographer unknown. Published between 1860 and 1870. *Courtesy of The Library of Congress.*

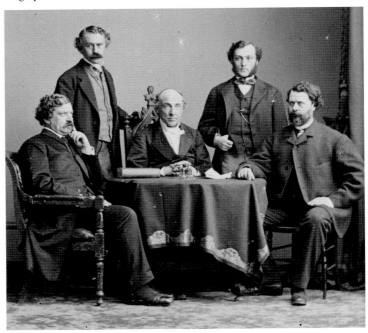

RIGHT: Portrait of Mary Todd Lincoln in a gown that was created for her by Elizabeth Hobbs Keckley, a brilliant designer who purchased her own freedom from slavery. Keckley established a popular business in Washington, D.C.; her earlier clients included the wives of Robert E. Lee and Jefferson Davis. Photograph, albumen print, Mathew Brady, photographer, 1861. BELOW: *Grounds at Andersonville, Georgia, where are buried fourteen thousand Union soldiers, who died in Andersonville Prison.* Sketched by I. C. Schotel. A large part of Clara Barton's chosen mission was to identify missing and dead soldiers, especially those who died in Confederate prisons. Her perseverance and the assistance of veteran and former prisoner Dorence Atwater led to the official marking of 12,000 graves at Andersonville, Ga., and its classification as a national cemetery on August 17, 1865. She can be seen here raising the flag at the cemetery. Print, wood engraving. *Both images courtesy of The Library of Congress.*

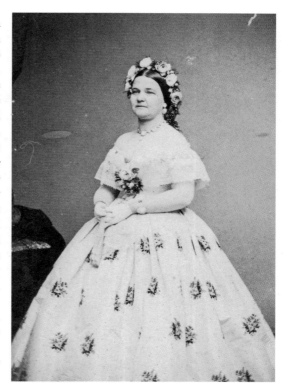

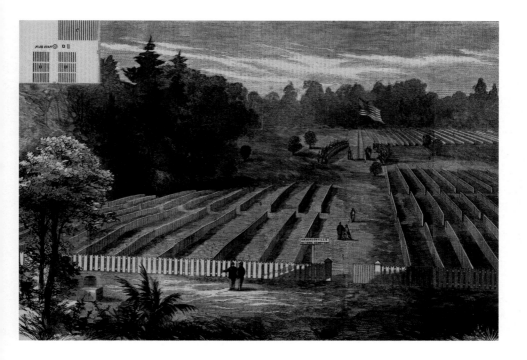

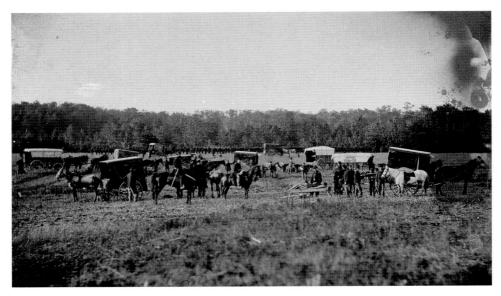

ABOVE: Removing Wounded. Ambulance drill of the 57th New York Infantry, 1864. At the beginning of the Civil War, the Union Army had no designated ambulance vehicles or trained personnel to transport the wounded men. Major Jonathan Letterman's Ambulance Corps created a reliable system to rescue and evacuate injured soldiers. Mathew Brady, photographer. War Department, Office of the Chief Signal Officer, 1866. *Courtesy of the National Archives.*

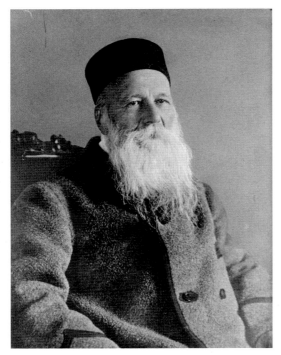

LEFT: Jean Henri Dunant of Geneva, Switzerland, conceived the idea of a society for the aid of wounded soldiers when he witnessed the terrible slaughter at the Battle of Solferino (Italy) in 1859. Dunant's vision led to the first Geneva Convention and the founding of the International Committee of the Red Cross. His work inspired relief worker and social reformer Clara Barton to establish the American Red Cross. Henri Dunant was a recipient of the first Nobel Peace Prize. Glass negative, American National Red Cross photograph collection. *Courtesy of The Library of Congress.*

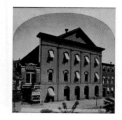

LEFT: *The Army Medical Museum and Library*, established during the Civil War by U.S. Army surgeon general William Hammond, was designed to house the Army Medical Museum, the Library of the Surgeon General's Office (later called the Army Medical Library), and some of the military's medical records. Hammond's design was intended as a collection center for specimens to be used in research for the improvement and advancement of military medicine and surgery. *From Wikimedia Commons.* BELOW: Group portrait of Civil War nurses Sarah ("Sallie") Elizabeth Dysart, Anna ("Annie") Bell Stubbs of 12th Army Corps, and Sarah ("Sallie") Chamberlin Eccleston, volunteer nurse, at Hospital No. 1, Nashville, Tenn. Albumen print on card mount, 1863. *Courtesy of The Library of Congress.*

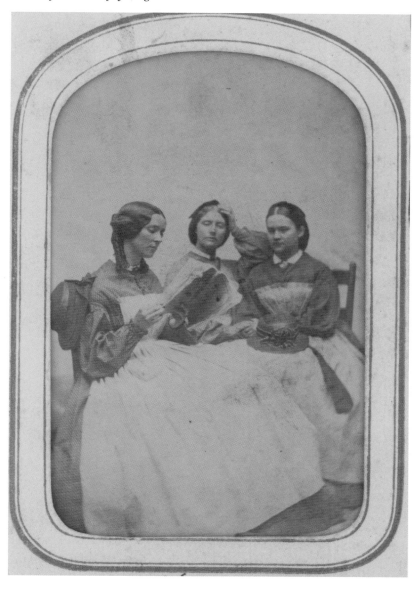

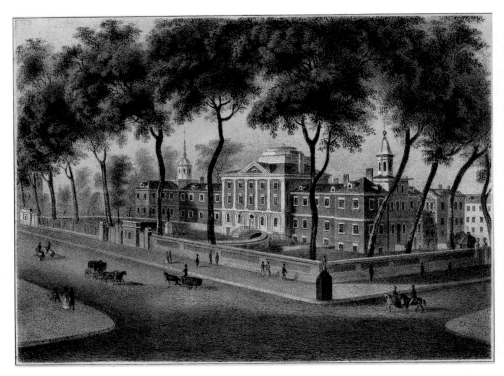

ABOVE: Pennsylvania Hospital, the nation's first hospital, was founded in 1751 to care for the indigent and homeless sick and insane of Philadelphia. It featured a deep "dry moat" so that mental patients could safely experience exercise outdoors. The Civil War inspired the establishment of hundreds more hospitals in America. Print lithograph, hand-colored. J. C. (John Caspar) Wild, artist. Published by J. T. Bowen at his Lithographic & Print Colouring Establishment, 94 Walnut Street, ca. 1840, 1848. *Courtesy of The Library Company of Philadelphia.* BELOW: *The Red Cross in Peace and War* is a 1912 reissue of Clara Barton's original 1898 book, *The Red Cross, A History of This Remarkable International Movement in the Interest of Humanity. Courtesy of the National Park Service.*

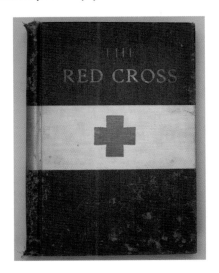

ACKNOWLEDGMENTS

I am profoundly grateful to the seven people who have been the architects of my knowledge in the field of Civil War medicine, introducing me to aspects of this 19th century phenomena in fascinating and eye-opening ways. They have shared their remarkable wealth of knowledge and given me the closest thing to a time warp experience, explaining much about a faraway time, the individuals, events and efforts of the people of a shattered America. It has been a remarkable privilege to experience their expert perspectives and to handle iconic pieces of our country's history. I hope you seven will all see your shared work in this story and please know that I am both proud and humbled to be presenting it. Michael, Jay, Pete, Robert, Sarah, Connie and Jim, thank you so much.

F. Michael Angelo, Alfred Jay Bollet, Peter J. D'Onofrio, Robert D. Hicks, Cornelia S. King, James G. Mundy Jr., Sarah Weatherwax.

A huge debt of gratitude and appreciation goes to my agent, Don Fehr of Trident Media Group Literary Agency for seeing the possibilities of this book, giving me the opportunity and encouragement and teaching me how to become a better writer in the process. I take great pride in being represented by you.

ACKNOWLEDGMENTS

I am very thankful for Claiborne Hancock and Jessica Case of Pegasus Books who saw the value in a work on this serious topic, believed in my ability to produce it and graciously welcomed me to this distinguished publishing house. It is truly an honor to be one of your authors.

It has been a great privilege and pleasure to work with the Pegasus team. My great gratitude to Maria Fernandez for her wonderful book design and for guiding me through the mysterious and very technical terrain of the publishing world. Peter Kranitz did an amazing copy edit that totally stunned me yet taught me so much. The cover art by Faceout Studio is thrilling and beautiful, and the exacting work of proofreader Drew Wheeler, and cold read by Madeleine Aitchison has made this a better book, for which I am very appreciative. Indexer Gina Guilinger has done a wonderful job of making the information in this book more accessible to the reader. Excellent editorial support from Victoria Wenzel helped to pull this entire project together. I am extremely grateful to all of you.

Many thanks to Grace Johnson, Don Fehr's stellar assistant, who has also really helped guide me through the Great Unknown of the publishing process with exceptional knowledge and charm.

There are some awesome friends and colleagues who deserve big thanks. You guys encouraged and cheered me on all the way through the writing, reviewed the legalities, read chapters and gave great feedback, or handled the technical and cyber end of things, and you all believed in me. I am so grateful to every one of you and promise to pass along your kindness and encouragement:

Richard J. Anthony Sr., Mary Bartlett, David Blistein, Tony Chan, Cynthia L. Dahl, Tris R. Fall, Rick Kiernan, Abbe Joan Klebanoff, Craig A. Meritz, Lisa Z. Meritz, Steven Polsky, Sy Rotter, J. M. Sullivan.

After stumbling upon the incredible story and implications of Civil War medicine, I spent several years researching the topic in order to create a documentary series, and met amazing people—curators, librarians, archivists, historians, teachers, and collectors—who shared a wealth of their information and primary source materials with me. They are an extraordinary group that dedicates its abilities and talents to ensure that the history of our country and its people is kept alive and supported. When the opportunity to write this book appeared, I drew directly on the foundation of knowledge they have shared with me. My extreme gratitude to the exceptional keepers of our history who staff these distinguished American institutions. I hope that you will enjoy this book and feel pride in your contributions to it.

American Dental Association, The Bio-Medical Library of the University of Pennsylvania, The Civil War Library and Museum, The College of the Physicians of Philadelphia, Drexel University Legacy Center Archives & Special Collections/College of Medicine, The Foard Collection of Civil War Nursing, The Free Library of Philadelphia, Grand Army of the Republic, Hollywood Cemetery, Kelman Library of Wills Eye Hospital, The Library Company of Philadelphia, The Library of Congress, Library of Virginia, MCP Hahnemann University Archives and Special Collections, Merck Archives, Museum of the Confederacy, The Mütter Museum, The National Museum of Civil War Medicine, The National Library of Medicine, The National Museum of Dentistry, The National Museum of Health and Medicine, Pennsylvania Hospital Historic Collections, Philadelphia Archdiocesan Historical Research Center, Philadelphia Orchestra Association Archives, Philadelphia VIP, Philadelphia Volunteer Lawyers for the Arts, Sisters of St. Joseph, The Society of Civil War Surgeons, Thomas Jefferson University Archives and Special Collections, The Union League of Philadelphia, United States Army Heritage and Education Center, University of Pennsylvania Archives, The University of Pennsylvania Carey Law School, Wood Library-Museum of Anesthesiology.

Special Thanks
J. P. Cummins

BIBLIOGRAPHY

Addison, Agnes, ed. *Portraits in the University of Pennsylvania*. University of Pennsylvania Press, Philadelphia, 1940.

Albin, Maurice S. "The Use of Anesthetics During the Civil War, 1861–1865." *Pharmacy in History*. Vol. 42, No. ¾, Civil War Pharmacy. Madison, Wisconsin, 2000.

——. "The Use of Anesthetics during the Civil War, 1861–1865." *Bulletin of Anesthesia History*. April 2001. Vol. 19, No. 2. Chicago.

Alexander, E. Porter, General. *The Confederate Veteran*. Address delivered on Alumni Day, West Point Military Centennial, June 9, 1902. Pub. The Burrows Brothers Company, Cleveland, Ohio, 1902.

American Association for the History of Nursing. *Nursing History Review*. Vol. 3. University of Pennsylvania Press, Philadelphia, 1995.

Angle, Paul M. *A Pictorial History of The Civil War Years*. Doubleday & Company, Inc., Garden City, N.Y., 1967.

Arnold, James R., and Roberta Wiener, editorial consultants. *The Timechart History of the Civil War*. Lowe & B. Hould Publishers, Ann Arbor, Michigan, 2001.

Asimov, Isaac. *Science Past-Science Future*. Doubleday & Company, Inc., New York, 1975.

Austin, F. E. Daniel. *Recollections of a Rebel Surgeon*. Von Boeckmann, Schutze and Co., Austin, Texas, 1899.

Avery, Derek, ed. *Fighting Forces: A Complete History of the United States Army-Marine Corps, Navy, Air Force*. Trodd, Brian Publishing, London, 1989.

Barnes, A. S. *A Brief History of the United States*. A.S. Barnes and Company, New York and Chicago, 1880.

Barnes, Joseph K., M.D. Surgeon General United States Army, J. J. Woodward, Assistant Surgeon United States Army: prepared under the direction of. *The Medical and Surgical History of the War of the Rebellion*. Government Printing Office, Washington, 1870.

Barton, Clara, president and treasurer of the American National Red Cross. *The Red Cross: A History of This Remarkable International Movement in the Interest of Humanity.* American National Red Cross, Washington, 1898.

Bell, George B. Tatum Jr., Whitfield J., Sellers, Charles Coleman. *The Art of Philadelphia Medicine.* Philadelphia Museum of Art, Philadelphia, 1965.

Billings, John S., M.D. *Medical Reminiscences of the Civil War. Remarks.* Transactions of the College of Physicians of Philadelphia. Third Series. 1905.

Bishop, Jim. *The Day Lincoln Was Shot.* Scholastic Book Services, New York, 1955.

Blay, John S. *The Civil War: A Pictorial Profile.* Thomas Y. Crowell Company, New York, 1958.

Bollet, Alfred Jay, M.D. *Civil War Medicine: Challenges and Triumphs.* Galen Press, Ltd., Tucson, Ariz., 2002.

Boos, Louis J., Late Sergeant 6th Pa. Cavy. *Civil War Papers.* 1870.

Botkin, B. A., ed. *A Civil War Treasury of Tales, Legends and Folklore.* Promontory Press, Victoria, Canada, 1960.

Bullough, Vern L., Lilli Sentz, and Alice P. Stein, eds. *American Nursing: A Biographical Dictionary, Vol. II.* Garland Publishing, Inc., New York & London, 1992.

Cashin, Joan E., ed. *War Matters: Material Culture in the Civil War Era.* University of North Carolina Press, Chapel Hill, 2018.

Catton, Bruce. *Grant Takes Command.* Little, Brown and Company, Boston, 1969.

Chambers, John Whiteclay II, ed. *The Oxford Companion to American Military History.* Oxford University Press, Inc., New York, 1999.

Channing, Steven A., and the editors of Time-Life Books. *Confederate Ordeal: The Southern Home Front.* Time-Life Books, Alexandria, Va., 1984.

Chisolm, J. Julian, M.D. *A Manual of Military Surgery, for the Use of Surgeons in the Confederate States Army.* Second edition. Richmond, Va., 1862.

Church News of the Diocese of Pennsylvania. *Obituary, Dr. S. Weir Mitchell.* Philadelphia, 1914.

Cohen, Daniel. *Civil War Ghosts.* Scholastic, Inc. New York, Toronto, London, 1999.

College of Physicians of Philadelphia. *Summary of the Transactions of the College of Physicians of Philadelphia. Vol. I.* New series. From November 1850 to April 1853, inclusive. Lippincott, Grambo, and Co., Philadelphia, 1853.

"Confederate Military Medicine." *JAMA Editorials. Journal of the American Medical Association.* February 4, 1961. Chicago.

Confederate States of America. Surgeon-General's Office. Confederate States of America Collection (Library of Congress), and Joseph Meredith Toner Collection (Library of Congress). *A Manual of Military Surgery: Prepared for the Use of the Confederate States Army.* Ayres & Wade, Illustrated News Steam Presses, Richmond, Va., 1863.

Cope, Doris K., M.D. "Anesthesia in Ante Bellum New Orleans." *AHA News.* April 1994. Vol. 112, No. 4. Presented at the Second Spring Meeting of the Anesthesia History Association, April 20, 1994, New York: 12–13.

Corner, George W., M.D., Sc.D., LL.D. *Two Centuries of Medicine: A History of the School of Medicine, University of Pennsylvania.* J.B. Lippincott Company, Philadelphia, 1965.

BIBLIOGRAPHY

Cowley, Robert, and Geoffrey Parker. *The Reader's Companion to Military History.* Houghton Mifflin Company, Boston, 1996.

Cox, Clinton. *Undying Glory: The Story of the Massachusetts 54th Regiment.* Authors Guild Backinprint.com, published by iUniverse, Inc., Lincoln, Neb., 1991, 2007.

Cross, Andrew Boyd. *The War and the Christian Commission.* Publisher not identified, possibly Baltimore, 1865.

Current, Richard N., T. Harry Williams, and Frank Freidel. *American History: A Survey. Volumes I and II.* Alfred A. Knopf. New York, 1961, 1979.

Davis, Kenneth C. *Don't Know Much About the Civil War.* William Morrow and Co., New York, 1996.

Davis, William C. *Rebels & Yankees: The Fighting Men of the Civil War.* Salamander Books, Ltd., London, 1999.

——. *Rebels and Yankees: The Commanders of the Civil War.* Salamander Books, Ltd., London, 1999.

——. *The Battlefields of the Civil War.* By Salamander Books, Ltd., London, 1999.

DeBarr, Candice M., and Jack A. Bonkowske. *Saga of the American Flag: An Illustrated History.* Harbinger House, Tucson, Ariz. and New York, 1990.

Denney, Robert E. *Civil War Medicine: Care & Comfort of the Wounded.* Sterling Publishing Co., Inc., New York, 1995.

Dodge, W. C., Late Examiner, U.S. Patent Office. *Breech-Loaders versus Muzzle-Loaders: Or, How To Strengthen Our Army and Crush the Rebellion, with a Saving of Life and Treasure.* Third Edition. Pamphlet. W.C. Dodge, Washington, 1865.

Drum, William. F., Lieutenant-Colonel, Twelfth U.S. Infantry. *Work of the Fifth Corps, Ambulance Train, Spring and Summer of 1864.* Glimpses of the Nation's Struggle. A series of papers read before the Minnesota Commandery of the Military Order of the Loyal Legion of the United States., D.D. Merrill Company, New York, St. Paul, Minn., 1893. Broadfoot Publishing Company, Wilmington, N.C., 1992.

Dunn, Richard Slator, and Mark Frazier Lloyd, eds. *A Pennsylvania Album: Undergraduate Essays on the 250th Anniversary of the University of Pennsylvania.* University of Pennsylvania, Philadelphia, 1990.

Dyer, Gwynne. *War.* Media Resources, Crown Publishers, Inc., New York, 1985.

Elkins, Stanley M. *Slavery: A Problem in American Institutional Intellectual Life.* University of Chicago Press, Chicago and London, 1968.

Ellsworth, Colonel Elmer. *Col. Ellsworth's Last Letter to His Parents.* Unpublished letter. Philadelphia, 1861.

Elson, Henry William. *History of the United States, Vol. V.* The Macmillan Company, New York, 1905.

Epps, Charles H. Jr., M.D., Davis G. Johnson, Ph.D., and Audrey L. Vaughan, M.S. *African-American Medical Pioneers.* Betz Publishing Co., Rockville, Md., 1994.

Ewing, James, M.D. (Formerly, Contract Surgeon, Army Medical Museum, Washington). *Experiences in the Collection of Museum Material from Army Camp Hospitals.* Cornell University Medical School, New York, 1922.

Farrar, Emmie Ferguson. *Old Virginia Houses Along the James.* Bonanza Books, New York, 1955.

Female Medical College of Pennsylvania. *Minute Book 1850–1864.* Philadelphia, 1864.

——. *Valedictory Address to the Graduating Class of the Female Medical College of Pennsylvania at the Twelfth Annual Commencement.* Philadelphia, March 16, 1864.

Fink, B. Raymond, ed. *The History of Anesthesia, Third International Symposium. Proceedings, Atlanta, Georgia, March 27–31, 1992.* Wood Library-Museum of Anesthesiology, Schaumburg, Ill., 1992.

Fogel, Robert William. *Without Consent or Contract: The Rise and Fall of American Slavery.* W.W. Norton and Company, New York, 1989.

Foreman, Amanda. *A World on Fire: Britain's Crucial Role in the American Civil War.* Random House, New York, 2010.

Franklin, William B., Major General, United States Army. *The Gatling Gun, For Service Ashore and Afloat: With a History of the Invention, Description of the Gun, Official Reports of Recent Trials, General Directions, and Engravings of the Gun, Carriages, Practice Targets, &c.* The Case, Lockwood and Brainard Co., Hartford, Conn., 1874.

Fritz, Jean. *Stonewall.* G.P. Putnam's Sons, New York, 1979.

Fussell, Paul. *Uniforms: Why We Are What We Wear.* Houghton Mifflin Company, Boston, New York, 2002.

Gardner, Alexander. *Gardner's Photographic Sketch Book of the Civil War.* Dover Publications, Inc., New York, 1959.

Garrison, Webb. *Civil War Curiosities: Strange Stories, Oddities, Events, and Coincidences.* Rutledge Hill Press, Nashville, Tenn., 1994.

Garrity, John A., and Mark Carnes. *American National Biography.* Oxford University Press, Oxford, UK, 1999.

Glatthaar, Joseph. *The Civil War's Black Soldiers.* Eastern National Park and Monument Association, Fort Washington, Penn., 1996.

Gleason, Michael P. *The Insiders' Guide to the Civil War: The Eastern Theater.* Richmond Newspapers, Inc., Richmond, Va., 1994.

Gordon, S. C., Major and Surgeon. *Reminiscences of the Civil War from a Surgeon's Point of View.* War Papers Read before the Commandery of the State of Maine, Military Order of the Loyal Legion of the United States. Volume 1. Portland, The Thurston Print, 1898. Broadfoot Publishing Company, Wilmington, N.C., 1992.

Graf, Mercedes. "Women Physicians in the Civil War." *Quarterly of the National Archives and Records Administration.* Summer 2001. Vol. 32, No. 2. Washington.

Grimsley, Mark. *The Hard Hand of War: Union Military Policy Toward Southern Civilians 1861–1865.* Cambridge University Press, Cambridge, UK, 1995.

Gross, S. G., M.D., LL.D., Professor of Surgery in the Jefferson Medical College, Philadelphia. *System of Surgery, Vol. 1.* Blanchard and Lea, Philadelphia, 1856.

——. *A Manual of Military Surgery; Or, Hints of the Emergencies of Field, Camp, and Hospital Practice.* J.B. Lippincott & Co., Philadelphia, 1861.

——. *A Manual of Military Surgery; Or, Hints on the Emergencies of Field, Camp and Hospital Practice.* J.B. Lippincott & Co., Philadelphia, 1862

Grun, Bernard. *The Timetables of History: A Horizontal Linkage of People and Events*. Simon & Schuster, New York 1999.

Hackett, Sir John, General. *The Profession of Arms*. Macmillan Publishing Company, New York, 1983.

Hammerton, Sir J. A., ed. *Concise Universal Biography, Vol. 3*. Amalgamated Press, London, 1936

Hammond, William A. "Excerpt." *The New York Medical Journal*, Vol. 5, No. 2, New York, May 1867.

Hand, Daniel, Colonel, Surgeon, U.S. Volunteers. *Reminiscences of an Army Surgeon*. Glimpses of the Nation's Struggle: A series of papers read before the Minnesota Commandery of the Military Order of the Loyal Legion of the United States. St. Paul Book and Stationery Company, 1887. Broadfoot Publishing Company, Wilmington, N.C., 1992.

Harper, Fletcher. *Harper's Weekly Journal of Civilization*. Volumes 5–9. Harper & Brothers, New York, 1861–1865.

Harvey, Eleanor Jones. *The Civil War and American Art*. Smithsonian American Art Museum, Washington, in association with Yale University Press, New Haven, Conn., 2012.

Hasegawa, Guy R., PharmD. "The Civil War's Medical Cadets: Medical Cadets: Medical Students; Serving the Union." *Journal of the American College of Surgeons*. July 2001. Vol. 193, No. 1. Chicago.

Hicks, Robert D., ed. *Civil War Medicine: A Surgeon's Diary*. Indiana University Press, Bloomington, 2019.

Hill, Sarah Jane Full. *Mrs. Hill's Journal: Civil War Reminiscences*. Edited by Mark M. Krug. The Lakeside Press, Chicago, 1980.

Holmes, Oliver Wendell Jr. "The Human Wheel, Its Spokes and Felloes." *Atlantic Monthly*, May 1863. Reprinted B. Frank Palmer, J.R. Osgood and Company, Philadelphia, Boston, 1872.

Holzer, Harold. *Lincoln at Cooper Union: The Speech That Made Abraham Lincoln President*. Simon & Schuster Paperbacks, New York, 2004.

Homeopathic Medical College. *Semi-Annual Report of the Ladies' Association of the Homoeopathic Hospital of Philadelphia for Sick and Wounded Soldiers*. Deacon & Peterson, Printers, Philadelphia, 1863.

Horgan, Kevin. *The March of the 18th: A Story of Crippled Heroes in the Civil War*. Xulon Press, Irving, Tx., 2013.

January, Brendan. *Fort Sumter (Cornerstones of Freedom)*. Children's Press, division of Grolier Publishing, New York, London, 1997.

Jenkins, J. Foster, M.D., President of the Society, New York. *Relations of the War to Medical Science*. The Annual Address delivered before the Westchester Co. [N.Y.] Medical Society, June 16, 1863. Bailliere Brothers, New York, 1863.

Jones, Buehring H., Col., 60th Virginia Infantry, *The Sunny Land; or, Prison Prose and Poetry, Containing The Productions of the Ablest Writers in the South, and Prison Lays of Distinguished Confederate Officers*. Houston, J. A., ed. Innes, Baltimore, 1868.

BIBLIOGRAPHY

Jordan, Robert Paul. *The Civil War.* Prepared by the Special Publications Division, National Geographic Society, Washington, 1969, 1983.

Katz, Harry L., and Vincent Virga. *Civil War Sketch Book: Drawings from the Battlefront.* W.W. Norton and Company, New York, 2012.

Kaufman, Martin, ed. *Dictionary of American Nursing Biography.* Greenwood Press, Westport, Conn., 1988.

Kavanagh, Jack, and Eugene C. Murdoch. *Robert E. Lee.* Chelsea Juniors, a division of Chelsea House Publishers, Broomall, Penn., 1995.

Keegan, John. *The Face of Battle.* The Viking Press, New York, 1976.

Keen, W. W., M.D., Professor of Surgery, Jefferson Medical College. "The Contrast Between the Surgery of the Civil War and That of the Present War." Philadelphia. Reprinted from the *New York Medical Journal Incorporating the Philadelphia Medical Journal and The Medical News.* New York, April 24, 1915.

——. *Military Surgery in 1861 and in 1918. The Annals of the American Academy of Political and Social Science.* No. 1234 (Reprint). Philadelphia, November 1918.

——. *Program Book: Celebration of the Ninetieth Birthday of William Williams Keen, M.D., January 19, 1927. A Service of Congratulation under the auspices of the First Baptist Church of Philadelphia.* Philadelphia, 1927.

——. *Surgical Reminiscences of the Civil War.* Transactions of the College of Physicians of Philadelphia. Third Series. 1905. Kelly, Howard A., M.D. *A Cyclopedia of American Medical Biography. Comprising the Lives of Eminent Deceased Physicians and Surgeons from 1610–1910.* W.B. Saunders Company, Philadelphia, 1912.

Kelly, Howard A., M.D., and Walter L. Burrage, A.M., M.D. *Dictionary of American Medical Biography. Lives of Eminent Physicians of the United States and Canada, from the Earliest Times.* Milford House, Boston, 1928.

Knauer, Kelly, ed. *Abraham Lincoln: An Illustrated History of His Life and Times.* Time Inc. Home Entertainment, New York, 2009.

Leslie, Frank. *Frank Leslie's Illustrated Newspaper,* Vols. 11–21. Frank Leslie, New York, 1861–1865.

Letterman, Jonathan, M.D. *Medical Recollections of the Army of the Potomac.* D. Appleton and Company, New York, 1866.

Library Company of Philadelphia. *The Citizens' Volunteer Hospital, Corners of Broad St., & Washington Ave., Opposite the Baltimore Depot.* Scrapbook, May 10, 1864.

——. *A Finished Picture of Philadelphia Women.* Editors' Table (Unsure of publication date, 19th Century.)

——. *Rules & Regulations, Citizen's Volunteer Hospital, Broad and Washington Streets.* Scrapbook c. 1866.

——. *Second Inaugural Address of the Late President Lincoln.* Scrapbook, Philadelphia, 1865.

Longmore, Sir Thomas, Esq., Deputy Inspector-General of Hospitals, Professor of Military Surgery at Fort Pitt, Chatham. *A Treatise on Gunshot Wounds, Authorized and Adopted by the Surgeon-General of the United States Army for the use of Surgeons in the Field and General Hospitals.* J.B. Lippincott & Co., Philadelphia, 1863.

Looney, Robert E. *Old Philadelphia in Early Photographs 1839–1914*. Published in Cooperation with the Free Library of Philadelphia by Dover Publications, Inc., New York, 1976.

Lowry, Thomas P., M.D. *The Story the Soldiers Wouldn't Tell: Sex in the Civil War*. Stackpole Books, Mechanicsburg, Penn., 1994.

Malone, Dumas, ed. *Dictionary of American Biography*. Under the auspices of the American Council of Learned Societies. Charles Scribner's Sons, New York, 1929, 1936.

Martin, James Kirby, Randy Roberts, Steven Mintz, Linda O. McMurry, and James H. Jones. *America and its People. Volumes One and Two*. Scott, Foresman and Company, Glenview, Ill., London, 1989.

Martin, R. W. *Thesis on Gun-Shot Wounds to Obtain the Degree of Doctor of Medicine of the Homoeopathic Medical College of Pennsylvania*. Philadelphia, Session 1864–1865.

Matusiak, Elizabeth. *The Battlefield Dead*. State of the Art, Ltd., Denver, 2000.

Medical and Surgical Reporter. *Vol. XII. News and Miscellany*. Philadelphia, July 19, 1864.

——. Philadelphia, September 3, 1864.

——. *No. 402 Vol. XII—No. 5*. Philadelphia, September 10, 1864.

——. Philadelphia, January 7, 1865.

——. Philadelphia, April 22, 1865.

Medical College of Virginia Bulletin. July 1954. Vol. LI, No. 4. Virginia.

Miller, Francis Trevelyan. *The Photographic History of the Civil War: Armies and Leaders, The Cavalry, The Decisive Battles*. Random House Value Publishing, Inc., New York, 1983.

Miller, Francis Trevelyan, ed. *The Photographic History of the Civil War: Part 8: Soldier Life and the Secret Service*. Castle Books, New York, 1957.

Mitchell, Reid. *Civil War Soldiers: Their Expectations and Their Experiences*. Viking Penguin, Inc., Fairfield, Penn., 1988.

Mitchell, S. Weir, M.D., LL.D., Corresponding Honorary Member of the French Academy of Medicine. "Some Personal Recollections of the Civil War". *Transactions of the College of Physicians of Philadelphia; Third Series*. College of Physicians of Philadelphia, Philadelphia, 1905.

Mitchell, S. Weir, M.D., George R. Morehouse, M.D., and William W. Keen, M.D., Acting Assistant Surgeons USA, in charge of USA wards for diseases of the nervous system, Turner's Lane Hospital, Philadelphia. *Gunshot Wounds and other Injuries of Nerves*. J.B. Lippincott & Co., Philadelphia, 1864.

Moore, Samuel Preston, Surgeon-General of the Confederate States of America. Letter to Dr. Monro Banister. November 27, 1862.

Morin, Isobel V. *Politics, American Style: Political Parties in American History*. Twenty-First Century Books, Brookfield, Conn., 1999.

Morison, Samuel Eliot. *The Oxford History of the American People*. Oxford University Press, Oxford, UK, 1965.

Morris, James M. *History of the U.S. Army*. Exeter Books, New York, 1986.

Morton, W.T.G., M.D. "The First Use of Ether as an Anesthetic. At the Battle of the Wilderness in the Civil War." *Journal of the American Medical Association*. 1904. Boston.

Murphy, Jim. *The Boys' War: Confederate and Union Soldiers Talk About the Civil War.* Clarion Books, New York, 1990.

Nash, Herbert M., M.D. "Some Reminiscences of a Confederate Surgeon." *Transactions of the College of Physicians of Philadelphia. Third Series.* Volume The Twenty-Eighth. College of Physicians of Philadelphia, Philadelphia, 1906.

Newland, Samuel J., Ph.D. *The Pennsylvania Militia: Defending the Commonwealth and the Nation: 1669–1870.* Commonwealth of Pennsylvania Department of Military and Veterans Affairs, Annville, Penn., 2006.

New York Public Library. *American History Desk Reference.* Stonesong Press, New York, 1997.

——. *Science Desk Reference.* Stonesong Press, New York, 1995.

Nicolas, John G., and John Jay. *Abraham Lincoln: A History, Vol. I.* The Century Co., New York, 1914.

Oxford Essential Dictionary of the U.S. Military. Berkeley Books, Oxford University Press, Inc., New York, 2001.

Palfrey, Francis Winthrop. *Have We the Best Possible Ambulance System?* Pamphlet reprint, *Christian Examiner,* Boston 1864.

Pelta, Kathy. *The U.S. Navy.* Lerner Publications Company, Minneapolis, 1990.

Pember, Phoebe. *A Southern Woman's Story: Life in Confederate Richmond.* G.W. Carleton, New York, 1879.

Pennsylvania Commission. *Fiftieth Anniversary of the Battle of Gettysburg: Report.* December 31, 1913. Revised edition, Philadelphia, April 1915.

Plarr, Victor. *Plarr's Lives of the Fellows of the Royal College of Surgeons of England.* John Wright & Sons, Ltd., Bristol, 1930.

Porcher, Francis Peyre, Surgeon, P.A.C.S. *Resources of the Southern Fields and Forests, Medical Economical and Agricultural. Being also a Medical Botany of the Confederate States.* Prepared and published by the order of the Surgeon General, Richmond, Va., Charleston, S.C., 1863.

Potter, William W., M.D. of the 57th New York. *One Surgeon's Private War.* White Mane Publishing Company Inc., Buffalo, N.Y., 1888.

Poynter, Lida. *Dr. Mary Walker: The Forgotten Woman.* Manuscript. Philadelphia, 2010.

Preston, Richard A., and Sydney F. Wise. *A History of Warfare and Its Interrelationships with Western Society, Second Revised Edition.* Praeger Publishers, Inc., Westport, Conn., 1970.

Ramachandran, V. S., M.D., PhD, and Sandra Blakeslee. *Phantoms in the Brain: Probing the Mysteries of the Human Mind.* William Morrow and Company, New York, 1998.

Reynolds, Richard, M.D., and John Stone, M.D., eds. *On Doctoring: Stories, Poems, Essays.* Simon & Schuster, New York and London, 2001.

Rhode, Michael. "'An enduring monument'; Philadelphia's Contributions to the Medical and Surgical History of the War of the Rebellion (1870–1888)." *Society for the History of Authorship, Reading and Publishing.* SHARP July 10–13, London, 2002.

Rifleman, A., Esq., Gent. *Prisoner of War, or Five Months Among the Yankees.* West & Johnson, Main Street, Richmond, Va., 1865.

Riordan, Leo. "Battlefield Medicine." *Thomas Jefferson University Alumni Bulletin*. Philadelphia, 1970.

Roberts, E. B., Norton, Frank H. "Twenty-five days in the Sanitary Commission." *New York Dental Journal*, Vol. 5, No. 3. New York, March 1863.

Roca, Steven Louis. *Presence and Precedents: The USS Red Rover during the American Civil War, 1861–1865*. Kent State University Press, Kent, Ohio, 1998.

Rodenbough, Theo. F., Robert S. Lanier, and Henry W. Elson. *The Photographic History of the Civil War: Three Volumes in One: Armies & Leaders, The Cavalry, The Decisive Battles*. Portland House, New York, 1997.

Schildt, John W. *Hunter Holmes McGuire: Doctor in Gray*. Privately printed, Maryland, 1986.

Schroeder-Lein, Glenna. *The Encyclopedia of Civil War Medicine*. M.E. Sharpe, Inc., Armonk, N.Y., 2008.

Schuppert, M., M.D. *A Treatise on Gun-Shot Wounds: Written for and Dedicated to the Surgeons of the Confederate States Army*. Printed at the Bulletin Book and Job Office. New Orleans, 1861.

Seitz, Ruth Hoover and Blair Seitz. *Pennsylvania's Historic Places: In Cooperation with Pennsylvania Historical and Museum Commission*. Good Books, Intercourse, Penn., 1989.

Serven, James E., ed. *The Collecting of Guns*. The Stackpole Company, Mechanicsburg, Penn., 1964.

Shea, William L. *The Campaign for Pea Ridge*. National Park Civil War Series. Eastern National, Fort Washington, Penn., 2001.

Sifakis, Stewart. *Who Was Who in the Civil War*. Facts On File Publications, Oxford, New York, 1988.

Sister of Charity. "Notes on Saterlee Military Hospital, West Philadelphia, Penna. From 1862 until its close in 1865." From the journal kept at the hospital by a Sister of Charity. *Records of the American Catholic Historical Society at Philadelphia*. Vol. 8, No. 4. American Catholic Historical Society, December 1897.

Slawson, Robert G., M.D., FACR. *Prologue to Change: African Americans in Medicine in the Civil War Era*. The NMCWM Press, Maryland, 2006.

Smith, Henry H., M.D. *A System of Operative Surgery: Based Upon the Practice of Surgeons in the United States: With a Bibliographic Index and Historical Record of Many of Their Operations, During a Period of Two Hundred and Thirty-Four Years*. Second edition. Vol. 1. Lippincott, Grambo and Co., Philadelphia, 1855.

Society of Civil War Surgeons. *The Journal of Civil War Medicine*. January/February/March 2001. Vol. 5, No. 1. Reynoldsburg, Ohio.

——. *The Journal of Civil War Medicine*. April/May/June 2001. Vol. 5, No. 2. Reynoldsburg, Ohio.

——. *The Journal of Civil War Medicine*. October/November/December 2001. Vol. 5, No. 2. Reynoldsburg, Ohio.

——. *The Journal of Civil War Medicine*. January/February/March 2002. Vol. 6, No. 1. Reynoldsburg, Ohio.

Soldier, 1st Conn Artillery, Company B. Letter to Miss Hattie. Unpublished letter. Fort Richardson, Va., 1862.

Surgeon General's Office. *Reports on the Extent and Nature of the Materials Available for the Preparation of a Medical and Surgical History of the Rebellion.* Circular No. 6. War Department, Washington, November 1, 1865. J.B. Lippincott & Co., Philadelphia, 1865.

Svenson, Peter. *Battlefield: Farming a Civil War Battleground.* Faber and Faber, Boston, London, 1992.

Taylor, Frank H. *Philadelphia in the Civil War 1861–1865.* Published by the City of Philadelphia, 1913.

Taylor, Susie King. *Reminiscences of My Life in Camp with the 33d United States Colored Troops, Late 1st S.C. Volunteers.* Self-published, Boston, 1902.

Taylor, William H., M.D. Surgeon De Jure, Assistant Surgeon De Facto, Nineteenth Regiment of Virginia Infantry, CSA. "Some Experiences of a Confederate Assistant Surgeon." *Transactions of the College of Physicians of Philadelphia.* Third Series. Volume The Twenty-Eighth, College of Physicians of Philadelphia, Philadelphia, 1906.

Time-Life Books, eds. *Antietam: Voices of the Civil War.* Time-Life, Inc., Alexandria, Va., 1996.

Tracey, Patrick Austin. *Military Leaders of the Civil War.* Facts on File, Inc., New York, 1993.

Trowbridge, J. J. *The South: A Tour of Its Battle-Fields and Ruined Cities, a Journey Through the Desolated States and Talks with the People.* L. Stebbins, Hartford, Conn., 1866.

Trumbull, Clay, formerly chaplain to the Tenth Regiment of Connecticut Volunteers. *War Memories of an Army Chaplain.* Charles Scribner's Sons, New York, 1898.

Union League of Philadelphia and Robert Wilson Torchia. *Portraits of the Presidents of the United States of America Vol. I.* The Collections of the Union League of Philadelphia, Philadelphia, 2005.

——. *125th Anniversary 1862–1987. Annual Reports of 1863, 1864, 1865, 1866.* Published by direction of The Library Committee, Robert M. Flood Jr., Chairman, and James G. Mundy Jr., Librarian and Archivist. The Winchell Company of Philadelphia, November 1987.

——. *While Lincoln Lay Dying: A Facsimile Reproduction of The First Testimony Taken in Connection with the Assassination of Abraham Lincoln and Recorded by Corporal James Tanner.* The Union League of Philadelphia, Philadelphia, 1968.

Union League of Philadelphia, Robert Wilson Torchia, and Maxwell Whiteman. *Paintings and Sculpture at The Union League of Philadelphia.* Union League of Philadelphia, Philadelphia, 1978.

United States Christian Commission. *Facts, Principles, and Progress.* Philadelphia, January 1864.

——. *United States Christian Commission for the Army and Navy. Work and Incidents. First Annual Reports.* Philadelphia, February 1863.

——. *United States Christian Commission for the Army and Navy. For the year 1864. Third Annual Report.* Philadelphia, 1865.

United States Government. *Duties of Elector Receiving a Soldier's Vote.* Extract from Section 5 of Chapter 253. Laws of 1864. Washington, 1864.

United States Sanitary Commission. *The Best Way to Aid the Sick and Wounded.* Pamphlet. Pittsburgh Branch, Pittsburgh, Pennsylvania, 1863.

——. *Commission No. 89. Extracts from the Quarterly Special Relief Report of the U.S. Sanitary Commission, Washington, D.C., April, 1865, Concerning the Rebel Hospitals at Richmond, Va., and the Provision Made for Their Patients, as Contrasted with the Supplies Furnished to Union Prisoners of War in Rebel Hands.* McGill & Witherow, Washington, 1865.

——. *The New York Metropolitan Fair.* New York, 1863.

——. *No. 40. A Report to the Secretary of War of the Operations of the Sanitary Commission and upon the Sanitary Condition of the Volunteer Army, its Medical Staff, Hospitals, and Hospital supplies.* McGill & Witherow, Washington, December 1861.

——. *No. 88, Address Delivered by Mrs. Hoge, of the North Western Sanitary Commission at a Meeting of Ladies, Held at Packer Institute, Brooklyn, L.I. March 1865 in Aid of the Great North Western Fair, To Be Held at Chicago, Illinois, May 30th, 1865.* Chicago, 1865.

——. *Our Daily Fare* (publication of the Great Sanitary Fair in Philadelphia). Philadelphia, June 1864.

——. *Report of a Committee of the Associate Medical Members of the Sanitary Commission on the Subject of Venereal Diseases, with Special Reference to Practice in the Army and Navy.* New York, 1862.

——. *A Report to the Secretary of War of the Operations of the Sanitary Commission and upon the Sanitary Condition of the Volunteer Army, Its Medical Staff, Hospitals and Hospital Supplies.* McGill and Witherow, Washington, 1861.

——. *The Sanitary Commission Bulletin.* January 1, 1864. Vol. 1, No. 5. New York.

——. *Sanitary Fair Held at the City of Poughkeepsie, From March 15 to March 19, 1864.* Platt & Schram, Poughkeepsie, N.Y., 1864.

——. *Speech of the Rev. Dr. Bellows, President of the United States Sanitary Commission, made at the Academy of Music.* C. Sherman, Son Co., Printers. Philadelphia. 1863.

——. *The State Fair Association of the Women of Maryland for the Benefit of the "Christian and Sanitary Commissions."* Baltimore, Dec. 18, 1863.

——. *To the Loyal Women of America.* Pamphlet. Washington, 1861.

——. *What They Have To Do Who Stay at Home.* Pamphlet. Washington, 1862.

United States Sanitary Commission North. *History of the North-Western Soldiers' Fair, Held in Chicago the Last Week of October and the 1st Week of November 1863.* Dunlop, Sewell & Spalding, Printers, Chicago, 1864.

Van Wyck, Edward Hunting. Committee on Pensions. Submitted. *Senate Report, 49th Congress, 1st Session. Report No. 351.* To accompany bill H.R. 700. Washington, D.C., March 31, 1886.

Warner, John Harley, and James M. Edmonson. *Dissection: Photographs of a Rite of Passage in American Medicine: 1880–1930.* Blast Books, New York, 2010.

Warren, Ruth. *A Pictorial History of Women in America.* Crown Publishers, Inc., New York, 1975.

Wawro, Geoffrey. *The Austro-Prussian War: Austria's War with Prussia and Italy in 1866.* Cambridge University Press, Cambridge, UK, 1996.

Webster's Biographical Dictionary. G. & C. Merriam Co., Springfield, Mass., 1961.

Weddle, Kevin J. *Lincoln's Tragic Admiral: The Life of Samuel Francis DuPont*. University of Virginia Press, Charlottesville, 2005.

Wert, Jeffrey D. *Gettysburg: Day Three*. Simon & Schuster, New York, London, 2001.

White, William C. *Papers*. Unpublished letters. Philadelphia, 1862–65.

Whitman, Walt. *Civil War Poetry and Prose*. Dover Publications Inc., Mineola, New York, 1995.

——. *Drum Taps: The Complete Civil War Poems*. Cider Mill Press, Kennebunkport, Me., 2015.

——. *Leaves of Grass*. Viking-Penguin, Inc., New York, 1998.

Wilbur, C. Keith, M.D. *Civil War Medicine 1861–1865*. The Globe Pequot Press, Guilford, Conn., 1998.

Wiley, Bell I. *The Life of Johnny Reb*. Louisiana State University Press, Baton Rouge, 1971.

Williams, T. Harry, and the Editors of Time-Life Books. *The Union Sundered: The Life History of the United States 1849–1865*. Time, Inc., New York, 1963.

Wilson, James Grant, and John Fiske, eds. *Appletons' Cyclopaedia of American Biography*. D. Appleton and Company, New York, 1887.

——. *Appletons' Cyclopedia of American Biography, Vol. IV*. D. Appleton and Company, New York, 1888.

Wilson, N. *Commencement Letter*. March 5, 1866. Matriculation Cards 1864–1866. Jefferson Medical College, 1866.

Wilson, Robert H. *Philadelphia Quakers 1681–1981*. Philadelphia Yearly Meeting of the Religious Society of Friends, Philadelphia, 1981.

Wittig, Ralph, Composer. "Jenny Wade, the Heroine of Gettysburg." Sheet Music. William R. Smith, Philadelphia, 1864.

Woman's Central Association of Relief. *How Can We Best Help Our Camps and Hospitals?* State and Correspondence, published by order of the WCAR, New York, 1863.

Woodward, Joseph Janvier, M.D. *Outlines of the Chief Camp Diseases of the United States Armies as Observed During the Present War: A Practical Contribution to Military Medicine*. J.B. Lippincott & Co., Philadelphia, 1863.

Woolsey, Jane Stuart. *Hospital Days*. D. Van Nostrand, New York, 1868.

Wormeley, Katharine Prescott. *The Cruel Side of War with the Army of the Potomac. Letters from the Headquarters of the United States Sanitary Commission During the Peninsular Campaign in Virginia in 1862*. Roberts Brothers, Boston, 1898.

Wright, Mrs. D. Giraud. *A Southern Girl in '61. The War-Time Memories of a Confederate Senator's Daughter*. Page & Company, Doubleday, New York, 1905.

Wright, Steven J. *The Irish Brigade*. Steven Wright Publishing, A Wright/Grenadier Production, Springfield, Penn., 1992.

Young, David M. *The Iron Horse and the Windy City: How Railroads Shaped Chicago*. Northern Illinois University Press, DeKalb, 2005.

INDEX

Dependent and Disability Pension
Act (1890), 112
Desmarres Hospital, 189
diarrhea, 14, 18, 19–20, 21, 27–28
disease: Civil War deaths from, xvii;
in civilian population, 29–30;
gastric and intestinal disorders,
26–28; germ theory, xi, xiv, 26,
143, 270; livestock, 35–37; mortality rates, 27–28; sexually transmitted, xvii, 32, 189–190. *See also
specific diseases*
dissection, 2, 61
District of Columbia Compensated
Emancipation Act (1862), 191
Dix, Dorothea, 86, 90–91, 121,
123–127, 133, 141, 204–207, 231,
254, 256
doctors and physicians: Confederate
Army, xiv, 61; demographics, 61;
female, xvi, 3–4, 82, 254; non-
combatant classification of, 70–71;
professionalization of, 278–279;
surgeons, 61–63, 278; Union
Army, xiv, 60–61
D'Onofrio, Peter J., 101
Douglas, H. Ford, 217
Douglas, Sattira "Sattie," 217
Douglass, Frederick, 74, 219
"drapetomania," 204
drug addiction, 19, 21
Drum Taps (Whitman), 138
Dufour, Henri, 245
Dunant, Jean-Henri, xxii, 241,
270–271

E

E. Remington and Sons, 58
Eakins, Thomas, 63
Eastern Lunatic Asylum, 204

Ebers Papyrus, 200
Elements of Pathological Anatomy
(Gross), 62
Elizabeth Blackwell Award, 87
Elizabeth Blackwell Medal, 87
Elliott Cresson Medal, 7
Ellis, William Baldwin, 82
Emancipation Proclamation, 76, 121,
216
erysipelas, 11–12
ether, 22–23, 95, 261
Ewing, James, 276

F

Female Education Society, 4, 88
Female Medical College of Pennsyl-
vania, xvi, 3–4, 82
Field, Betty, 97
Fifteenth Corps of the Army of the
Tennessee, 132
Fifty-Fourth Massachusetts Volun-
teer Infantry Regiment of African
Americans, 92, 196
Finley, Clement Alexander, 66
First Carolina Volunteers of African
Descent, 113
First Regiment of South Carolina
Volunteers, 91
First World Y.M.C.A. Conference, 243
Flint, Austin, Jr., 211
food supply, 150–151
Fort Hill Cemetery, 112
Fort Leavenworth (hospital), xix
Fort Riley, 67
Fort Sumter, Battle of, 55, 60
Fort Wagner, Battle of, 92
Franco-Prussian War, 157, 241
Frank Leslie's Illustrated Newspaper, 214
Fredericksburg, Battle of, xxii, 96,
135, 226, 238

Stuart, J.E.B., 59
Stuart, Mary, 70
Summit House Hospital, 196
Sumner, Charles, xv, 78
Surgeon General's Library, 71, 73
surgeons, 61–63, 278
"The Surgical Examination of Epilepsy" (Billings), 71
surgical practices: amputation, 10–11, 173, 181, 262, 266; anesthetics, 22–24, 167–169, 260–262; chest wounds, 265–266; dental, 35; facial and jaw, 169–170, 190, 264–265, 268; instruments for, 5–6, 10; orthopedics, 190
syphilis, xvii, 32, 189–190
Syracuse Medical College, 254
A System of Surgery (Gross), 62

T
Taylor, Charles H., 82
Taylor, Russell, 114
Taylor, Susannah Baker King, 112–114
Taylor, William H., 26–27, 61, 149–150
telegraph, 38, 213
Tenth General Hospital, 195–196
Third New York Light Artillery, 266
Thirty-Third United States Colored Infantry, 113
Thomas Jefferson University Center City Archives and Special Collections, 10, 178
Thomson, William, 98
Tompkins, Sally Louisa, 115–117, 199, 200
Toronto City Hospital, 76
torpedoes, 55–56
Towne, Laura, 136

trains, as ambulances and hospitals, 154–158, 252–253
transport of wounded soldiers: ambulance corps, 67, 151, 152–154, 176, 181, 257–260; boats and ships, 158–163, 226, 227, 251–252; railroad, 154–158, 252–253; stretcher-bearers, 152, 182, 257, 259
Treatise on Gunshot Wounds (Longmore), 63
A Treatise on Gun-Shot Wounds (Schuppert), 74
A Treatise on Hygiene (Hammond), 67
Trinity Medical College, xv
Triumph Over Pain (Fülöp-Miller), 97
Trumbull, Henry Clay, 207–209
Tubman, Harriet, 110–112
Tubman, John, 111
Tulane University, 68
Turner, Nat, 75
Turner's Lane Hospital, xx, 187–188, 250, 263–264
turpentine, medicinal use of, 16–17
typhoid fever, 27–28

U
Under the Guns (Wittenmyer), 234
Underground Railroad, 79, 110–111
Union Army: African American troops, 195–196; dentists in, 33–34, 93–94, 268; disease mortality, 27–29; doctors in, xiv, 60–61; nurses in, 140–141; smallpox cases, 26; supply system, 151–152; surgeons general, 64, 66–68
Union Army Medical Department, 234
Union Hospital, 209

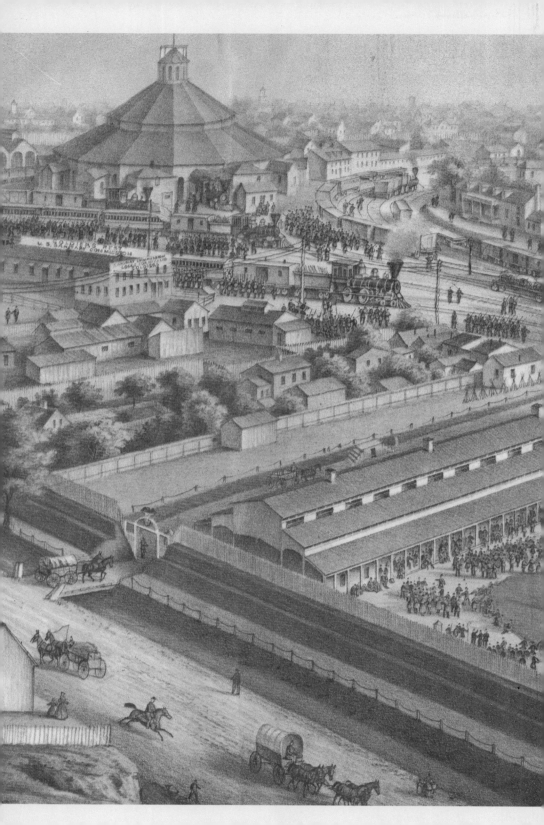